ABC of
Transfer and Retrieval Medicine

ABC series

An outstanding collection of resources for everyone in primary care

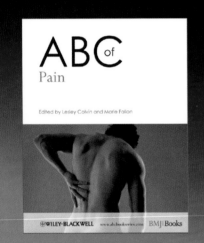

ABC of
Pain

Edited by Lesley Colvin and Marie Fallon

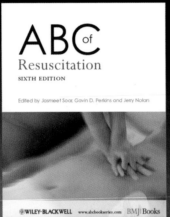

ABC of
Resuscitation

SIXTH EDITION

Edited by Jasmeet Soar, Gavin D. Perkins and Jerry Nolan

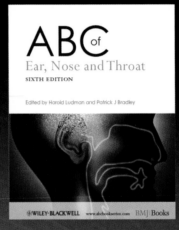

ABC of
Ear, Nose and Throat

SIXTH EDITION

Edited by Harold Ludman and Patrick J Bradley

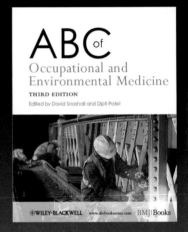

ABC of
Occupational and
Environmental Medicine

THIRD EDITION

Edited by David Snashall and Dipti Patel

The *ABC* series contains a wealth of indispensable resources for GPs, GP registrars, junior doctors, doctors in training and all those in primary care

▶ **Highly illustrated, informative and a practical source of knowledge**

▶ **An easy-to-use resource, covering the symptoms, investigations, treatment and management of conditions presenting in day-to-day practice and patient support**

▶ **Full colour photographs and illustrations aid diagnosis and patient understanding of a condition**

For more information on all books in the *ABC* series, including links to further information, references and links to the latest official guidelines, please visit:

www.abcbookseries.com

WILEY Blackwell

BMJ|Books

ABC of

Transfer and Retrieval Medicine

EDITED BY

Adam Low

Specialist Registrar in Anaesthetics
West Midlands Deanery
West Midlands Central Accident Resuscitation & Emergency (CARE) Team
West Midlands Ambulance Service NHS Foundation Trust Medical Emergency Response Incident Team (MERIT), UK
AMREF Flying Doctors, Kenya

Jonathan Hulme

Consultant in Intensive Care Medicine and Anaesthesia, Sandwell and West Birmingham Hospitals NHS Trust
Honorary Senior Clinical Lecturer, University of Birmingham, Birmingham
West Midlands Ambulance Service NHS Foundation Trust Medical Emergency Response Incident Team (MERIT)
Medical Director, West Midlands Central Accident Resuscitation & Emergency (CARE) Team
Mercia Accident Rescue Service (MARS) BASICS, UK

WILEY Blackwell

BMJ Books

This edition first published 2015, © 2015 by John Wiley & Sons Ltd.

BMJ Books is an imprint of BMJ Publishing Group Limited, used under licence by John Wiley & Sons.

Registered office: John Wiley & Sons, Ltd, The Atrium, Southern Gate, Chichester, West Sussex, PO19 8SQ, UK

Editorial offices: 9600 Garsington Road, Oxford, OX4 2DQ, UK

The Atrium, Southern Gate, Chichester, West Sussex, PO19 8SQ, UK

111 River Street, Hoboken, NJ 07030-5774, USA

For details of our global editorial offices, for customer services and for information about how to apply for permission to reuse the copyright material in this book please see our website at www.wiley.com/wiley-blackwell

Library of Congress Cataloging-in-Publication Data

ABC of transfer and retrieval medicine / edited by Adam Low, Jonathan Hulme.
       p. ; cm.
   Includes bibliographical references and index.
   ISBN 978-1-118-71975-6 (pbk.)
   I. Low, Adam, 1982- editor. II. Hulme, Jonathan, 1974- editor.
   [DNLM: 1. Critical Care – methods. 2. Transportation of Patients. 3. Monitoring, Physiologic. 4. Patient Care Team. 5. Patient Transfer.
WX 218]
   RT87.T72
   616.02′8 – dc23

2014020562

A catalogue record for this book is available from the British Library.

Wiley also publishes its books in a variety of electronic formats. Some content that appears in print may not be available in electronic books.

Cover image: 12-03-13 © Paolo Cipriani. Medical emergency team arrives at street accident. Stock Photo: 31074458

Set in 9.25/12 MinionPro by Laserwords Private Ltd, Chennai, India
Printed and bound in Singapore by Markono Print Media Pte Ltd

1   2015

Contents

Contributors

Anders Aneman

Senior Staff Specialist, Intensive Care Unit, Liverpool Hospital, South Western Sydney Local Health District
Conjoint Associate Professor, University of New South Wales, NSW, Australia

Oliver Bartells

Lieutenant Colonel Royal Army Medical Corps, Consultant Anaesthetist, Ministry of Defence Hospital Unit Northallerton, UK

Hannah Bawdon

Anaesthetic registrar, West Midlands Deanery
West Midlands Central Accident Resuscitation & Emergency (CARE) Team
West Midlands Ambulance Service NHS Foundation Trust Medical Emergency Response Incident Team (MERIT), UK

Jon Bingham

Consultant in Trauma, Resuscitation and Anaesthesia, Department of Anaesthesia, University Hospital of North Staffordshire, Stoke-on-Trent
Midlands Air Ambulance, Cosford
West Midlands Ambulance Service Medical Emergency Response Incident Team (MERIT)
North Staffordshire BASICs
West Midlands Central Accident Resuscitation & Emergency (CARE) Team, UK

Clare Bosanko

Specialty Doctor, Emergency Medicine, University Hospital North Staffordshire, Stoke-On-Trent; West Midlands Ambulance Service NHS Foundation Trust Medical Emergency Response Incident Team (MERIT), UK

Michael Büeschges

Resident, Universitätsklinikum Schleswig Holstein Campus Lübeck, Abteilung für Plastische Chirurgie, Intensiveinheit für Schwerbrandverletzte, Lübeck, Germany

Andrew Cadamy

Consultant in Intensive Care Medicine and Anaesthetics, NHS Greater Glasgow and Clyde, Glasgow, UK

Felicity Clarke

Specialist Registrar Intensive Care & Anaesthetics, University Hospital of North Staffordshire, NHS Trust, Stoke on Trent
PHEM Doctor, West Midlands Ambulance Service NHS Foundation Trust Medical Emergency Response Incident Team (MERIT), UK

Alasdair Corfield

Consultant, Emergency Medicine & Emergency Medical Retrieval Service
Honorary Clinical Associate Professor, University of Glasgow, Glasgow, UK

Stuart J Cox,

Senior Nurse, Critical Care and Aeromedical Transfer CEGA Air Ambulance, Dorset
Senior Charge Nurse, General Intensive Care Unit, University Hospital Southampton NHS Foundation Trust, Southampton, UK

James Cuell

Anaesthetic Registrar, West Midlands Deanery, Birmingham School of Anaesthesia, Birmingham, UK

Zoey Dempsey

Consultant Anaesthetist, Department of Anaesthesia and Pain Medicine, Royal Infirmary of Edinburgh, UK

Joep M. Droogh

Consultant in Intensive Care Medicine
Medical Coordinator Mobile Intensive Care Unit, Department of Critical Care, University Medical Center Groningen, University of Groningen, Groningen, The Netherlands

Catriona Duncan

Consultant in Anaesthesia, Timaru District Hospital, Timaru, New Zealand

Daniel Ellis

Director, MedSTAR Emergency Medical Retrieval Service, South Australian Ambulance Service, Australia
Deputy Director of Trauma and Senior Consultant in Emergency Medicine, Royal Adelaide Hospital, Australia
Associate Professor, School of Public Health and Tropical Medicine, James Cook University, Queensland, Australia

George Evetts

Specialist Registrar Intensive Care & Anaesthesia, Royal Air Force, Imperial College School of Anaesthesia, UK

Rob Fenwick

Charge Nurse, Emergency Department, Shrewsbury and Telford Hospitals NHS Trust, UK.

Anna Fergusson

Anaesthetic Registrar, Peninsula Deanery, South West School of Anaesthesia, Plymouth, UK

Karel Habig

Position
Greater Sydney Area Helicopter, Emergency Medical Service, Ambulance
Service NSW Rescue, Helicopter Base, Bankstown Airport, NSW, Australia

Tim Harris

Professor Emergency Medicine, QMUL and Barts Health NHS Trust
London, UK

Chris Harvey

Adult and Paediatric ECMO Consultant, ECMO Department, University
Hospitals of Leicester, Leicester, UK

Stephen Hearns

Consultant in Emergency Medicine, Royal Alexandra Hospital, Paisley
Lead consultant Emergency Medical Retrieval Service, Scotland, UK

Jo Hegarty

Consultant Neonatologist, Newborn Services, National Women's Health,
Auckland City Hospital, Auckland, New Zealand

Matthias Helm

Assistant Professor, Head Section Emergency Medicine, Department of
Anaesthesiology and Intensive Care Medicine, Federal Armed Forces
Medical Centre, Ulm, Germany

Scott Hepburn

Consultant in Emergency Medicine and EMRS
EMRS Lead for Risk Management, Department of Emergency Medicine,
Western Infirmary, Glasgow, UK

Craig Hore

ICU Staff Specialist, Liverpool Hospital ICU/ Retrieval Staff Specialist,
Ambulance Service of New South Wales, Sydney, Australia

Martin Horton

Immediate Care Practitioner-nurse, Royal Air Force Emergency and pre
hospital specialist MERT practitioner, Emergency Department, Heartlands
Hospital, Birmingham, UK

Amy Hughes

Clinical Academic Lecturer in Emergency Response, Humanitarian and
Conflict Response Institute, University of Manchester
Emergency Medicine Registrar, Derriford Hospital
Honorary Physician in Pre Hospital Care, London's Air Ambulance, Barts
and The Royal London NHS Trust, UK

Jonathan Hulme

Consultant in Intensive Care Medicine and Anaesthesia, Sandwell and West
Birmingham Hospitals NHS Trust
Honorary Senior Clinical Lecturer, University of Birmingham, Birmingham
West Midlands Ambulance Service NHS Foundation Trust Medical
Emergency Response Incident Team (MERT), UK
Medical Director, West Midlands Central Accident Resuscitation &
Emergency (CARE) Team, UK
Mercia Accident Rescue Service (MARS) BASICS, UK
Midlands Air Ambulance, UK

Lesley Jackson

Consultant Neonatal Medicine and Regional Director, West of Scotland
Neonatal Transport Service, Yorkhill Hospital, Glasgow, UK

Emma L. Joynes

Retrieval registrar, Careflight Darwin, NT, Australia

Damian D. Keene

Major, Specialist trainee Anaesthesia and Pre-Hospital Emergency Medicine,
Department of Military Anaesthesia and Critical Care

Minh Le Cong

Assistant Professor in Retrieval Medicine, Royal Flying Doctor Service
Queensland Section, Australia

Fiona Lecky

Clinical Professor and Honorary Consultant in Emergency Medicine,
University of Sheffield and Salford Royal NHS Foundation Trust, Greater
Manchester, UK

Ian Locke

Critical Care Paramedic, West Midland Ambulance Service, NHS Trust,
Midlands Air Ambulance, UK

David Lockey

Consultant, North Bristol NHS Trust, Bristol, & London's Air
Ambulance, UK
Hon. Professor University of Bristol, Bristol, UK

Adam Low

Specialist Registrar in Anaesthetics, West Midlands Deanery
West Midlands Central Accident Resuscitation & Emergency (CARE) Team,
UK
West Midlands Ambulance Service NHS Foundation Trust Medical
Emergency Response Incident Team (MERIT), UK
AMREF Flying Doctors, Kenya

Stefan Mazur

Chief Medical Officer, South Australian Ambulance Service
Senior Consultant, PreHospital and Retrieval Medicine, MedSTAR
Emergency Medical Retrieval Service
Senior Consultant in Emergency Medicine, Royal Adelaide Hospital
Associate Professor, School of Public Health and Tropical Medicine, James
Cook University, Australia

Russell D. MacDonald

Attending Staff, Emergency Services, Sunnybrook Health Sciences Centre,
Toronto, Ontario, Canada
Associate Professor and Co-Director, Emergency Medicine Fellowship
Program, Department of Medicine, University of Toronto, Toronto, Ontario,
Canada
Medical Director and Chair, Quality Care Committee, Ornge Transport
Medicine, Mississauga, Ontario, Canada

Terry Martin

Consultant in Anaesthesia and Intensive Care Medicine, Royal Hampshire
County Hospital, Winchester
Medical Director, Capital Air Ambulance, Exeter, UK, Director, CCAT
Aeromedical Training, UK
Board Director, AMREF Flying Doctors, Nairobi, Kenya
Board Director, European Aeromedical Institute (EURAMI), Tuebingen,
Germany

Heather Mcneilly

Paediatric Registrar, West Midlands Deanery, Birmingham, UK

Michael McCabe

Consultant in Anaesthesia, Anaesthetic Department, Worcester Royal Infirmary, Worcester, UK

Carl McQueen

PHEM Doctor, Midlands Air Ambulance; West Midlands Ambulance Service, Medical Emergency Response Incident Team (MERIT), UK &NIHR Doctoral Research Fellow, University of Warwick, UK

Mary Montgomery

Consultant, Kids Intensive Care & Decision Support, Birmingham Children's Hospital, West Midlands, Birmingham, UK

Patrick Morgan

Specialist Registrar, North Bristol NHS Trust, Bristol

Thomas Muehlberger

Associate Professor, Department of Plastic & Reconstructive Surgery, DRK-Kliniken, Berlin, Germany

Blair Munford

Senior Specialist Anaesthetist, Liverpool Hospital
Senior Retrieval Physician, CareFlight
Conjoint Lecturer in Anaesthetics, UNSW, and Senior Lecturer in Physiology, UWS Medical School
Sydney, Australia

Tim Nutbeam

Consultant in Emergency Medicine, Derriford Hospital, Plymouth Hospitals NHS Trust, Plymouth
West Midlands Ambulance Service NHS Foundation Trust Medical Emergency Response Incident Team (MERIT), UK

William O'Regan

Senior Staff Specialist, Intensive Care Unit, Liverpool Hospital, South Western Sydney Local Health District
Consultant for Careflight International Retrieval Service, Sydney, Australia

Christian Ottomann

Associate Professor, Universitätsklinikum Schleswig, Holstein Campus Lübeck, Sektion für Plastische Chirurgie und Handchirurgie, Intensiveinheit für, Schwerbrandverletzte, Lübeck, Germany

Peter Paal

Associate Professor, Department of Anaesthesiology and Critical Care Medicine, Medical University Innsbruck, Innsbruck, Austria
Helicopter Emergency Medical Service Christophorus 1, Innsbruck, Austria

Eithne Polke

Retrieval coordinator, Children's Acute Transport Service, Great Ormond Street Hospital for Children NHS Trust, London, UK

Richard Protheroe

Consultant in Critical Care Medicine and Neuro-Anaesthesia, Salford Royal NHS Foundation Trust, Salford, Greater Manchester, UK

David Quayle

Chief Flight Nurse, Air Medical Ltd, London Oxford Airport, UK

Samiran Ray

Consultant, Children's Acute Transport Service, Great Ormond Street Hospital for Children NHS Trust, London, UK

Cliff Reid

Senior Staff Specialist and Director of Training, Greater Sydney Area Helicopter Emergency Medical Service, NSW Ambulance, Australia
Clinical Associate Professor in Emergency Medicine, University of Sydney, Australia

Sanjay Revenna

Consultant, Kids Intensive Care & Decision Support, Birmingham Children's Hospital, West Midlands, Birmingham, UK

Gareth Roberts

Department of Anaesthesia, University Hospital of Wales, UK

Mark Ross

Specialist Trainee Registrar in Anaesthesia, Department of Anaesthesia and Pain Medicine, Royal Infirmary Edinburgh, UK

Mark Sheils

Flight Doctor, Careflight NT, Nightcliff, Darwin, Australia

Charlotte Small

Research Fellow, Anaesthesia and Critical Care, University Hospitals Birmingham NHS Foundation Trust (Queen Elizabeth Hospital) Birmingham, UK

Helen Simpson

Consultant Obstetrician, James Cook University Hospital, South Tees Foundation Trust, Middlesbrough, UK

Stephen J. M. Sollid

Dean, Norwegian Air Ambulance Academy, Norwegian Air Ambulance Foundation, Drøbak, Norway;
Consultant Anaesthetist, Air Ambulance Department, Oslo University Hospital, Oslo, Norway
Associate professor, University of Stavanger, Stavanger, Norway

Karl Thies

Consultant Anaesthetist Birmingham Children's Hospital, Birmingham
West Midlands Ambulance Service NHS Foundation Trust Medical Emergency Response Incident Team (MERIT)
Mercia Accident Rescue Service (MARS) BASICS, UK

Robert Tipping

Consultant Anaesthetist, Queen Elizabeth Hospital, Birmingham, UK,
West Midlands Ambulance Service NHS Foundation Trust Medical Emergency Response Incident Team (MERIT), UK
University Hospitals Birmingham NHS Foundation Trust (Queen Elizabeth Hospital), Birmingham, UK

Oddvar Uleberg

Consultant anaesthetist, Norwegian Air Ambulance Foundation, Drøbak, Norway
Department of aeromedical and clinical emergency services, St Olavs University Hospital, Trondheim, Norway

Bettina Vadera

Chief Executive and Medical Director of AMREF Flying Doctors, Kenya
Vice-President of EURAMI (European Aeromedical Institute)
Member of AMPA (Air Medical Physician Association), USA

Mathew Ward

Head of clinical practice, West Midlands Ambulance Service; Immediate
Care Practitioner, West Midlands CARE Team, UK

Jon Warwick

Consultant Anaesthetist, Oxford University Hospitals NHS Trust, UK
Medical Director, Air Medical Ltd, London Oxford Airport, UK

Anne Weaver

Consultant in Emergency Medicine & Pre-Hospital Care, London's Air
Ambulance, Royal London Hospital, UK

Claire Westrope

Consultant PICU/ECMO, University Hospital Leicester NHS Trust,
Leicester, UK

Yashvi Wimalasena

Consultant in Emergency Medicine, Retrieval/HEMS Fellow, Greater Sydney
Area HEMS, Ambulance Service of NSW Rescue Helicopter Base
Bankstown, NSW, Australia

Jan G. Zijlstra

Professor in Intensive Care, Department of Critical Care, University Medical
Center Groningen, University of Groningen, Groningen, The Netherlands

Preface

The introduction of the Diploma in Transfer and Retrieval Medicine by the Royal College of Surgeons of Edinburgh in 2012 was the catalyst for ABC of Transfer and Retrieval Medicine. Reviewing the recommended reading for the Diploma, it was clear that there was no single revision guide to aid candidates' preparation; by using the Diploma curriculum as a framework, we could provide a useful addition to the highly acclaimed "ABC of … " series. Transfer Medicine is also a recognised component of anaesthetic training in the United Kingdom, with dedicated learning outcomes highlighted in the curriculum from the Royal College of Anaesthetists. On this background, we aim to provide a useful point of reference for all healthcare practitioners involved in the field of transfer and retrieval medicine.

We are indebted to all the individuals who have contributed their expertise to the book. As you will see, we have a distinctly multi-national contributor list from a range of healthcare backgrounds, with the specific aim of producing a text of relevance to all practitioners within the field, irrespective of country of practice. All the contributors have a wealth of experience and we are extremely grateful to them for sharing their expertise.

We would like to thank all the team at Wiley for their invaluable guidance, realistic timelines and patience with this project; our families for their unwavering support and tolerance, and our authors for agreeing to contribute to the book, adhering to timelines and stringent word counts!

Whilst on paper, the aim of "maintaining the same standard of care as the patient would receive in hospital throughout the course of the transfer" may sound straight forward, the reality is that it rarely is. This text is dedicated to all of you who move critically ill or injured patients to, or from, health care facilities at all hours of the day and night in often challenging circumstances.

Adam Low
Jonathan Hulme

List of Abbreviations

AAGBI	Association of Anaesthetists of Great Britain and Ireland
ACCM	American College of Critical Care Medicine
AC	Alternating current
ACT	Activated clotting time
ALS	Advanced life support
ANZCA	Australian & New Zealand College of Anaesthetists.
ATC	Acute trauma coagulopathy
ATLS	Advanced trauma life support
ARDS	Adult respiratory distress syndrome
BMI	Body mass index
BP	Blood pressure
CAA	Civil Aviation Authority
CAT	Combat application tourniquet
CCF	Congestive cardiac failure
CCNs	Critical care networks
CCP	Critical care paramedic
CBRN	Chemical, biological, radiological or nuclear
CAMTS	Commission on accreditation of medical transport systems
CCAST	Critical Care Air Support Team
CDR	Cognitive dispositions to respond
CDH	Congenital diaphragmatic hernia
CO	Cardiac output
CO (burns)	Carbon monoxide
CO_2	Carbon dioxide
COPD	Chronic obstructive pulmonary disease
CNS	Central nervous system
CPD	Continued professional development
CPR	Cardio-pulmonary resuscitation
CQC	Care Quality Commission
CSF	Cerebrospinal fluid
CVA	Cerebrovascular accident
CVC	Central venous catheter
CVP	Central venous pressure
CVS	Cardiovascular system
CXR	Chest X-ray
DBD	Donation after brain-stem death
DCD	Donation after circulatory death
DC	Direct current
DCR	Damage control resuscitation

ECG	Electrocardiogram
ECLA	Extracorporeal lung assist
ECLS	Extracorporeal life support
ECMO	Extracorporeal membrane oxygenation
ECT	Enhanced care teams
ED	Emergency Department
EMS	Emergency medical services
$ETCO_2$	End tidal carbon dioxide
ETT	Endotracheal tube
EURAMI	European Aero-Medical Institute
FAST	Focussed assessment with sonography in trauma
FFP	Fresh frozen plasma
FiO_2	Fractional inspired oxygen concentration
FRC	Functional residual capacity
FWAA	Fixed-wing air ambulance
GCS	Glasgow Coma Score
GMC	General Medical Council
GPS	Global positioning system
HAFOE	High air flow oxygen enrichment
HCPC	Health and Care Professionals Council
HDU	High dependency Unit
HEMS	Helicopter emergency medical system
HICAMS	Helicopter intensive care medical services
HIE	Hypoxic ischaemic encephalopathy
HIV	Human immunodeficiency virus
HLS	Helicopter landing site
HME filter	Heat moisture exchange filter
HR	Heart rate
HSE	Health and Safety Executive
IABP	Intra-aortic balloon pump
IBW	Ideal body weight
ICP	Intracranial pressure
ICU	Intensive Care Unit
ICS	Intensive Care Society
IFR	Instrumental flight rules
IM	Intramuscular
IN	Intranasal
iNO	Inhaled nitric oxide
IO	Intraosseus
ISS	Injury Severity Score
IUGR	Intra-uterine growth restriction
IUT	In utero transfer

IV	Intravenous
IVC	Inferior vena cava
IVH	Intra-ventricular haemorrhage
kPa	Kilopascals
km	Kilometres
LA	Left atrium
LCD	Liquid crystal display
LV	Left ventricle
MAD	Mucosal atomising device
MAP	Mean arterial pressure
MAS	Meconium aspiration syndrome
MCN	Managed clinical networks
MHRA	Medical and Healthcare Regulatory Agency
MRSA	Methicillin resistant staphylococcus aureus
MTC	Major trauma centre
MV	Minute volume
NACA	National Advisory Committee for Aeronautics
NAI	Non-accidental Injury
NEC	Necrotising enterocolitis
NIBP	Non-invasive blood pressure
NICE	National Institute for Health and Care Excellence
NICU	Neonatal intensive care unit
NiMH	Nickel metal hydride
NMBD	Neuromuscular blocking drugs
NMC	Nursing and Midwifery Council
NTS	Non-technical skills
NVG	Night vision goggles
O_2	Oxygen
O_3	Ozone
OR	Operating room
PACs	Picture Archiving & Communication system
PDA	Patent ductus arteriosus
PEEP	Positive end expiratory pressure
PHEM	Pre-hospital emergency medicine
PPHN	Persistent pulmonary hypertension of the newborn
POCT	Point of care testing
PPH	Post-partum haemorrhage
PRBC	Packed red blood cells
PRF	Patient record form
PTC	Patient transport compartment
PVR	Pulmonary vascular resistance
RDS	Respiratory distress syndrome
REBOA	Resuscitative endovascular balloon occlusion of the aorta.
RR	Respiratory rate
RS	Respiratory system
RTD	Regional trauma desk
RSI	Rapid sequence induction
SAR	Search and rescue
Sats	Saturations
SIRS	Systemic inflammatory response syndrome
SOPs	Standard operating procedures
SV	Stroke volume
SVC	Superior vena cava
SVR	Systemic vascular resistance
TB	Tuberculosis
TBSA	Total body surface area
TETRA	Terrestrial trunked radio
TPN	Total parenteral nutrition
TRM	Team resource management
TU	Trauma unit
TUC	Time of useful consciousness
TV	Tidal volume
UK	United Kingdom
UK-DMS	United Kingdom Defence Medical Services
UPS	Universal power supply
UV	Ultraviolet
V	Volts
VFR	Visual flight rules
VHF	Very high frequency
WHO	World Health Organization
°C	Degrees Celsius
<	Less than
>	Greater than

CHAPTER 1

Introduction

A. Low[1,2,3] *and J. Hulme*[1,2,4,5,6,7]

[1] West Midlands Central Accident Resuscitation & Emergency (CARE) Team, UK
[2] West Midlands Ambulance Service NHS Foundation Trust Medical Emergency Response Incident Team (MERIT), UK
[3] AMREF Flying Doctors, Kenya
[4] Intensive Care Medicine and Anaesthesia, Sandwell and West Birmingham Hospitals NHS Trust, UK
[5] University of Birmingham, UK
[6] Mercia Accident Rescue Service (MARS) BASICS, UK
[7] Midlands Air Ambulance, UK

Intensive care beds are a limited and often pressurised resource within any healthcare setting. As the complexity and breadth of surgical interventions increases, alongside longevity and associated co-morbidities, the requirement for critical care is expanding worldwide. In the developed world many healthcare systems are moving towards networked care: with tertiary centres for specialist care, meaning patients presenting to their local hospital may subsequently need to be transferred for definitive intervention (e.g. neuro/cardiothoracic/transplant surgery or an intervention such as hyperbaric oxygen therapy). Neonatal and paediatric intensive care facilities are becoming centralised, increasing the need for 'Retrieval Teams' who will travel to the patient, assist local health care professionals in resuscitation and stabilisation before transporting the patient back to base facility. The development of trauma networks may mean patients are transported longer distances from point of injury to Major Trauma Centres (MTCs), or stabilised at Trauma Units before onward transfer to a MTC for definitive multidisciplinary care. Regional Enhanced Care Teams (ECTs) are becoming increasingly common to assist in the primary management and transfer of these polytrauma patients. Figure 1.1 illustrates an example of a critically ill patient undergoing numerous transfers.

The increase in worldwide travel and business networks means people risk ill health while abroad. They may want or require repatriation for healthcare, family support or financial reasons. This request may be instigated by their medical insurance company, resulting in international transportation.

It is inevitable that critically ill patients will need to be moved at some point in their illness. This may be from point of injury or small healthcare facility to specialist care, or from one area of a healthcare facility to another. Pressures on critical care beds may necessitate movement of patients in order to manage local resources. In the UK, the NHS has created Critical Care Networks on a regional basis to facilitate this aspect of resource management. The principles and risks associated with moving any critically ill patient are discussed in depth in this book.

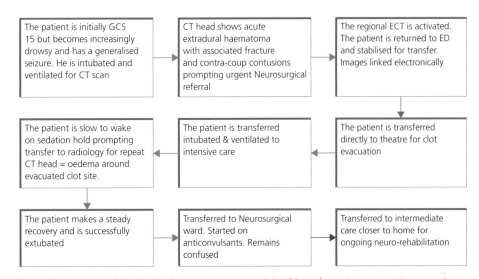

Figure 1.1 A 20-year-old male is assaulted and hits his head on the pavement with brief loss of consciousness. He is assessed on scene by paramedics who stabilise him and transfer him to the nearest Emergency Department. Green arrow, intra-hospital transfer; red arrow, secondary retrieval; blue arrow, repatriation.

ABC of Transfer and Retrieval Medicine, First Edition.
Edited by Adam Low and Jonathan Hulme.
© 2015 John Wiley & Sons, Ltd. Published 2015 by John Wiley & Sons, Ltd.

The following definitions and concepts are important to understand:

- *Retrieval*: deployment of a specialist team of appropriately trained health care professionals to the patient's location to resuscitate and stabilise prior to transfer to definitive care.
- *Transfer*: the movement of a patient (not necessarily critically ill), from one location (or healthcare facility) to another.
- *Primary retrieval*: from a pre-hospital location to hospital.
- *Secondary retrieval*: movement from a healthcare facility with limited resources/expertise to a specialist care facility.
- *Tertiary retrieval*: movement from one specialist care facility to another, or for bed availability.
- *Repatriation*: retrieval from distant or international health care facility to patient's local hospital or specialist care unit.
- *Inter-hospital transfer*: movement of a patient from one hospital facility to another.
- *Intra-hospital transfer*: movement of a patient from one department to another within the same hospital buildings.

Movement of critically ill patients can be achieved via a variety of transport modalities, selection of which requires clinical, financial and logistical consideration.

The movement of critically ill patients is not without risks to patient and team (summarised in Box 1.1). Historical data have suggested that retrievals and transfers may be associated with increased mortality and length of hospital stay, with increased incidence of hypoxaemia and hypotension, persisting upon arrival at the receiving facility (see Further reading).

Box 1.1 Potential risks encountered during patient transfers

Environmental exposure
Road traffic collision
Equipment failure
Physiological instability

- hypoxaemia
- arrhythmias
- hypotension
- hypertension
- raised intracranial pressure
- death during transfer

Acknowledgement of these factors has resulted in the development of dedicated transfer and retrieval teams with associated clinical governance/training schemes, standardised equipment and standardised operating procedures to optimise patient safety (Box 1.2). All these factors will help to ensure 'the rule of RIGHT':

The RIGHT patient is taken at the RIGHT time, by the RIGHT people to the RIGHT place, using the RIGHT transport modality and receiving the RIGHT clinical care throughout.

Box 1.2 Key components to being a part of an effective retrieval team

Understanding of the physiological consequences of moving critically ill patients
Good clinical acumen and skill to assess and stabilise critically ill patients
Familiarity and understanding of equipment utilised
Familiarity and understanding of commonly used drugs
Good communication between the team, base hospital and receiving hospital
Good management and leadership skills
Appreciation of ethical and legal issues surrounding patient transfers and retrievals
Working within ones scope of practice and clinical governance scheme

---

This book aims to introduce the reader to all these different aspects of transfer and retrieval medicine. It is no substitute for hands-on clinical experience, but we hope it will provide a useful reference for any practitioner (paramedic, nurse or doctor) involved in the transfer and retrieval of critically ill patients.

Further reading

Flabouris A, Hart GK, George C. Outcomes of patients admitted to tertiary intensive care units after interhospital transfer: comparison with patients admitted from emergency departments. Crit Care Resusc 2008;10(2): 97–105.

Flabouris A, Hart GK, George C. Observational study of patients admitted to intensive care units in Australia and New Zealand after interhospital transfer. Crit Care Resusc 2008;10(2):90–6.

Section 1

Physiology of Transfer Medicine

CHAPTER 2

Acceleration, Deceleration and Vibration

M. Sheils[1] and C. Hore[2]

[1]Careflight NT, Australia
[2]Ambulance Service of New South Wales, Austalia

OVERVIEW

This chapter will enable the reader to:

- discuss gravity in relation to the flight environment
- list the origins of negative, positive, linear accelerations and radial accelerations
- understand the value of appropriate positioning and orientation of patients for transfers
- discuss the key fundamentals of crashworthiness in road and air modes of patient transport
- discuss the physics of vibration, harmonics and resonance and the physiological/physical consequences
- list the sources of mechanical vibration in road and air modes of patient transport.

Introduction

Any patient being moved will experience acceleration and vibration, irrespective of mode of transport. In the critically ill, these can have significant physiological impact that the transferring team must be aware of. This chapter will discuss the physics, sources and physiological consequences of acceleration and vibration. The importance of crashworthiness in reducing exposure to short-duration acceleration and protective strategies in limiting the effects of long-duration accelerations and vibration will also be considered.

Acceleration

Physics of acceleration

- *Speed*: The distance travelled in a given unit of time regardless of direction, usually measured as miles/kilometres per hour or metres per second. Air travel is measured as nautical miles per hour (knots).
- *Velocity*: Speed applied to a given direction, e.g. 300 knots West.
- *Force*: Newton's first law states that an object will remain at a constant velocity or state of rest unless a force is applied to it. Force therefore causes acceleration. The standard international (SI) unit

for force is a newton (N): a force that will accelerate a mass of $1 \, kg \times 1 \, m/s^2$. The gravitational pull of the earth exerts 9.81 N on any mass. That is, if an object with a mass of 1 kg is dropped from a height, gravity would cause it to accelerate at $9.81 \, m/s^2$ until terminal velocity is reached. The 9.81 N force of gravity is better known as 1 G. Inhabitants of this planet have evolved so that our physiological performance is optimised under the gravitational force of 1 G.

- *Weight*: When the force of gravity is applied to a mass it gives rise to the force we sense as weight. If an 80-kg patient is subjected to an accelerative force of 2 G they would weigh 160 kg.
- *Acceleration*: A rate of change of velocity measured in metres per second squared. Acceleration can be a positive number or a negative number (deceleration). Newton's second law states that acceleration is directly related to the force applied to it and inversely proportional to the mass of the object.

Newton's third law states that for every action or force, there is an equal and opposite reaction. Therefore when we are accelerated by one force in one direction, we will be exposed to a force in the opposite direction, known as the reactive or inertial force. The reactive force felt during acceleration is known as G force and is labelled according to the magnitude (in multiples of Gs) and the direction it is applied in relation to the body (Figure 2.1).

G force along the vertical axis of the body is labelled Gz, with a positive vertical G force (+Gz) when the body is accelerated upwards and the reactive force pushes down. This is felt as an increased weight. A negative vertical G force (–Gz) occurs when the body is accelerated downwards with the reactive force pushing upwards. G force along the anteroposterior axis is labelled Gx. Positive anteroposterior G force (+Gx) occurs when the body is accelerated forward and the reactive force pushes the body backwards. Negative anteroposterior G force (–Gx) occurs as the body decelerates or accelerates in a backwards direction with the reactive force pushing the body forward. G force applied laterally is labelled Gy. Positive lateral G force (+Gy) occurs when the body is accelerated to the right and negative lateral G force (–Gy) when the body is accelerated to the left.

Sources of acceleration

Broadly speaking acceleration can be defined as long-duration accelerations, lasting greater than 2 seconds in excess of 1 G, or short

ABC of Transfer and Retrieval Medicine, First Edition.
Edited by Adam Low and Jonathan Hulme.

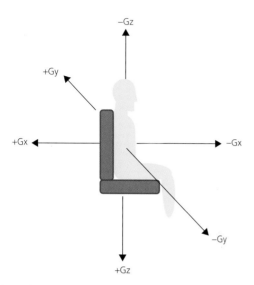

Figure 2.1 G force nomenclature.

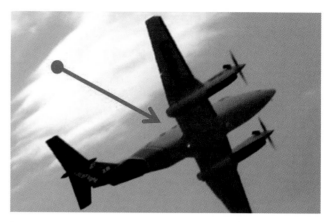

Figure 2.3 Mid-flight the craft changes course. The radial accelerative forces will be applied from the point at which the plane is turning. This would push a seated patient into their seat, sensed as an increase in weight.

duration accelerations, lasting less than 1 second. Long-duration accelerations can be due to a change of rate of movement (linear acceleration) or change of direction (radial acceleration) or a combination of both (angular acceleration).

Linear accelerations include the increase in forward velocity as a fixed wing aircraft prepares for take-off or a land ambulance leaves the scene of retrieval (Figure 2.2). Negative linear acceleration occurs as a fixed wing aircraft decelerates following a landing or a land-based ambulance decelerates on arrival. In a seated patient the reactive G forces will be applied along the anteroposterior axis (Gx) with little physiological effects. However if supine, the linear acceleration will act along the vertical axis with greater displacement of organs and fluid volumes in response to the vertical G force (Gz). In rotary wing aircraft, lift off will cause the linear acceleration along the vertical axis (Gz) in the seated patient and anteroposterior axis in (Gx) in the supine patient.

Radial accelerations occur when an aircraft is turning at a constant speed (Figure 2.3). The reactive force is applied from the point around which the turn is occurring. As the plane tilts into the turn

the G force is applied in the positive vertical axis (+Gz) of the seated occupant, felt as an increase in weight as the occupant is pushed into their seat.

Examples of short-duration accelerations include the impact of a crash, an extremely heavy landing or the deployment of a parachute, resulting typically in linear accelerations.

Physiological effects of acceleration
Long-duration acceleration

During transportation, patients are exposed to forces greater than 1 G. If acceleration is sustained, the reactive forces can lead to significant shifts in fluid volumes and organs leading to physiological changes.

Hypoxia, hypoglycaemia, hypovolaemia and acidosis all affect the efficiency of compensatory mechanisms, reducing tolerance to sustained G force. Other factors determining tolerance are rate of onset, magnitude, duration and direction of acceleration.

Acceleration is tolerated least, when applied to the vertical axis of the body (Gz). In this axis there is more space for the organs to shift, and greater hydrostatic pressures are produced as the G force is applied across a longer column. Physiological effects of acceleration along the vertical axis depend on whether it is applied as a positive (+Gz) or negative G force (−Gz).

Effects of sustained high positive vertical G force (+Gz)

As +Gz increases, hydrostatic forces causes the blood pressure to fall in the head and increase in the feet. The capacitance vessels of the lower extremities are dilated and blood pools reducing venous return. At +5Gz blood flow to the brain ceases, resulting in loss of consciousness.

After 6 seconds of exposure to +Gz, baroreceptors in the carotid artery initiate compensatory mechanisms in response to the drop in carotid blood pressure. Heart rate, contractility and peripheral vasoconstriction can increase blood pressure; however, it rarely returns to pre-exposure levels. In hypovolaemic and septic patients, these mechanisms are quickly overwhelmed.

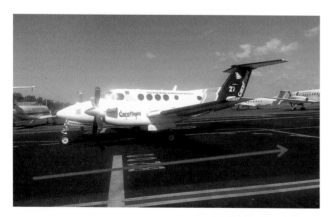

Figure 2.2 An Aeromedical King Air fixed-wing accelerating in a straight line down the runway prior to take-off. The linear accelerative force will be felt along the anterior-posterior aspect of the craft.

During high +Gz the abdominal viscera and diaphragm are pulled down. This results in an increase in residual capacity of the lung. The descent of lung tissue causes distension of apical alveoli and compression of basal alveoli leading to preferential ventilation of the lung apices. Simultaneously perfusion to the apical alveoli is reduced, with resultant ventilation perfusion (V/Q) mismatch (exaggerated in hypovolaemic patients).

Effects of sustained high negative vertical G force (–Gz)

- Gz is poorly tolerated. Hydrostatic pressures will increase venous return leading to a reflex bradycardia. After sustained exposure peripheral vessels in the lower body dilate reducing blood pressure. Pooling of blood in the cerebral circulation will lead to raised intracranial pressure and reduced cerebral perfusion pressure.
- Gz forces the abdominal organs and diaphragm to be pushed up reducing the residual capacity and causing a V/Q mismatch equal and opposite to that described in +Gz.

Short-duration accelerations

Short duration accelerations are usually unplanned and have the potential to cause serious injury or even death dependant on multiple factors (Box 2.1).

Box 2.1 **Factors that predict injury in short-duration accelerations**

1 *Magnitude and duration:* The greater the magnitude and the longer this is applied the higher the incidence of injury.
2 *Rate of onset:* If the rate of onset of the deceleration can be buffered, survivability is increased.
3 *Direction of force:* Forces along the Gz axis cause the greatest organ displacement and hydrostatic effects. These are applied to a smaller surface area to spread the force.
4 *Site of application:* A site with a larger surface area (buttocks) or stronger bony structure (skull) will provide greater protection from injury.

Limiting the effects of acceleration

Long-duration accelerations

In hypovolaemic patients it may be beneficial to position the supine patient feet first during the acceleration at the start of the retrieval in a fixed wing or land-based ambulance. This will increase venous return. In patients with fluid overload, high ventilation pressures, suspected head injury or penetrating eye injury it may be advantageous to position the supine patient head first at the start of the journey to prevent the physiological changes described when exposed to –Gz.

When considering patient positioning, it is important to note that due to the limited space of retrieval vehicles, the patient's position cannot be changed during the retrieval. Therefore during deceleration the patient will be exposed to the force, which was risk managed at the start of the journey. For this reason the best

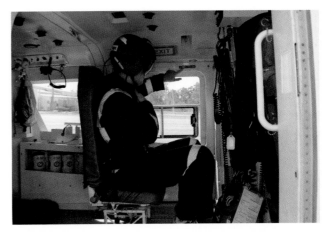

Figure 2.4 CREEP acronym of crashworthiness applied to a BK117 rotary-wing craft. Container – the structure must be of sufficient strength to prevent intrusion into the allocated survival area. It must prevent penetration of external objects. Restraint – the 4 point harness provides sufficient strength to maintain the crewman in the allocated survival area. Energy attenuation – crumple zones attenuate energy, reducing exposure to the deceleration forces. The skids and crumple seat provide added protection from +Gz forces in this craft. Escape – failure to escape will cause morbidity and mortality in an otherwise survivable crash. The jettison door to the left of the crewman is designed to fall away with a simple pull of the red handle. Post-crash factors – Life jackets, survival packs, EPOS masks and fire extinguishers are stored on this craft.

strategy for protecting patients from long-duration accelerations is to request a smooth transit. When transporting a head injury patient by fixed wing aircraft, request the pilot use the full length of the runway on landing rather than rapidly decelerate to make the shortest taxi route.

In fixed-wing aircraft more consideration should be placed on the effects of tilt as the aircraft climbs at take off and descends for landing. If the flight path of the fixed-wing aircraft is unobstructed by land masses, buildings or flight plan restrictions, it would be sensible to ask for a shallow gradient during take-off and landing to reduce the effect of tilt.

It is important to ensure we prevent any harm which may be caused from equipment subjected to acceleration. High-magnitude accelerations may cause equipment to fall if not securely fastened. Equipment resting on the patient will increase in weight when subjected to +Gz such as during a turn in a fixed-wing aircraft.

Short-duration accelerations

During the rapid deceleration of a crash the severity of injuries may be reduced by the crashworthiness of the vehicle involved. Crashworthiness can be described as vehicle factors that determine the level of exposure to the short duration acceleration suffered by the occupants, this can be summarised by the 'CREEP' acronym (Figure 2.4).

Vibration

Physics of vibration

Vibration: any form of movement which is repeatedly alternating in direction. Everything has a 'natural frequency' that it will oscillate at dependent on its mass and spring tension. Vibration can be transmitted from one body to another if they come into direct contact. If a source of vibration is oscillating close to the natural frequency of a second body, it will cause maximal oscillation of the second body (its resonant frequency).

Sources of vibration

Vibration during retrieval is unavoidable. The most common source is a turning land-based ambulance at low frequencies (0–2 Hz). In rotary-wing craft, vibration is marked, the main sources being transmitted from the main rotor (12–15 Hz) and tail rotor (23–25 Hz). Vibration in fixed wing aircraft comes from turbulence (0–4 Hz). Engine vibration (20 Hz to 20 kHz) is dampened as a design feature of the aircraft.

Physiological effects of fibration

Vibrations with a frequency of 0.1–100 Hz are likely to have adverse effects. The area of the body affected is dependent on the body part whose resonant frequency is closest to the source of vibration (Table 2.1).

Vibration causes pain and fatigue to muscles as they work to maintain body position and dampen the vibration, consequently increasing metabolic rate. Vibration causes vasoconstriction and impaired sweating, which coupled with the increased muscle activity impairs thermoregulation. Vibrations with a frequency close to the heart rate can potentially cause fluctuations in blood pressure and induce dysrhythmias. Exposure to high levels of vibration has the potential to disrupt clot formation.

Interference with monitoring, malfunctioning of pacemakers and dislodgement of IV access/endotracheal tubes are additional risks.

Limiting the effects of vibration

Most vibration reduction occurs as a design function of the vehicle/aircraft. Further reductions are achieved by avoiding direct contact between the patient and airframe, using padding to dampen the vibration, and ensuring the crew, the patient and the equipment

are adequately secured. Route planning is another important tool for protecting patients from vibration forces, e.g. avoiding turbulence in fixed-wing retrieval and excessive turning in road retrieval (Box 2.2 case scenario).

Box 2.2 **Case scenario highlighting strategies to protect the patient from acceleration at take-off and the vibrational forces caused by turbulence in fixed wing retrieval**

15-year-old male injured in a motor vehicle roll over in a rural location
Transport modality: Fixed wing
Flight time: 90 minutes
Location: transferred to airfield for retrieval

Primary survey

A: Patent. B: Sats 95%, RR 17 on 02 via Hudson mask. Reduced air entry to the left base noted, percussion is equivocal. C: HR 95, BP 100/65, warm peripherally. No external haemorrhage. D: GCS 15, crying due to severe left thigh pain. E: deformed left femur, closed.

Resuscitation

Despite the reduced air entry to the left base the patient has been stable since injury. For this reason you decide not to place a chest drain but ensure access by positioning the patient head first as the stretcher is situated on the right side of the aircraft. Two peripheral cannula are sited and 1 L of 0.9% saline is primed to pre-empt a significant drop in blood pressure during take-off. Analgesia is given and the leg splinted.

You request a slow acceleration and shallow gradient at take-off, and a cruising altitude of 16,000 feet, allowing the cabin to be pressurised to sea level.

Progression

Take off occurs without incident or the need to provide a fluid bolus. 45 minutes into the flight your pilot advises that there is an area of storm clouds ahead at this altitude. He provides you with three options:

1 He advises that he can fly through but there will be at least moderate turbulence.
2 He requests permission to fly above the storm cloud.
3 He advises that he has sufficient fuel to fly around the storm cloud but this will add a further 30 minutes to the journey.

Which option do you feel is most appropriate?

Table 2.1 Effects of vibration according to its frequency.

Frequency (Hz)	Effect
0–2	Motion sickness
3–4	Hyperventilation (caused by resonance of air in trachea)
3–8	Abdominal contents
4–8	Leg muscles
12–15	Differential head/torso movement
15–20	Soft facial muscles
60–90	Eyes
20–100	Muscle contraction

Further reading

Glaister DH, Prior ARJ. The effects of long duration acceleration, in Ernsting J, Nicholson AN, Rainford DJ (eds) *Aviation Medicine* (3rd ed.). Arnold: London, 2003.

Harding RM, Mills FJ. Acceleration, in Harding RM, Mills FJ (eds) *Aviation Medicine* (3rd ed.) BMJ: London, 2003.

Stott JRR. Vibration, in Ernsting J, Nicholson AN, Rainford DJ (eds) *Aviation Medicine* (3rd ed.) Arnold: London, 2003.

http://ftp.rta.nato.int/public/PubFullText/RTO/EN/RTO-EN-HFM-113/EN-HFM-113-07.pdf.

CHAPTER 3

Environmental Exposure and Noise

P. Paal[1,2] and M. Helm[3]

[1]Department of Anaesthesiology and Critical Care Medicine, Medical University Innsbruck, Austria
[2]Helicopter Emergency Medical Service Christophorus 1, Austria
[3]Department of Anaesthesiology and Intensive Care Medicine, Federal Armed Forces Medical Centre, Germany

---

OVERVIEW

- Retrieval medicine is practised in environments highly varying in geography, weather conditions, transfer facilities and time frames. Stakeholders of retrieval services should adapt transport modalities to the idiosyncrasies of a given area
- Noise may adversely affect a transfer. To overcome problems with hearing loss and communication by both patients and crew during air transport, a proper pre-flight brief should occur, equipment be available (e.g. intercom and headsets) and communication discipline during transport agreed. During transport, adequate monitoring (with acoustic and visual alarms) has to be guaranteed continuously
- Discrepancies between sensory stimuli can lead to spatial disorientation, with potentially dire consequences. Specifically developed night vision goggles may improve night vision
- Extreme environmental conditions can negatively impact on the patient, equipment and crew.

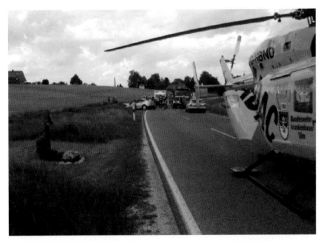

Figure 3.1 Airborne transport of multiple trauma patient in a rural civilian setting to a level I trauma centre after pre-hospital stabilization (Source: Matthias Helm. Reproduced with permission).

Introduction

Retrieval medicine is practised in environments highly varying in geography (e.g. urban, rural or remote areas), weather conditions and transfer facilities. Retrieval in urban areas usually will be over a short distance and transport time (typically <2 hours). In rural areas (Figure 3.1) the transport time may exceed 2 hours, while in remote areas distances may exceed 100 km with associated prolonged transportation and careful consideration for transport modality. This is important because distance, weather and transport facilities may substantially impact on the transport time and quality. On retrieval missions, compared to the hospital environment, equipment, personnel and space are constrained. Cold and moisture may negatively impact on the durability of battery-driven and functionality of electrically hardware. Similarly, operations may be difficult without proper equipment (e.g. night goggles).

The retrieval of patients may be greatly influenced by the demography of a given area. For instance, rural areas may have more transfers due to accidents through construction, recreation and traffic and environmental influences (e.g. hypothermia, lightning, snake bites). In urban areas internal medicine cases (e.g. myocardial infarction, sepsis, stroke) and intoxication may prevail. In wilderness areas the diagnostic and therapeutic possibilities in medical facilities may be very limited and the hospital network will be sparse. Trauma and environment-linked pathologies may dominate; airborne transfers are recommended.

Weather conditions and time of the day will substantially influence the retrieval possibilities. For example, many countries in continental Europe provide an airborne retrieval service during the day. During night, most bases will not be staffed, which makes organisation of airborne retrieval time-consuming or impossible. Some countries, e.g. Switzerland, offer retrieval service on a 24/7 basis because helicopter emergency medicine systems (HEMS) are equipped with night goggles and helicopter bases are staffed 24/7.

Stakeholders of retrieval services should adapt transport modalities to the idiosyncrasies of a given area. For instance, in rural and remote areas it may be sensible to transport patients with need of urgent intervention (e.g. coronary angiography and stenting) by air.

The patient and transfer crew may be faced with a number of adverse environmental conditions. Slow changes may be better compensated than extreme changes.

Equipment

In an in-hospital environment several resources are taken for granted when caring for a seriously ill or injured patient. Common problems or shortages during retrieval missions may include:

- equipment: faulty, inadequate, missing or unfamiliar
- oxygen depletion
- power failure.

Equipment in vehicles should be flight-tested to ensure compatibility with the aircraft's avionics systems, secured and selected on the basis of ease of use, compatibility, robustness, size and weight. The safety and well-being of the team and the patient are paramount (Table 3.1).

Reliable communication systems and equipment are fundamental for effective and safe patient retrieval. Retrievals are unique in presenting clinical and transfer logistical challenges (e.g. terrestrial vs. airborne). Rarely does everything go as planned. Senior clinicians, with specific skills and training, should therefore be in charge of retrieval missions.

Noise

Noise is defined as sound that bothers and may harm the medical crew and patient (Table 3.2). Noise may adversely affect a transfer. During ground missions, noise may be generated by traffic, the engine and sirens. In airborne missions, noise is mainly generated by the engines of the aircraft. The noise level is measured in decibels. Humans discern sound waves of the same noise level but with differing frequencies as distinctly loud (e.g. high- compared with low-frequency noise is perceived louder). To overcome problems with hearing loss and communication by both patients and crew during air transport, a comprehensive pre-flight brief should occur detailing available equipment (e.g. intercom and headsets) and communication discipline during transport. During transport communication and adequate monitoring (e.g. with acoustic and visual alarms) have to be guaranteed continuously (Figure 3.2).

Table 3.1 Strategies to increase safety of crew and patient.

Health and safety policies and procedures
Training
Protective equipment, which is appropriate and personal
Personal injury insurance
Retrieval system organised and well governed

Table 3.2 Harmful effects of noise.

Irritation of and central nervous system
Increase of blood pressure, heart rate and respiratory rate
Release of stress hormones
Impairment of psychological wellbeing
Decreased level of concentration/distraction
Sensorineural hearing loss

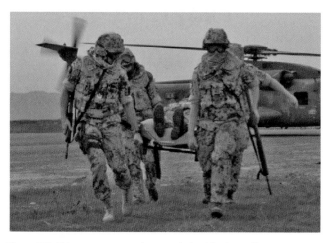

Figure 3.2 Airborne transport of a wounded soldier in a military setting from the battlefield to a field hospital (tactical evacuation care) (Source: Matthias Helm. Reproduced with permission).

Spatial disorientation

Spatial orientation in flight may be difficult because a multitude of sensory stimuli (proprioceptive, vestibular and visual) affect the crew. Discrepancies between sensory stimuli can lead to spatial disorientation. Between 5% and 10% of all general aviation accidents are attributable to spatial disorientation; 90% are lethal. Spatial disorientation can also be caused by a disease within the vestibular system. Poor weather conditions and low visibility may exacerbate spatial disorientation. For instance, low visibility may deprive a pilot of the external visual horizon.

Visual flight rules (VFR) are a set of regulations under which a pilot operates an aircraft in weather conditions generally good enough to direct an aircraft. If visibility is too low for VFR, pilots are required to rely on instrument flight rules (IFR). Operation of the aircraft will be primarily through referencing the instruments rather than external visibility. Heavy fog, torrential rain and snowfall are major causes of poor visibility, limiting visual acuity, especially in HEMS missions.

The ability to see in low light conditions (i.e. night vision) is poorly developed in humans compared to many animals. Specifically developed devices may improve night vision. These devices convert invisible to visible light, thus a dimly lit scene can be appreciated. Night vision goggles (NVG) are equipped with a dual eyepiece. In HEMS missions NVG are used to improve flight safety.

Harsh environmental conditions

Obtunded and unconscious patients are unable to protect themselves from harsh environments and probably deteriorate without medical support. Retrieval teams should safeguard the patient throughout the transport. Therapeutic issues in obtunded and unconscious patients are given in Table 3.3.

The operability of the equipment and the survival of the patient should ideally be guaranteed regardless of the harsh environment. Retrieval of patients should take into account transport distance,

Table 3.3 Therapeutic issues in obtunded and unconscious patients.

Airway protection
Analgesia
Continuous monitoring
Maintenance of anaesthesia and lines
Normocapnia
Normothermia
Normoxygenation
Protection from dust, fumes, light and noise
Stable circulation

geographic peculiarities, transport modalities (e.g. terrain-bound vs. airborne), weather and temperature. In a temperate climate the environmental impact may be less, but temperatures may still change quickly by >40°C over a single day.

Extreme dry and moist conditions

Extreme dry and moist conditions can affect the operability of the equipment. The crew must be prepared to improvise in case of equipment failure (e.g. clinical monitoring with LCD monitor failure). To avoid patient overheating, core body temperature monitoring is mandatory and active cooling may need to be considered if equipment is available. Dehydration may be a serious challenge for both crew and patient. Care should be take to avoid direct exposure to constant direct sunlight.

Extreme cold conditions

With extreme cold the life-time of batteries may be reduced by more than 80%; spare battery capacity is essential. Fluids in infusion bags and in syringe pumps may freeze. Patients may cool rapidly, especially if they are wet and exposed to wind. Progressive hypothermia increases the risk of haemorrhage and arrhythmias, and when <30°C of cardiac arrest. In mountainous areas, altitude (Figure 3.3) and concomitant hypobaric hypoxia have to be considered (see Chapter 2). Hypobaric conditions may set patients with trapped

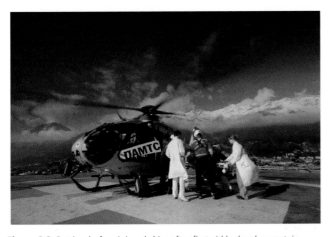

Figure 3.3 Retrieval of an injured skier after first aid by local mountain rescuers in alpine winter conditions (Source: Thomas Widerin, leading HEMS crew member Christophorus 1, Innsbruck, Austria. Reproduced with permission).

air in body cavities at risk. For example, when patients are lifted to higher altitudes a tension pneumothorax may develop and tracheal tube cuff pressure will increase. At sea, all conditions discussed for temperate, hot and cold climates can be found. Humidity and wind may be considerably stronger than on dry land.

Weather

Weather is the day-to-day state of the atmosphere. It is driven by air pressure differences between different regions on Earth. Owing to varying sun exposure, moisture and temperature gradients build up, which cause air pressure difference variation by latitude. Air pressure and density diminish with altitude. Only the most internal layer of the atmosphere, the troposphere, is relevant for retrieval medicine. It commences at the Earth's surface and depending on the latitude it extends ~9 (at the poles) to 14.5 km (at the equator) into the atmosphere. The troposphere is mainly heated by energy transfer from the Earth's surface. Hence, on average, the lowest part of the troposphere (i.e. at sea level) is the warmest and temperature decreases with altitude. The energy and moisture transfer from the Earth's surface into the troposphere favours vertical air mixing.

Mass air movements are triggered by gradients in atmospheric pressure (defined by moisture and temperature). Warmer and drier air is less dense than cool air, this causes warmer and drier air to act and appear "lighter". If warmer air is beneath cool air, air currents will develop as the air layers of different temperatures exchange positions. Mass air movements may be dangerous to airborne retrieval missions (Box 3.1).

> Box 3.1 **The main types of turbulence**
>
> *Convective turbulence*: ranges from simple rising bubble of warm air to thunderstorm (with lightning, hail, air turbulence, icing and downburst)
> *Mechanical turbulence*: air currents develop around mountain ranges and tall buildings
> *Wind shear*: a rapid change of wind speed or direction over a short distance. May be critical during take-off or landing
> *Clear-air turbulence*: the turbulent movement of air masses in the absence of any visual cues (e.g. clouds). It is caused when layers of air, moving at varying speeds, collide
> *Jet streams*: fast flowing narrow air currents in the upper troposphere. They lie between the cold polar air and the warm tropical air

The upper troposphere (7000–12000 m) is prone to clear air turbulence. In the lower troposphere mountain ranges may cause clear-air turbulence. It is almost impossible to detect with the naked eye but can be detected with optical techniques. Thin cirrus clouds can indicate clear-air turbulence. Clear-air turbulences may be located in the vicinity of jet streams.

Other conditions that may affect aviation include i.cing due to super-cool water droplets, which freeze on objects they come in contact with; visibility may be limited due to fog, haze, mist, sandstorm or rain- and snowfall (Figure 3.4).

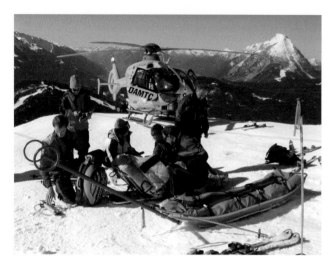

Figure 3.4 HEMS crew and hospital staff cooperate in the fast transfer to the trauma department (Source: Thomas Widerin, leading HEMS crew member Christophorus 1, Innsbruck, Austria. Reproduced with permission).

Further reading

Hearns S, Shirley PJ. Retrieval medicine: a review and guide for UK practitioners. Part 2: safety in patient retrieval systems. Emerg Med J 2006;23(12): 943–7.

Helm M, Kulla M, Birkenmaier H, Lefering R, Lampl L. Traumamanagement unter militärischen Einsatzbedingungen. Der Chirurg 2007;78:1130–8.

Hossfeld B, Lampl L, Helm M. Notfallmedizin in Krisengebieten – Einsatzkonzepte der Bundeswehr. Notfallmedizin up2date 2008;3:1–7.

Hossfeld B, Lampl L, Helm M. Die Bedeutung des Sekundärtransports in der Luftrettung. Notfall & Rettungsmedizin 2008;11:252–7.

Shirley PJ, Hearns S. Retrieval medicine: a review and guide for UK practitioners. Part 1: clinical guidelines and evidence base. Emerg Med J 2006; 23(12):937–42.

Taylor CB, Stevenson M, Jan S, et al. A systematic review of the costs and benefits of helicopter emergency medical services. Injury 2010;41(1):10–20.

Weber U, Reitinger A, Szusz R, et al. Emergency ambulance transport induces stress in patients with acute coronary syndrome. Emerg Med J 2009;26: 524–8.

http://www.caa.co.uk/homepage.aspx?catid=3

CHAPTER 4

Altitude Physiology

Y. Wimalasena[1,2] and C. Duncan[3]

[1] Emergency Medicine, Retrieval/HEMS Fellow, Greater Sydney Area HEMS, Australia
[2] Ambulance Service of NSW Rescue Helicopter Base Bankstown, NSW, Australia
[3] Department of Anaesthesia, Timaru District Hospital, New Zealand

---

OVERVIEW

- The structure and composition of the atmosphere
- The Gas Laws and the relationship of pressure and altitude
- Causes and effects of decompression
- Strategies for prevention of hypoxia
- Low altitude aeromedical transport.

KEY LEARNING POINTS

- Working knowledge of the gas laws, the relationship between pressure and altitude and physiological consequences of these are important for aeromedical work
- Recognition of decompression sickness is important for both flying and diving injury
- When planning an aeromedical transfer think about the consequences of reduced pressure, the consequences of loss of pressure and the possibilities of worsening their acute problem and the practicalities involved.

Introduction

Most of the medical issues that occur at high altitude are due to the low partial pressure of oxygen in the atmosphere. This chapter aims to explore the composition of the atmosphere, the relationship between different gases and its effect on the human body.

The atmosphere

Atmospheric structure

The atmosphere can be divided into a series of concentric shells of varying depths around the earth, defined by their thermal features and divided by 'pauses', where one gives way to the next. Successive layers are the troposphere, stratosphere, mesosphere, thermosphere and exosphere (Box 4.1).

ABC of Transfer and Retrieval Medicine, First Edition.
Edited by Adam Low and Jonathan Hulme.
© 2015 John Wiley & Sons, Ltd. Published 2015 by John Wiley & Sons, Ltd.

Box 4.1 The layers of the atmosphere

Troposphere

0–14.5 km
Consistent temperature fall as altitude increases (up to −52°C)
Water vapour is present
Large-scale air turbulence/movements which cause weather changes

Stratosphere

14.5–50 km
Progressive rise in temperature up to −3°C (absorption of UV radiation)
Ozone is present here

Mesosphere

50–85 km
Coldest layer with a rapid decline in temperature to −93°C

Thermosphere

85–600 km
Continuous temperature increase (due to absorption of solar radiation)

Exosphere

Uppermost layer
Extends out to the distance where particles are still gravitationally bound to earth, to 190000 km
Atmosphere thins out and merges with interplanetary space

Atmospheric composition

Atmospheric composition is relatively constant from sea level to 300,000 feet as is gas composition, shown in Table 4.1.

Table 4.1 Composition of gases in the atmosphere.

Gas	% Composition
Nitrogen	78%
Oxygen	20.90%
Argon	0.90%
Carbon dioxide	0.04%
Water vapour	0.25–1%
Other	1%

Gas laws

Understanding the laws that govern the behaviour of gases is essential when studying the effects of altitude on the human body (Box 4.2).

Box 4.2 Summary of the gas laws

Boyle's law

At a constant temperature, volume is inversely proportional to pressure

Charles' law

At a constant pressure, volume is directly proportional to temperature

Dalton's law

Total pressure exerted by a mixture of gases is equal to the sum of the pressures exerted by each of its components

Henry's law

At a constant temperature, the mass of gas dissolved in a liquid is directly proportional to the partial pressure of the gas above the liquid and its solubility coefficient

---

Changes in atmospheric pressure with altitude

We live at the bottom of an ocean of air, which by unquestioned experiments is known to have weight Evangelista Torricelli, 1644

As so eloquently explained by Torricelli, atmospheric pressure (and density) falls exponentially with ascending altitude (Figure 4.1). In keeping with Dalton's law, so does the partial pressure of oxygen, the resulting 'hypobaric' hypoxia leads to many of the pathophysiological changes experienced by the human body at altitude (Figure 4.2).

Atmospheric radiation, ozone and the earth's magnetic fields

Ozone (O_3) is found in the stratosphere, protecting the Earth from ultraviolet radiation. It is produced when oxygen absorbs UV radiation causing the molecule to split into free atoms, which can then combine with O_2 to form O_3. This reduces the amount of UV radiation reaching the Earth's surface.

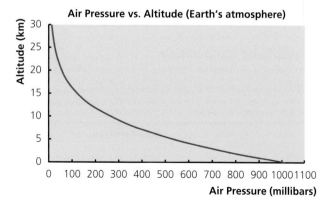

Figure 4.1 Changes in partial pressure with increasing altitude as described in Dalton's law.

Infrared radiation is also partly absorbed in the upper atmosphere, but much of it reaches the Earth's surface.

Primary ionising radiation comes from our own sun and other stars. It consists of protons, alpha particles and nuclei of heavier atoms. Secondary radiation is produced when primary particles collide with atoms in the atmosphere and consists of protons, electrons, neutrons and gamma rays. Both are capable of significant ionisation, the power of which reduces as they descend through the atmosphere and collide with other molecules.

At sea level, the ionizing effect of cosmic radiation is only one-seventieth of that encountered at 70,000 feet. Hence long hours of flying at altitude can increase an individual's lifetime dose of ionising radiation; however, its clinical significance is unclear.

Decompression

Decompression occurs when there is a breach in the airframe of a pressurised aircraft at altitude.

Box 4.3 Factors affecting rate of cabin decompression

The rate of decompression depends on

the volume of the cabin
the size of the breach
the absolute pressure in the cabin at the beginning of the decompression
the absolute pressure outside the cabin

Decompression can be rapid or slow (Box 4.3). Rapid decompression occurs with a sudden loss of hull integrity (e.g. a cargo door loss).

Rapid decompression is associated with:

- a loud noise on the release of pressure
- rushing air
- rapid temperature drop
- misting from condensing of water vapour.

Slow decompression occurs with a low-volume leak (e.g. a door seal failure), causing a gradual drop in cabin pressure and temperature.

Box 4.4 Factors affecting the physiological response to decompression

The physiological effect of decompression depends on

- the rate of the decompression
- the pressure change during the decompression
- the pressure in the cabin after the decompression.

Clinical effects of decompression
Hypoxia

Hypobaric hypoxia is the most dangerous hazard in decompression. In rapid decompression, hypoxia occurs extremely quickly as

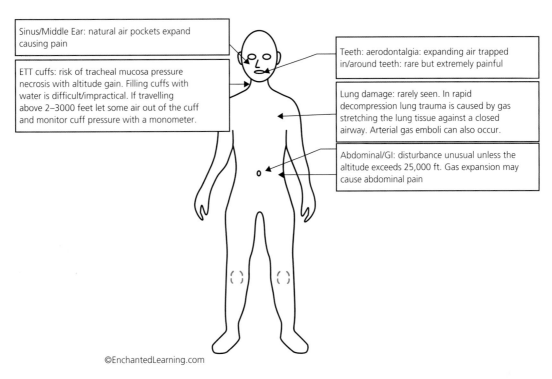

Sinus/Middle Ear: natural air pockets expand causing pain

ETT cuffs: risk of tracheal mucosa pressure necrosis with altitude gain. Filling cuffs with water is difficult/impractical. If travelling above 2–3000 feet let some air out of the cuff and monitor cuff pressure with a monometer.

Teeth: aerodontalgia: expanding air trapped in/around teeth: rare but extremely painful

Lung damage: rarely seen. In rapid decompression lung trauma is caused by gas stretching the lung tissue against a closed airway. Arterial gas emboli can also occur.

Abdominal/GI: disturbance unusual unless the altitude exceeds 25,000 ft. Gas expansion may cause abdominal pain

©EnchantedLearning.com

Ventilator –Ventilator performance at altitude varies, a recent RFD study at altitude unto 3000m showed that:
Oxylog 1000-Tidal volume increased by 68% and respiratory rate decreased by 28%.
Oxylog 2000 Tidal volume increased by 29%
Oxylog 3000 - No change
So closely monitor Tv and resp rate to ensure the vent is delivering what its meant to with altitude changes.

Figure 4.2 The consequences of reduced pressure of altitude that warrant consideration by retrieval teams.

Table 4.2 An illustration of how TUC reduces with increasing altitude in the case of sudden cabin decompression.

Altitude (ft)	TUC (mean) seconds
25,000	270
26,000	220
27,000	201
28,000	181
30,000	145
32,000	106
34,000	84
36,000	71

oxygen rapidly diffuses out of the venous system into alveoli, leading to complete deoxygenation of blood in the circulation (Box 4.5).

Time of useful consciousness (TUC) is the period of time between exposure to hypoxia and impairment in cognitive performance. The TUC for various altitudes is demonstrated in the Table 4.2.

Expansion of gases
Boyle's Law affects any gas inside the body; hence as the pressure drops, the gases will expand.

Hypothermia
Temperature at cruising altitude of 34,000 feet is less than −50°C: rapid exposure will result in profound hypothermia.

Box 4.5 **Factors affecting physiological response to acute hypoxia**

Factors that affect an individual's response to acute hypoxia are:

- genetic
- intensity of hypoxia
- physical activity: exercise exacerbates hypoxia
- ambient temperature: cold reduces tolerance to hypoxia
- inter-current illness
- iatrogenic, including alcohol.

Decompression sickness

Decompression sickness is a group of effects produced by exposure to altitude that are not due to expansion of trapped gas or hypoxia. The aetiology is believed to be due to supersaturation of body tissues with nitrogen, which then precipitates out on decompression, producing bubbles in various sites that produce characteristic symptoms (Box 4.6). The same process occurs in diving decompression sickness (the bends – symptoms summarised in box 4.6).

> **Box 4.6 Clinical symptoms of decompression sickness**
>
> Symptoms of decompression sickness:
>
> - limb and joint pain
> - respiratory disturbances
> - skin irritation
> - disturbances of the central nervous system
> - visual disturbances
> - CVS collapse.

Symptoms usually improve on descent.

Factors that influence decompression sickness incidence are:

- altitude: it is rare below 18,000 ft
- the change in absolute pressure to which the individual has been exposed
- time at altitude
- recent altitude exposure
- exercise at altitude
- cold
- hypoxia
- genetic susceptibility
- age
- obesity
- lower physical fitness.

Strategies for prevention of hypoxia (Box 4.7)

As humans gain altitude, the partial pressure of oxygen in their blood slowly declines but usually only causes physiologically effects once above 3000 metres (8000 ft).

> **Box 4.7 Strategies for prevention of hypoxia**
>
> The main strategies to prevent hypoxia in aircraft are
>
> - low altitude flying: rotary aircraft tend to fly at altitudes well below hypoxic levels
> - increasing inspired oxygen: by carrying oxygen or oxygen production equipment
> - pressurisation of the cabin

Pressurisation of the cabin

The cabin is artificially pressurised so occupants are not exposed to the hypobaric external environment. Most modern aircrafts achieve cabin pressurisation by tapping high-pressure air off the engines, conditioning it and feeding it into the cabin (Figure 4.3). The cabin pressure is controlled by outflow valves, which open to reduce pressure and close to increase pressure. Cabin pressurisation is a compromise between pressurisation to a physiologically acceptable

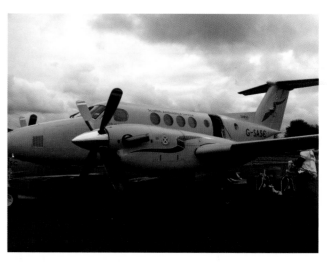

Figure 4.3 Scottish Ambulance Service Beechcraft B200C King Air, used for long haul retrievals from remote isles.

level and the drawbacks of the pressurisation system. These include additional weight carriage (compressors), fuel consumption and the structural safety hazard of a large pressure differential across an airframe. Commercial cabin pressures are kept between 5,000 and 8,000 feet.

Every country has regulations that govern oxygen carriage depending on flying altitudes and cabin pressurisation of an aircraft.

Oxygen is most commonly carried as gas in high-pressure cylinders. In pressurised fixed-wing aircraft, the delivery system involves pressure regulators and separate 'ring mains' for the flight deck and the cabin areas. The pressure in the system is controlled automatically so that if the cabin altitude increases above a set level, the pressure in the system rises causing the masks to be activated.

Air transport at low altitude

The decision to request transport by air at low altitude needs to be deliberated carefully, as it can significantly reduce the safety, increase the cost and prolong the transfer.

Clinical reasons for low altitude transfer:

- diving bends/decompression illness is the most common reason for low altitude transport:
  - As discussed above, divers who ascend too fast suffer from the same "decompression illness" as occurs in the event of decompression at altitude
  - Any further reduction in pressure by flying at altitude will worsen symptoms
  - Transfer of patient by air with "the bends" after diving is a common request, as definitive treatment is recompression in a pressure chamber. Recompression chamber facilities are few in number, thus requiring long distance transfer
  - Advice should always be obtained from the specialist at the centre but usually transfer involves transport on high flow oxygen and at the lowest practicable cabin altitude

○ Gold standard in rotary wing is to remain under 500 feet and in fixed wing to maintain cabin pressure at sea level, although not all aircraft are capable of this.
- Lung/chest injuries
  ○ In patients with pneumo-pericardium or pneumo-mediastinum, expansion of these would be life threatening
  ○ Simple untreated pneumothoraces may tension with gas expansion.
- Post lung surgery:
  ○ In patients with anastamoses in lung tissue, exposure to altitude risks suture rupture.
- Post ophthalmic surgery or penetrating eye injury:
  ○ Residual air or other gases left within the orbit can cause severe damage on expansion.
- Facial/Base of skull fractures:
  ○ Air expansion within the cranium could cause secondary intracranial injury.
- Abdominal:
  ○ Large unreduced hernias, volvulus or intersusception can have air trapped within the obstructed bowel

○ The circulation of an involved loop may be severely compromised if expansion occurs, threatening irreversible ischaemia or perforation.

Further reading

Klein, Vuylesteke, Nashef. *Core Topics in Cardiothoracic Critical Care*. Cambridge University Press 2008.

Mohler A. Sudden high altitude cabin decompression immediately threatens the safety of aircraft passengers and crew. Flight Safety Foundation 1994;41:6.

Rainford DJ, Gradwell DP. *Ernsting's Aviation Medicine*. CRC Press. 4th ed.

Stephenson J. Pathophysiology, treatment and aeromedical retrieval of SCUBA. J Military Veterans Health 17(3).

Sinclair TD, Werman HA. Transfer of patients dependent on an intra-aortic balloon pump using critical care services. Air Med J 2009;28:40–6.

Smith RPR, McArdle BH. Pressure in the cuffs of tracheal tubes at altitude. Anaesthesia 2002;57:374–8.

Van Horn J, Hatlestad D. Air transport of the IABP patient. Air Med J 2002;21:42–8.

Section 2

Clinical Considerations

CHAPTER 5

Resuscitation and Stabilisation

C. Reid[1,2] and K. Habig[1,3]

[1]Greater Sydney Area Helicopter, Emergency Medical Service, NSW Ambulance, Australia
[2]University of Sydney, Australia
[3]Ambulance Service NSW Rescue, Helicopter Base, Bankstown Airport, NSW, Australia

OVERVIEW

- The degree of resuscitation and stabilisation that is appropriate prior to transfer depends on clinical, environmental and logistical factors and therefore is case-specific

- Generally, the ability to provide procedural interventions during transport is limited by space and safety concerns, so where possible, they should be completed prior to moving the patient

- A structured <C>ABCDE approach to assessment and resuscitation is recommended in line with other clinical resuscitation settings

- The time-critical nature of many retrieval missions combined with limited equipment and personnel and unfamiliar environments require retrieval practitioners to have strong leadership and communication skills to manage effective resuscitation

- The stabilisation phase requires predicting and preparing for eventualities in transport, and protecting the patient from the adverse effects of the transport environment.

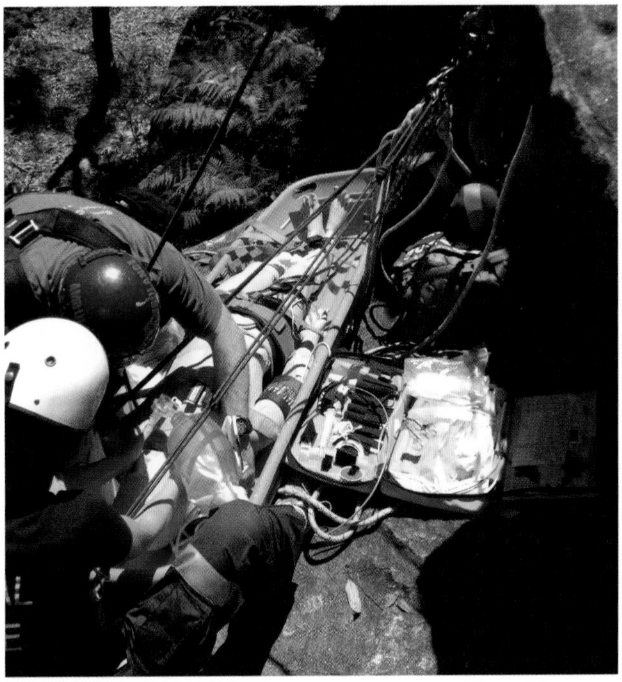

Figure 5.1 Environmental and logistic factors can affect the degree of resuscitation appropriate prior to transport.

Introduction

The retrieval medicine practitioner may have to resuscitate patients in environments as diverse as a canyon floor (Figures 5.1 and 5.2) and an intensive care unit. The amount and type of intervention appropriate to the mission therefore varies according to clinical, environmental and logistical factors (Box 5.1). For example, at a pre-hospital trauma case, the need for transport to hospital for surgical control of non-compressible haemorrhage may override the need for advanced airway intervention. During a secondary retrieval of a patient requiring transfer for urgent neurosurgery, incoming adverse weather conditions may require that non-invasive blood pressure monitoring be used in lieu of invasive monitoring, if instituting the latter will cause delays in departure and render helicopter evacuation impossible.

Box 5.1 **Factors that influence level of resuscitation prior to transfer**

- Immediate resuscitation needs
- Urgency of receiving unit care (e.g. craniotomy)
- What can be done en route (limited by vehicle size, type and personnel)
- Weather/daylight (influences air transport)
- Expertise of team
- Availability of equipment, drugs and oxygen supplies
- Safety (hostile civilian or military scene).

Nevertheless, general principles can be applied to the assessment, resuscitation and stabilisation of all patients following the establishment of personal and scene safety (Figures 5.3 and 5.4). When communication with on-scene personnel is achievable, it is

ABC of Transfer and Retrieval Medicine, First Edition.
Edited by Adam Low and Jonathan Hulme.
© 2015 John Wiley & Sons, Ltd. Published 2015 by John Wiley & Sons, Ltd.

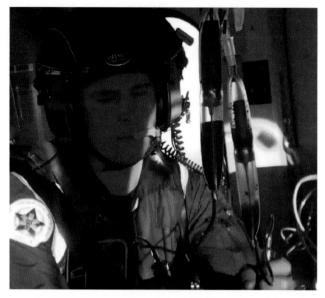

Figure 5.2 In critical patients who cannot be stabilised outside the receiving facility, some resuscitation must take place en route.

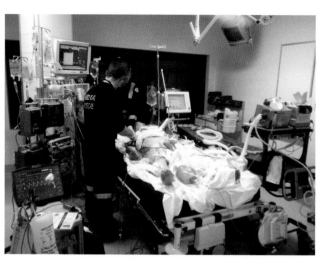

Figure 5.4 A systematic approach is required to assess and resuscitate a retrieval patient.

often possible to plan initial resuscitation prior to the arrival of the retrieval team. Advice and guidance to medical staff at referring hospitals is an essential role of a retrieval coordination centre. Such advice is best guided via tele-health connections where possible.

Handover

On arrival, a structured handover should be obtained, preferably according to a standardised system appropriate to the healthcare setting (Box 5.2). The handover may need to be truncated or postponed if there are immediate resuscitation needs, such as

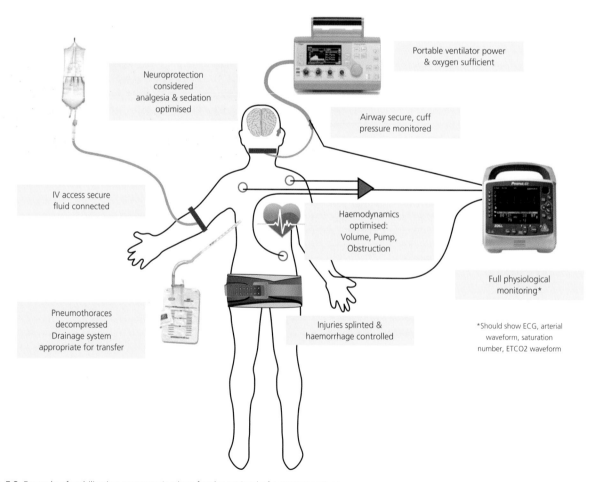

Portable ventilator power
& oxygen sufficient

Neuroprotection
considered
analgesia & sedation
optimised

Airway secure, cuff
pressure monitored

IV access secure
fluid connected

Haemodynamics
optimised:
Volume, Pump,
Obstruction

Full physiological
monitoring*

Pneumothoraces
decompressed
Drainage system
appropriate for transfer

Injuries splinted &
haemorrhage controlled

*Should show ECG, arterial
waveform, saturation
number, ETCO2 waveform

Figure 5.3 Example of stabilisation measures in place for the retrieval of a trauma patient.

control of catastrophic haemorrhage or relief of airway obstruction. Verbal handover can simultaneously be supplemented by visual information regarding the appearance of the patient, interventions being delivered and vital signs on charts or monitor screens. A history of comorbidities, medications and allergies is crucial since they may have a significant bearing on the clinical and logistic aspects of the retrieval (Box 5.3).

Airway

The airway should be assessed for patency and protective reflexes. The possibility of a loss of, or threat to patency of the airway in transport, should be managed by pre-emptively establishing a definitive airway prior to retrieval. In the vast majority of cases this will be achievable after rapid sequence induction (RSI) of anaesthesia and orotracheal intubation. Retrieval RSI can be made safer and more efficient with the use of standard operating procedures that employ pre-drawn medications in standardised doses, standardised equipment layout and the use of checklists. Attention to patient positioning, peri-intubation oxygenation techniques and minimising haemodynamic disturbance can maximise first-pass laryngoscopy success rates and reduce complications. Full monitoring including the use of waveform capnography is mandatory.

Patients in whom direct laryngoscopy is anticipated to be difficult may be assessed using an 'awake' look with direct or video laryngoscopy after airway topicalisation and sedation. If oral access to the airway is impaired, then flexible optic airway devices may be guided nasally (provided compliance is achievable, oxygenation is adequate and airway visualisation is not impeded by blood or secretions). In the event of failed laryngoscopy retrieval practitioners should be equipped and prepared to administer effective bag-mask ventilation and utilise supraglottic airways and transtracheal airways (surgical cricothyroidotomy). In urgent cases in which difficulty is anticipated, a 'double set-up' can be employed in which the preparation for a surgical airway is undertaken prior to RSI.

Intubated patients should have the size and depth of tracheal tube recorded and correct placement confirmed with waveform capnography and bilateral lung expansion. Tracheal cuff pressure should be monitored and maintained within recommended limits (using high-volume, low-pressure cuffs) during retrieval. Tracheal tubes and attached ventilator tubing should be adequately secured to resist tension forces generated during movement.

Breathing

Oxygenation should be assessed using pulse oximetry, and consideration given to the adequacy of vehicle oxygen supplies and any effect of altitude on oxygenation. Insufficient oxygenation via facemask after optimising other medical therapies necessitates positive pressure ventilation, either non-invasively or after tracheal intubation.

Adequacy of ventilation should be assessed by attention to rate and depth of respiration, their effects on lung expansion and carbon dioxide balance. End-tidal capnography should be used to monitor trends in the mechanically ventilated patient but should wherever possible be calibrated to arterial pCO_2 in the intubated patient undergoing secondary/tertiary transfer. Patients with inadequate spontaneous ventilation associated with single system disease (e.g. COPD exacerbation) may be transferable on non-invasive ventilation if vehicle oxygen supplies are sufficient. Patients with diseases causing high respiratory system resistance (e.g. asthma) or decreased compliance (e.g. ARDS) may be difficult to ventilate on transport ventilators. An appropriate ventilation strategy should be applied and the patient trialled on the retrieval service ventilator for a period prior to transfer. Continued difficulty may result in transferring the patient with permissive hypercapnoea, providing inhaled nitric oxide during transport, or instituting extracorporeal carbon dioxide removal strategies such as extracorporeal membrane oxygenation (ECMO).

A heat–moisture exchange (HME) filter should be used for all intubated patients, and is especially important in air medical transport where altitude-associated changes in temperature and water vapour can be significant.

Significant pneumothoraces should be drained prior to air medical transport. Traditional diagnostic modalities such as radiography can be replaced by thoracic ultrasound for this diagnosis where equipment and training allow, with the significant advantage of allowing serial assessment during the transport phase. Tension pneumothoraces may be managed temporarily with simple (open) thoracostomy in mechanically ventilated patients. The risk of retensioning due to reapposition of thoracic wall tissues is prevented by intercostal tube insertion. Endotracheal tubes have been used for this purpose but are not intended to be used in this manner. Proprietary large bore cannula devices with a release valve are available for insertion through the thoracic wall and may also offer a temporary but less invasive method. If time allows or there is significant haemothorax, an intercostal drain can be placed. It is often preferable for handling and transport to replace underwater sealed drainage systems with a drainage bag incorporating a Heimlich valve.

Circulation

Vascular/intra-osseous access should be attained, checked and secured. A dedicated line should be available and labelled for emergency use, preferably with crystalloid attached to maintain vessel patency and to provide a medication flush. In significant abdomino-pelvic trauma, vascular access should be obtained above the diaphragm. It is advisable to have at least two points of access.

The heart rate, rhythm and the blood pressure should be assessed. Circulatory insufficiency may be evident through impaired cerebration, decreased skin perfusion, oliguria or hyperlactataemia. A trial of volume therapy may be appropriate if hypovolaemia is suspected. In the patient with fluid refractory hypotension, clinical assessment of volume responsiveness is unreliable and may be augmented

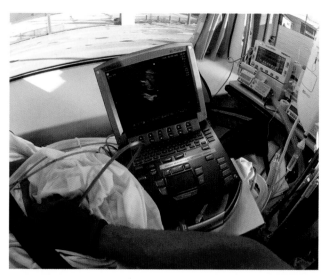

Figure 5.5 Point of care ultrasound can assist in directing resuscitative intervention.

by various portable imaging and monitoring modalities such as sonographic assessment (Figure 5.5) of inferior cava collapsibility or echocardiographic cardiac output measurement before and after a fluid bolus or passive leg raise. Permissive hypotension may be indicated in missions of short duration for bleeding patients with non-compressible haemorrhage that is not manageable locally.

In non-volume-responsive hypotensive patients, obstructive causes of shock (e.g. tension pneumothorax/massive pulmonary embolism/pericardial tamponade) should be considered. Alternatively, the cause may be failure of the heart pump (e.g. brady- or tachydysrhythmias, acute valvular disease, myocardial ischaemia, cardiomyopathy, myocarditis, and toxic or metabolic suppression (Figure 5.6)). Portable sonography can rapidly delineate obstructive causes from pump failure thereby guiding therapy in the retrieval patient.

Vasoactive infusions may be running or need to be commenced. Catecholamines such as noradrenaline (norepinephrine) and adrenaline (epinephrine) ideally should be infused via a central venous catheter, although dilute solutions may be used through reliable proximal peripheral lines if other factors render central vascular access unachievable. In critically ill patients this is often preferable to intermittent boluses of vasopressors, such as metaraminol or phenylephrine, which may raise blood pressure at the expense of cardiac output and peripheral perfusion. Continuous invasive blood pressure monitoring is advised while on vasoactive infusions, but there is probably no role for routinely monitoring central venous pressure during transport. Patients with cardiogenic shock refractory to vasoactive therapy may require the institution of mechanical circulatory support prior to retrieval, such as intra-aortic balloon counterpulsation or veno-arterial ECMO.

Actively bleeding patients should be managed with haemorrhage control measures, supported by haemostatic resuscitation with balanced blood products (Box 5.4). Owing to limitations of blood products, surgical expertise and interventional radiology facilities in the retrieval environment, the care of the bleeding patient remains one of the most challenging areas of retrieval medicine.

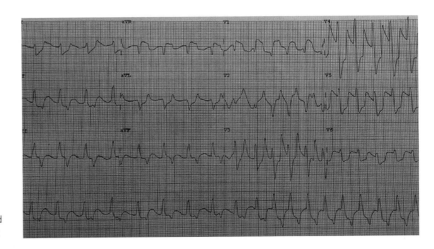

Figure 5.6 Hyperkalaemic ECG in a patient with acute kidney injury. Potassium-lowering measures were required prior to helicopter retrieval for renal replacement therapy.

Box 5.4 **Management of the bleeding patient**

1. Optimise haemostatic function (availability of blood products/other adjuncts may be limited)

Balanced resuscitation with packed red cells and plasma (or whole blood)

Early tranexamic acid

Correct deficits (e.g. platelets for thrombocytopenia, factor VIII for haemophilia A, calcium)

Reverse anticoagulants (e.g. prothrombin complex concentrate for warfarin)

Minimise haemostatic dysfunction (desmopressin for uraemic bleeding)

Optimise haemostatic environment (normothermia, avoid acidaemia)

Deep anaesthesia to reduce adverse sympathetic drive

2. Reduce blood loss

Splint long bone and pelvic fractures

Sutures, staples and pressure bandages with elevation to skin/scalp wounds

Haemostatic dressings for arterial wounds

Tourniquets for exsanguinating extremity trauma

Balloon tamponade

- junctional zone penetrating wounds (especially neck): Foley catheter
- variceal haemorrhage: Sengstaken–Blakemore tube or equivalent
- post-partum haemorrhage: Rusch balloon or equivalent
- life-threatening epistaxis and maxillofacial trauma: Epistat® or equivalent
- resuscitative endovascular balloon occlusion of the aorta (REBOA)

Resuscitative surgical methods

- thoracotomy with hilar twist or clamping for unilateral thoracic haemorrhage
- thoracotomy with aortic pressure for abdominopelvic haemorrhage (extreme short-term measure pending immediate surgical control)
- damage control laparotomy (requires more advanced surgical skills and facilities than those generally available to retrieval teams).

Rarely a patient who remains in cardiac arrest requires transport, usually to receive an intervention to treat a reversible cause (such as percutaneous coronary intervention for myocardial infarction or rewarming for severe hypothermia) or to support the patient with ECMO pending recovery or transplantation (such as myocarditis). The safety and effectiveness of manual chest compressions are severely compromised during transport and in such cases the patient should be established on a mechanical CPR device.

Disability: the central nervous system

Minimum assessment prior to retrieval should include pupil size, symmetry, reactivity, level of consciousness and any lateralising signs. In patients with spinal cord pathology the neurological level of any deficit should be assessed and documented.

In patients with central nervous system (CNS) pathology, efforts should be aimed at minimising secondary injury from the disease and from the effects of transfer, and a neuroprotective strategy should be employed (Box 5.5).

In the event of cerebral herniation, emergency strategies to lower intracranial pressure include osmotherapy (hypertonic saline or mannitol), hyperventilation as a short-term measure, and if present a pre-existing ventricular shunt reservoir or external ventricular drain can allow drainage of cerebrospinal fluid. If a traumatic extra-axial collection is present (extradural or subdural haematoma) and logistical circumstances entail a significant delay to neurosurgical operative intervention, consideration should be given to evacuation at the referring site pre-retrieval by a local surgeon, emergency physician or retrieval physician via a burr hole.

Patient eye protection (e.g. tape) during transfer is important but must not discourage regular papillary assessment. If the patient has had poorly controlled seizures, it may be advisable to avoid long-acting neuromuscular blocking drugs that may mask ongoing seizure activity, although this must be weighed against the risk of intracranial pressure surges if movement of the intubated patient stimulates a cough reflex.

Exposure and environmental protection

Examination of the patient is completed with an assessment of abdomen and limbs. Presentations such as penetrating trauma and

Box 5.5 **Neuroprotective measures for patients with acute CNS pathology**

1. Optimise blood flow

Support mean arterial pressure to maintain cerebral perfusion
Avoid hypertension in uncontrolled CNS bleeding (e.g. acute sub-arachnoid haemorrhage)
Optimise pCO_2
30 degree head-up position if not contraindicated
Avoid excessively tight cervical collars and tracheal tube ties

2. Optimise metabolism

Protect the airway from aspiration risk
Avoid hypoxaemia (and hyperoxia), hyperthermia and hyponatraemia
Maintain normoglycaemia

3. Minimise ICP

Prevent ICP surges: adequate analgesia, sedation, muscle relaxation
Control of seizures
Osmotherapy if indicated: hypertonic saline or mannitol
Allow CSF drainage (if ventricular drain *in situ*, although clamp during movements between beds and stretchers or during turbulent flight).

burns may also warrant visualisation of the patient's back. Existing vascular lines, gastric tubes, bladder catheters and drains should be identified, checked, secured, documented and if necessary emptied prior to transfer.

Any therapies and infusions not required for immediate management during primary, or delayed primary, tranfers (e.g. nutrition, thromboprophylaxis, stress ulcer prophylaxis) should be discontinued to minimise clinical and logistic complications.

Protection of the patient from the stresses of the transport environment includes thermal protection with appropriate wrapping, and hearing protection when using helicopter transport. In air medical retrieval, gas expansion in physiological and pathological air spaces should be anticipated. Adequate analgesia, sedation and splintage of injuries should minimise the noxious effects of movement and acceleration on comfort, haemodynamics, mechanical ventilator synchrony and intracranial pressure.

Documents/investigations and imaging

To facilitate seamless care on arrival at the receiving hospital it is vital to ensure that relevant documentation, imaging and investigations are transported with the patient or are available by linked electronic medical record and PACS (picture archiving and communication systems). In addition, a range of blood tests can be essential adjuncts to the initial resuscitation and stabilisation of patients undergoing retrieval, including blood gas measurements, haemoglobin, glucose, potassium and calcium. Correction of severe anaemia, hypoglycaemia, hyperkalaemia or acid–base disturbances can be life-saving in some patients and needs to be achieved as

early as possible. Blood testing may be obtainable prior to arrival of the retrieval team by on-site pathology services but if not it can be measured by portable point-of-care testing equipment which should be accessible, as a minimum standard, to any retrieval staff managing patients in small centres without these facilities.

Planning ahead

Ongoing resuscitation needs must be anticipated and prepared for prior to departure. These include sufficient quantities of infusion medications, fluid and drugs for resuscitation and ongoing anaesthesia, taking into account any possible delays or logistical challenges. Adhesive defibrillator pads should be applied prior to packaging if electrical therapy for dysrhythmia or transthoracic pacing may be required.

Human factors

Resuscitation of a retrieval patient often requires working with unfamiliar professionals in austere environments on a patient whose clinical needs by definition cannot be completely met by the referring facility. Logistical factors may add to the time criticality, and normally used resuscitation protocols, equipment and therapies may not be applicable or appropriate. These factors add to the challenge of the mission. Retrieval practitioners require leadership and communication skills to delegate tasks optimally to achieve concurrent activity towards clearly verbalised treatment goals.

Limiting resuscitation

Occasionally a retrieval team may be deployed to a patient in whom resuscitation attempts fail or are futile. Further information from family members or the production of advanced directive paperwork may lead to this conclusion, or it may be that referring clinicians underappreciated the futility or were not comfortable managing end-of-life care alone. Any decision to limit support or discontinue resuscitation should be ideally discussed with the referring and receiving clinicians, family members and when possible the patient.

It may be appropriate for the retrieval team to remain and coordinate end-of-life care locally. In some situations transport of a patient recognised to be dying should still take place to facilitate intensive care pending family arrival and consultation, to allow a second opinion or to move to a dedicated palliative care facility. On occasion this may result in the additional benefit of allowing organ donation to be an option.

Further reading

AAGBI Safety Guideline: Pre-hospital Anaesthesia. The Association of Anaesthetists of Great Britain and Ireland. London, 2009 http://www.aagbi.org/sites/default/files/prehospital_glossy09.pdf (accessed 30/9/2013).

Mackenzie R, French J, Lewis S, Steel A. A pre-hospital emergency anaesthesia pre-procedure checklist. Scand J Trauma Resusc Emerg Med 2009; 17(Suppl 3):O26.

NSW Aeromedical & Medical Retrieval Service Helicopter Operating Procedure: Neuroprotection. 2011 http://nswhems.files.wordpress.com/2011/09/c-14-neuroprotection.pdf (accessed 30/9/2013).

NSW Health Policy Directive PD2012_019: Retrieval Handover (Adults) http://www0.health.nsw.gov.au/policies/pd/2012/PD2012_019.html (accessed 30/9/2013)

Spahn DR, Bouillon B, Cerny V, Coats TJ, Duranteau J, Fernández-Mondéjar E, et al. Management of bleeding and coagulopathy following major trauma: an updated European guideline. Crit Care 2013;19; 17(2):R76.

CHAPTER 6

Patient Packaging and Nursing Care

C. Small[1] *and F. Clarke*[2,3]

[1] Anaesthesia and Critical Care, University Hospitals Birmingham NHS Foundation Trust (Queen Elizabeth Hospital), UK
[2] Intensive Care & Anaesthetics, University Hospital of North Staffordshire NHS Trust, UK
[3] West Midlands Ambulance Service NHS Foundation Trust Medical Emergency Response Incident Team (MERIT), UK

> **OVERVIEW**
> • Patients are vulnerable to clinical deterioration and environmental hazards during transfer
> • A logical system, such as head-to-toe or ABC, will ensure all aspects of patient preparation are considered
> • Consideration of current and potential patient needs should be considered during patient preparation

Introduction

Patient packaging is a process whereby current support and systematic monitoring continues, with consideration of additional support that may be required during transportation. The patient should be resuscitated and stabilised prior to transfer. A standardised approach with meticulous attention to detail, aided by a checklist, reduces the risk of adverse events mid-transfer. Packaging must ensure that monitoring, infusion and therapeutic devices are adequately secured, and the patient is secured to the stretcher or bed, which is itself fixed (depending on transport modality). Vehicle layout and access must be considered (Figure 6.1). It is the transfer team's responsibility to protect patients from environmental hazards, especially when patients are unable to protect themselves. Motion and acceleration forces predispose the patient to risks including equipment dislodgement, motion sickness and cardiovascular instability (see Section 1).

Airway and breathing

Airway management depends on patient factors and transfer type. Any self-ventilating patient who is considered to be at risk of significant airway compromise or ventilatory insufficiency during transfer should be electively intubated and ventilated prior to departure.

Likewise, careful consideration should be made before extubating patients prior to transfer. The airway must be secured with a firmly fixed endotracheal tube (and cuff pressure checked pre-departure); laryngeal mask airways are not acceptable unless used as a rescue technique. Endotracheal tube position should be confirmed

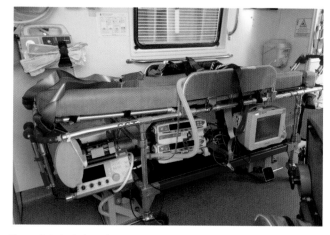

Figure 6.1 Ambulance layout.

and adequacy of ventilation and oxygenation established. Adequate monitoring is vital. Minimum standards of monitoring are recommended for all mechanically ventilated patients (Box 6.1).

> Box 6.1 **AAGBI minimum monitoring for anaesthetised patients**
>
> Attentive suitably trained healthcare provider
> Checked equipment with suitable alarm limits
> Oxygen supply and failure alarms
> Pulse oximeter
> End tidal carbon dioxide
> Airway gases and pressures
> Non-invasive blood pressure
> ECG
> Stethoscope
> Available: means of measuring temperature/peripheral nerve stimulator

---

Circulation

ECG monitoring should continue for all patients. Non-invasive blood pressure monitoring uses a lot of battery power and invasive monitoring should be instituted in those patients requiring high-frequency blood pressure monitoring. Consider placing

---

ABC of Transfer and Retrieval Medicine, First Edition.
Edited by Adam Low and Jonathan Hulme.
© 2015 John Wiley & Sons, Ltd. Published 2015 by John Wiley & Sons, Ltd.

defibrillation pads or pacing pads on unstable patients prior to mummy wrapping, as applying these en route will be difficult.

Disability and exposure

Critically ill patients may have impaired temperature homeostasis and are unable to adapt to the changes in ambient temperature, which may be difficult to control. Exposed patients may develop hypothermia, though many have SIRS and become hyperthermic (Box 6.2). Normothermia should be sought prior to transfer and equipment to monitor and maintain body temperature utilised wherever feasible. Active warming is difficult to achieve during transfer; many systems require a power supply or are too cumbersome to use in a vehicle. Therefore, packaging must ensure that heat loss is minimised.

Box 6.2 Modes of heat loss during transfer

Radiation: accelerated by patient exposure
Convection: accelerated by exposure to air flow, e.g. wind, air conditioning
Conduction: accelerated by patient contact with cold surfaces
Wrapping a sheet securely around the patient or 'mummy wrapping' will help to minimise environmental exposure for the patient while improving the security of intravenous lines, tubes and cables. Mummy wrapping should be undertaken such that accessibility to injection ports and vital monitoring are not compromised. For land transfer it is recommended that at least one IV line is on the side adjacent to the caregiver for ease of access (Figure 6.2).

Undertaking a basic neurological assessment should be feasible throughout transfer. Such an assessment, including pupil response, should be completed and documented as part of the packaging process. While pupillary response must be monitored, protection of the eyes in ventilated cases includes lubricant, padding and tape.

Immobility can cause discomfort in awake patients and they should be allowed to mobilise where it can happen safely. Mobility assessment should be undertaken prior to transfer. Ventilated patients are at increased risk of pressure skin necrosis 'pressure sores' and such areas should be protected as part of their preparation for transfer. Patient positioning should be carried out meticulously, checking that sheets under patients are smoothed, pressure points are protected and barrier cream or absorbent dressings are used in damp areas in contact with skin. These patients, especially those with hypercoagulability due to trauma or sepsis, are at a significantly increased risk of venous thromboembolism, and thromboprophylaxis should be used both prior to and during the transfer unless specifically contraindicated.

Vibration and movement, coupled with anxiety can lead to increased pain levels in patients whose pain is well controlled before transfer. Pain management must be optimised using a multimodal model, with anticipation of the potential for increased pain during the transfer. Those at risk of motion sickness should receive precautions such as antiemetics and intravenous fluid.

Trauma patients must be packaged with particular care. Spinal boards must not be used for transfers; patient spines can be immobilised adequately using a hard cervical collar with head blocks. Vacuum mattresses assist immobilisation (Figure 6.3), but may cause the patient temperature to rise so should be used with caution. Injured limbs may swell in transfer; thus plaster casts should be bivalved and non-circumferential casts loosened. These patients require regular neurovascular monitoring during the transfer.

Feeding and fluids

It is advisable to insert nasogastric tubes into all intubated patients, though feeding should be discontinued for all but the longest transfers due to the risk of vomiting and aspiration. Awake patients can be offered food during long-distance transfers if not nauseated. Unless the patient can reliably maintain his or her own oral fluid intake, intravenous crystalloid fluid can be used for fluid maintenance.

Elimination can be facilitated by a urinary catheter and collection bag, with absorbent pads under the patient. Loose stools or diarrhoea should be managed with a rectal tube and collection

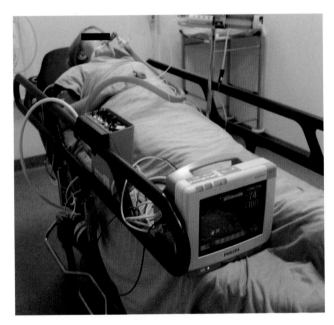

Figure 6.2 Patient packaged prior to transfer.

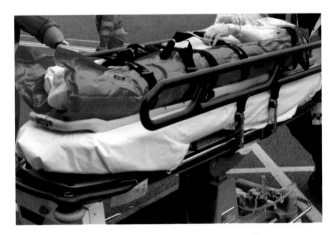

Figure 6.3 Use of vacuum mattress for transfer. (Source: Mike Greenway. Reproduced with permission).

system, which will also serve to reduce infection risk to other contacts.

Infection control

Where feasible, a microbiological screen should be carried out in the discharging unit and appropriate antimicrobial prophylaxis or treatment instituted. Infection control measures, such as hand decontamination and waste disposal, must be carried out in transfer. Nonetheless, a standard transfer environment will not allow for strict patient isolation, and other patients, passengers and crew will be placed at risk if a patient with a highly contagious or virulent pathogen is not adequately isolated. Such cases are extremely rare but include viral haemorrhagic fevers and multidrug-resistant tuberculosis. Transfer of such patients requires specialist input (see Section 7).

Nursing care

Most aspects of standard nursing care should continue, where feasible, during a transfer. Depending on the transfer timeframe, medication can be given prior to departure. Access to give drugs, such as intravenous and nasogastric ports, must be available. Recording of observations and drug administration should continue throughout.

An important aspect of nursing care is ensuring continued protection for the patient during the transfer. Considerations include basic comfort, such as pillows and clean sheets as well as minimisation of the effect of environmental hazards. Earplugs or noise reduction headsets may be warranted for some air transfers, alongside patient advice on the avoidance of otic barotrauma.

Communication between the patient and escorting staff can be challenging, particularly in areas of restricted space or increased noise. The patient can be briefed prior to departure on methods of communication, such as hand signals. Nonetheless, staff vigilance during transfer remains important.

Briefing the awake patient as part of the pre-departure protocol will identify patient concerns and fears as well as potential risks, such as travel sickness.

Air transfers

Considerations for air transfers reflect environmental changes of increasing altitude, as discussed in Section 1, such as reduced oxygen availability, gas expansion and reduced humidity. Pneumothoraces must be drained and underwater seals replaced by a one-way device, such as a Heimlich or flutter valve. Nasogastric tubes should be placed under free drainage and laparotomy wounds may be left open to allow intestinal distension. Endotracheal cuff pressure must be checked regularly in flight. Cuff air can be replaced with saline or cuff pressures monitored.

Any patient with respiratory deficiency, reduced oxygen tissue delivery or increased oxygen requirement will require supplemental oxygen in flight. The requirement during transfer may be increased if the patient deteriorates. The reduction in ambient humidity can lead to drying of respiratory secretions, risking endotracheal tube blockage, thus humidity and moisture exchangers should be used in the breathing circuit. It may be difficult to provide humidified oxygen or nebulisers in flight, but should be provided where required prior to departure.

The physics of flight subjects the patients to alterations in gravitational forces, particularly during take off, landing and turbulence (see Section 1). This leads to fluid shifts within the body compartments, the most important being the intravascular space, with consequential alterations in perfusion and pressure, particularly in the brain. This effect is exaggerated when intravascular volume is reduced, thus fluid status should be optimised prior to transfer and then managed meticulously in flight. Patient positioning in the aircraft must follow local protocol with consideration of injury pattern.

In common with oxygen requirements, the transfer teams must calculate drug requirements for the transfer, including contingency supplies for use during unexpected delays. Drug infusions and blood products should be labelled to the standard used in the critical care unit and stored appropriately.

Further reading

Brokalaki HJ, Brokalakis JD, Digenis GE, et al. Intrahospital transportation: monitoring and risks. Intensive Crit Care Nurs 1996;12(3):183–6.

Driscoll P, Macartney I, Mackway-Jones K, et al. *Safe Transfer and Retrieval: The Practical Approach. Group ALS*, editor: Blackwell Publishing; 2006.

Intensive Care Society (UK). Guidelines for the transport of the critically ill adult. ICS 2002 http://www.ics.ac.uk/intensive_care_professional /standards_and_guidelines/transport_of_the_critically_ill_2002

CHAPTER 7

Mode of Transport

A. Cadamy[1] and T. Martin[2,3,4,5]

[1] Intensive Care Medicine and Anaesthetics, NHS Greater Glasgow and Clyde, UK
[2] Anaesthesia and Intensive Care Medicine, Royal Hampshire County Hospital, UK
[3] Capital Air Ambulance, UK
[4] AMREF Flying Doctors, Kenya
[5] European Aeromedical Institute (EURAMI), Germany

OVERVIEW

- Modes of transport for transferring and retrieving patients are diverse
- Options are often constrained by a service's parameters, and by cost
- Selection of mode of transport involves balancing risks and benefits
- Knowledge and familiarity with the benefits and limitations of each available mode is essential
- Good communication and team working is necessary across all platforms.

Box 7.1 Factors determining mode of transport

Operational characteristics

Range
Point to point speed
Susceptibility to weather conditions
Need for inter-vehicular transfers

Patient environment

Temperature
Humidity
Noise
Vibration
Accelerations
Ambient air pressure
Privacy

Working environment

Space and access to patient
Noise
Vibration

Introduction

The mode of transport is a key consideration when planning a patient transfer or retrieval, and also for designing a transport service. Historically, patients have been moved using every conceivable mode of transport, by air, land and water. In the context of modern patient transport, the options still encompasses a broad range of modalities according to the clinical needs, geographical area, ambient conditions and the defined role and economic circumstances of the service.

As with all decision-making in patient transportation, the process comes down to balancing risks and benefits. Those who transport ill and injured patients therefore require detailed knowledge of the specific advantages and limitations of each modality in order to weigh the associated advantages and disadvantages for their patient (Box 7.1). Any need for moving patients between different vehicles in the course of a single transfer is also an important consideration. Inter-vehicular transfers can add significantly to the duration of transport and also increase potential exposure to hazards.

Ground transport

Road vehicles are, perhaps, the most common and familiar mode of ground transport. However, most forms of land-based transport

have been adapted historically for patient transport: passenger vehicles such as coaches have been converted to carry multiple stretchers, so called 'jumbulances', and trains and underground systems have been utilised to evacuate multiple casualties (Figure 7.1).

Road ambulances are found in most health systems and are familiar to all health professionals. In addition to their independent use for patient transport, road ambulances almost always act as an intermediate mode of transport linking transfers with other platforms, such as aircraft.

Although transport by road is perhaps the slowest of the commonly used modes of transport while in motion, for short distance or duration transfers a single road journey can often be more straightforward and faster than a flight requiring multiple inter-vehicular transfers and loading/unloading operations.

Road ambulances generally provide a quieter and more spacious environment. Acceleration forces and vibration however remain significant, making interventions quite difficult while moving. For team safety reasons it remains best to adhere to the principles of good transfer and retrieval practice by assessing, optimising and

---

ABC of Transfer and Retrieval Medicine, First Edition.
Edited by Adam Low and Jonathan Hulme.
© 2015 John Wiley & Sons, Ltd. Published 2015 by John Wiley & Sons, Ltd.

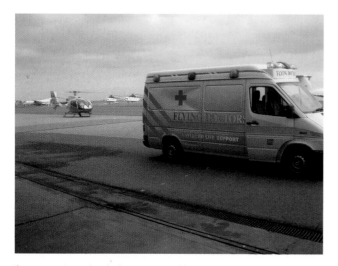

Figure 7.1 Ground ambulances are used for many primary transfers, as well as providing 'ground' transfers for fixed wing aero-medical transports.

packaging patients appropriately so as to avoid having to carry out procedures en route. Nevertheless, a major advantage of road transport is the ability to stop the vehicle at the roadside if an emergency intervention is required.

Across the globe, ground ambulances differ enormously in their capabilities. They may have a good level of basic equipment that may be useful in planning a transfer – items such as defibrillator, monitors and airway devices. The term 'ambulance' can, however, also refer to minimally equipped patient transport vehicles as well as the acute 'front-line' vehicles. In some countries, an ambulance may simply be the empty back of a van or pick-up truck. When planning a transfer it is essential to be cognisant of the type of vehicle available and its capabilities. However, it is important not to rely on equipment that is not included within the governance systems of the transfer and retrieval service, and the medical team should ideally be self-sufficient for all essential items. Modern vehicles are often equipped with DC/AC invertors that allow operation of mains powered equipment and chargers (see Section 3), but this is not standard in many services.

Emergency driving under 'lights and sirens' is governed by specific regulations and laws in many countries and only trained drivers can do so in situations of genuine clinical urgency. There are significant risks associated with 'rapid response' driving, both for the team and general public. The accelerations and motion associated with fast driving create an even more difficult environment for all vehicle occupants. It goes without saying that, outside of genuinely time-critical situations, these risks are unjustifiable. However, the use of legal exemptions in order to facilitate smooth passage through congested traffic, while not driving at maximum speed, is a practical compromise that most trained drivers are familiar with. In genuinely time-critical situations a police escort will add an extra margin of safety but should be requested in good time.

Air transport

Transport of a patient by air offers the obvious advantage of covering a large distances in a short time. However, as already mentioned,

the need for ground transfers and the time required for loading and unloading should be considered. Equipment should be flight-tested to ensure compatibility with the aircraft's avionics systems, secured and selected on the basis of ease of use, compatibility, robustness, size and weight.

Broad categorisation of air transport is according to the general type of airframe: fixed wing or rotary wing (helicopter). However, within these categories there is further variation according to the primary intended purpose of the aircraft, and the associated configuration. Aircraft operated by an air ambulance service, the military, a search and rescue service or commercial passenger aircraft will each vary both in equipment levels and in important operational restrictions (Figures 7.2 and 7.3).

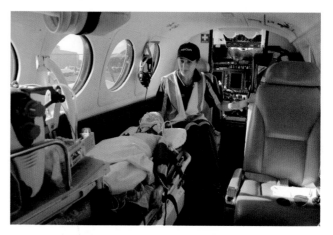

Figure 7.2 The interior of a Kingair air ambulance.

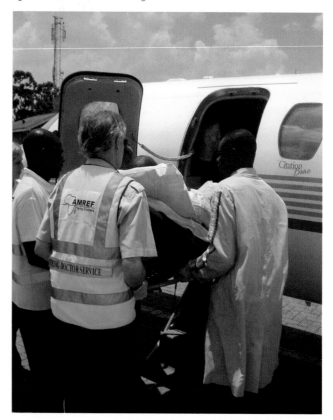

Figure 7.3 A patient being loaded into a Citation Bravo air ambulance.

Flying operations are influenced by weather, daylight, air traffic restrictions and aviation authority regulations. For example, large fixed-wing aircraft operating from airports with instrument landing systems, and which cruise at high altitude are minimally affected by weather and can fly at any time of day. On the other hand smaller single-pilot helicopters without weather radar or de-icing capability are far more restricted by weather conditions and daylight. Visibility is the major factor for helicopters as flying is often required to be below the height of surrounding features such as buildings, masts, hills and mountains.

Although helicopters may be equipped with radar and night-vision equipment to increase their operational versatility, without de-icing capability it may not be possible to fly a helicopter through cloud to an altitude that clears the aircraft of any near obstructions. Routes around, rather than through or over, bad weather need to be considered. Often the weather may therefore preclude access to certain locations. Aviation rules regarding minimal safe altitude are different for civilian and military aircraft, and according to type of flight designation, further influencing the operational limitations.

There appears to be a strong case for using ground ambulances with transfer distances of less than 100 km and helicopters for greater distances, depending on local geography. In some 'middle-distance' missions (150–300 km) either helicopters or fixed-wing aircraft could be used interchangeably, and this is often decided according to availability. However, in general, there are relatively different roles for helicopters and fixed-wing aircraft in terms of range and cost. Thus the greater cost per kilometre (at least twice) of helicopters often precludes them from standard ambulance activities and results in their being reserved predominantly for critical care and rescue operations.

Fixed-wing aircraft are obviously limited to flying from and to airfields and airports, often not conveniently situated near to either the patient's location or the destination. Rotary-wing aircraft are less limited but, unless they are flying in a military, search and rescue or primary 'HEMS' role, they are still restricted to operating from surveyed landing sites. However these sites are more versatile in their location, and may be, for example, in a designated area of a hospital.

The internal environment of an aircraft presents challenges to both patients and clinical teams. Noise and vibration are particular hazards which may affect patients (communication difficulties, increased pain and motion sickness). Acceleration forces may be considerable, especially at take-off and landing, and may cause problems such as haemodynamic instability, mechanical respiratory compromise or changes in intracranial pressure according to physical orientation within the aircraft and the clinical state of the patient.

The effects of altitude are a major consideration for aeromedical transfers. Even the airline standard cabin pressure is equivalent to around 7,000 ft (~2,000 m) above sea level and this is sufficient to cause expansion of gas by a factor of 1.4, which can certainly be clinically significant, in terms of both volume expansion and the hypoxic environment that the gas expansion causes. Most fixed-wing aircraft are capable of being pressurised to counter this effect, but some smaller fixed-wing aircraft and all helicopters are unpressurised. Helicopters invariably operate at much lower altitudes, where gas expansion effects are less significant, and unpressurised aircraft must be limited to cruise altitudes below 10,000 ft (~3000 m) whenever possible. In most parts of the world, unpressurised aircraft are only used on short flights, in which climbing to high altitude is not feasible. Hence there is simply no cabin altitude advantage to the majority of unpressurised flights. Table 7.1 details the benefits and disadvantages of pressurised versus unpressurised aircraft.

For financial reasons, air ambulances (Figure 7.4) are commonly small or medium-sized aircraft and, in terms of the working environment, space is often very limited, even in what appear to be large aircraft. To perform medical care in flight, the crew need to be able to access the patient's whole body. In an ideal situation, the stretcher should be located to enable free access to both sides of the patient but this is an uncommon luxury, as is standing room. Finding the space for medical equipment, the patient's luggage and sometimes an accompanying family member is a challenge.

Table 7.1 The benefits and disadvantages of pressurised vs. unpressurised aircraft.

Pressurised jet/turboprop aircraft	Unpressurised piston aircraft
They fly at higher altitudes because of independent cabin conditioning	They fly at lower altitudes to prevent adverse effects of hypobaric atmosphere
Often quieter than piston aircraft	Often noisier than jets
May be subject to clear air turbulence at high altitudes	May be subject to turbulence at lower levels especially in mountainous regions and in high temperatures
No weather or terrain route restrictions	Higher likelihood of route restrictions due to weather or terrain
Cabin pressurisation level may be altered by the aircrew to compensate for the patient's hypoxia at altitude (in dedicated air ambulances)	The reduced ambient/cabin pressure necessitates that the patient's oxygen status will require closer monitoring and often continuous supplementation
Cabin conditioning includes better temperature control than in unpressurised aircraft, and some degree of control over humidity and circulation of clean air (in commercial airliners)	Since the doors do not have to be sealed against depressurisation, they are often 'drafty'.
Require long paved runways runway for take-off and landing	They require much less runway for take-off and landing
In the event of a rapid decompression at high altitude the time of useful consciousness may be only 15 seconds - a significant risk to the crew who will become unconscious rapidly. They are then dependent on the pilot's ability to descend the aircraft rapidly to 10,000 ft	They can be flown from unpaved surfaces
	They are ideal for small hops during which there is little time to climb to high altitude
Pressurised aircraft are expensive to lease or purchase	The occupants of an unpressurised aircraft will never be exposed to the risks of a rapid decompression
They can benefit from reduced fuel costs and higher speeds	They cost less to lease or purchase
When distances are long, they are the only choice	They cost less to operate over short distances
	When budgets are tight the only choice might be 'unpressurised'

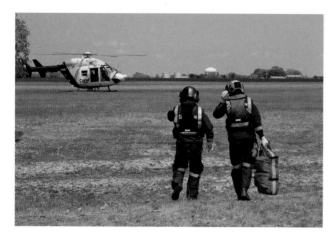

Figure 7.4 A HEMs retrieval mission.

For longer missions, space on large commercial airliners can be purchased, but the medical team is often confined to a small section around a stretcher placed in the area of six to nine seats in the economy class cabin, and often completely surrounded by fare-paying passengers. One airline (Lufthansa) has a complete and fully equipped ICU Patient Transport Compartment that can be installed on their Boeing 747 and Airbus A340-600 aircraft flying routes to and from Frankfurt: an expensive but very comfortable mode of long-haul transport for critical care patients (Box 7.2).

Box 7.2 **Considerations determining appropriate aircraft**

Distance

Helicopter and unpressurised fixed-wing aircraft are suitable for shorter distance missions, ranging to large commercial or military aircraft for long haul international scale retrievals.

Accommodation

Access to patient for medical team
Space for medical equipment
Luggage and escorts

Loading/unloading requirements

Fixed-wing aircraft inevitably require inter-vehicle transfer of patients and secondary transfers by road from airfields; helicopters may be able to land on designated hospital landing sites negating need for secondary transfers.

Ease of loading unloading varies: some aircraft have systems to facilitate this reducing need for manual lifting and reducing risk to patients and crew.

Cost

Cost will depend on contractual arrangements with aircraft operator. Mile for mile costs of rotary wing flights are greater than fixed wing.

Cabin pressure

See Table 7.1

Other modes of transport

Transfer and retrieval of patients between sites across bodies of water or from ocean-going vessels occurs commonly around the world (Figure 7.5). Water transfer may make the difference in some geographical settings between a road transfer of several hours and one of only minutes. Many patients will require retrieval from water-based locations such as oil platforms, merchant ships or leisure vessels: transferring patients by boat may be necessary in these circumstances. Commercial ferry boats are commonly used to transport road ambulances in many geographical locations and this may sometimes be the most appropriate means of moving a patient rather than an air transfer or an overly long road transfer. Coastguard vessels or lifeboats are often used to transfer patients in emergencies and may be the only means to get medical teams to islands in cases of extreme weather. Hovercraft are sometimes used to access patients in remote or hostile environments. Passenger vessels, such as cruise ships, may use tenders to transfer passengers ashore and these can also be used for medical transfers. Each of these modalities has particular demands and challenges (Box 7.3). Air transport may be preferable, using helicopters operating either from helipads built onto ships and oil platforms or through winching operations. The complexity of winching should not be

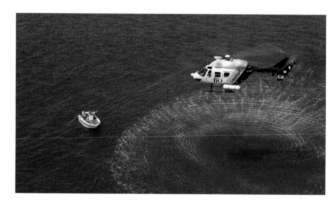

Figure 7.5 A HEMs mission over open water.

Box 7.3 **Maritime operations**

Tender/lifeboat/ferry transfer

Environmental exposure
Motion sickness
Isolation of team
Potential for water contamination of equipment
Hazardous embarkation/disembarkation
Slow: but may be faster than by road according to geography.

Winching operations

Risk to aircraft
Risk to vessel from ditching
Risk from static charge from winch cable
Physiological insult to patient from positional changes during winching
Inability to monitor or treat patient during transfer
Loss of continuity of care

underestimated as it is hazardous not only for the aircraft and crew, but also to the vessel involved. Most vessels have standard operating procedures for air–sea operations that are intended to mitigate the risks and put contingencies in place should a problem occur. For example, cruise ships may evacuate passengers from several decks below winching operations and muster primary and secondary fire crews in case of a ditching incident.

Summary

The various modes of transport available to transfer and retrieval teams each carry their own benefits and limitations. Adequate knowledge and training is required to facilitate good decision-making and effective operation in the particular environment and the parameters of each service. Close liaison with the operational crew, be it of road ambulance, aircraft or other mode, is routinely necessary in order to weigh various options and integrate their operational considerations with clinical and logistical factors. Good communication and team working are key to providing safe and effective patient care.

Further reading

CAMTS (Commission on Accreditation of Medical Transport Systems). 9th Edition Accreditation Standards. Anderson, SC, USA: 2013. http://camtsshelley.homestead.com/04FINAL_9th_EditionStds_9-5-12.pdf

Martin TE. Under pressure to comply. AirMed & Rescue 2012;June:38.

Martin TE. *Aeromedical Transportation: A Clinical Guide*. Aldershot: Avebury, 2006.

Martin TE. *Handbook of Patient Transportation*. London: Cambridge University Press, 2001.

CHAPTER 8

International Repatriations

B. Vadera[1,2,3]

[1] AMREF Flying Doctors, Kenya
[2] European Aeromedical Institute (EURAMI), Germany
[3] Air Medical Physician Association (AMPA), USA

OVERVIEW

- Repatriation involves returning the patient to their domiciliary country or local health resource
- Planning and logistics play a significant role in the smooth running of a repatriation
- The patient must be as medically stable as possible
- Different transport modes may be considered depending upon patient factors and distances travelled.

Introduction

The history of aero-medical transportation is almost as long as the history of flying itself: its concept rooted in military history.

As aviation technology progressed, so did the awareness of the potential use of aircraft as airborne ambulances. Today, air-medical transportation plays a vital role in the care of critically ill or injured patients as well as repatriating patients over long distances.

Definition

'International repatriation' refers to the process of returning a patient back to their home country. It is usually carried out by air, once the patient is stable enough to endure the transfer.

Unlike 'medical evacuation', where the patient is transported to the nearest centre of medical excellence for initial treatment and stabilisation, a decision for international repatriation is irrespective of whether or not the patient can be treated locally. It is a *planned* event in which a number of stakeholders are involved.

Criteria for international repatriation

International repatriation is an expensive undertaking and most medical insurances offer repatriation as an optional cover to their medical policies. Patients who have repatriation cover have the right to be repatriated back home and can insist on it. For those

who are not covered, a decision for international repatriation will depend on the following:

- the patient's insurance is not valid overseas, therefore limiting medical services overseas to emergency care only
- hospitalisation and convalescence are expected to be of long duration
- there is significant language barrier with negative consequences on the patient's care and/or prognosis
- there is good evidence that the surroundings and support of the patient's home environment would positively influence recovery
- on humanitarian grounds in cases of terminal illness.

Determining whether or not the above criteria apply can be challenging and requires good communication between the patient, relatives, the treating doctor, the receiving doctor and the medical insurers.

Selecting the mode of transport

Once the decision for international repatriation has been made, the right mode of transport has to be selected. Important considerations include the patient's diagnosis, clinical condition, mobility, requirement for medical equipment, drugs and general assistance before and during the flight. The costs differ significantly (Box 8.1).

> Box 8.1 **Transportation options for international repatriation, with increasing associated cost**
>
> - Repatriation on commercial flight: seated (usually in Business or First class)
> - Repatriation on commercial flight: stretcher (likely use of a 'high loader')
> - Repatriation on commercial flight: patient transport compartment
> - Repatriation by air ambulance.

Repatriation on commercial airline

For all repatriations on commercial flights, medical clearance has to be endorsed by the airline's medical department prior to departure. Most airlines request that a Medical Information form based on the International Air Travel Association Medical Information Form for

ABC of Transfer and Retrieval Medicine, First Edition.
Edited by Adam Low and Jonathan Hulme.
© 2015 John Wiley & Sons, Ltd. Published 2015 by John Wiley & Sons, Ltd.

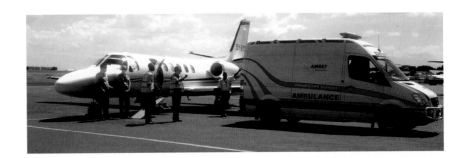

Figure 8.1 Cessna Citation Bravo private air ambulance receiving a patient at the airport.

Air Travel (IATA MEDIF) document is completed by the patient's treating doctor to assess the patient's medical condition and special needs (e.g. wheelchair, stretcher, 'high loader', oxygen, etc.).

It is the airline's prerogative to approve/reject the transfer request. Depending on their condition, patients need to be accompanied by a doctor and/or nurse. For stretcher patients a medical escort team of not less than two people is recommended to provide the necessary care and manual handling assistance. The same is recommended for psychiatric patients who have to be observed at all times before, during and after the flight. Patients travelling in First or Business class have to be able to sit during take-off and landing.

Medical escort crews will carry equipment that enables them to provide medical treatment to the patient during the flight. Common equipment for medical escort services includes:

- basic medication
- monitoring unit
- CPR equipment

Other items depending on the patient's individual needs.

It is advisable to declare the medical items carried in the hand luggage officially at check in to avoid unexpected restrictions.

Medical conditions that are likely to be rejected on commercial airlines are summarised in Box 8.2.

> Box 8.2 **Potential reasons for refusal of medical repatriation on a commercial airline**
>
> Contagious illness
> Illness or disease that negatively impacts on the comfort of other passengers, i.e. bad smell, irritating noise or unpredictable and disturbing patient behaviour.
> Requirement of a wide range of medical equipment during flight
> Patient condition that is unstable and could result in an aircraft diversion.

Long-distance international transportation of intensive care unit patients is extremely costly and logistically challenging. Only a few airlines accept patients in unstable or critical conditions. An exception is the Patient Transport Compartment (PTC), a specially installed unit with comprehensive intensive care capabilities and a wide range of medical supplies offered by Lufthansa on special routes (see Chapter 6). The airframes are configured in a way that provides access to power outlets and large amounts of oxygen inside the PTC. The compartment can be closed allowing privacy

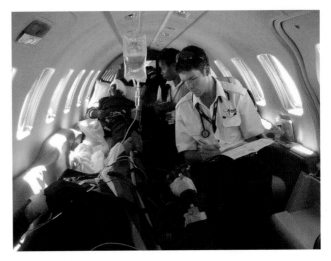

Figure 8.2 Cabin of an air ambulance.

and ensuring other passengers are not inconvenienced. Using the PTC for critically ill patients on long-distance repatriations offers some advantages compared to the use of an air ambulance in terms of cost-effectiveness, shorter transport times and reduced acceleration/deceleration trauma as a result of multiple fuel stops (Figures 8.1 and 8.2).

Repatriation by air ambulance

Using an air ambulance for international repatriation is extremely expensive, but has many important advantages (Box 8.3).

> Box 8.3 **Advantages of repatriation using an air ambulance**
>
> Flexibility of flight schedule
> Wide variety of patients can be transported
> The interior is configured to meet the patient's needs with full intensive care capabilities
> Specialised equipment like a neonatal incubator can be installed allowing the transport of neonates
> Additional stretcher systems can be fitted, allowing repatriation of multiple patients.

The type of air ambulance aircraft will determine the speed and the number of fuel stops en route. Generally, the bigger the airframe, the longer the range with fewer stops, but the higher the costs.

Patients on air ambulance flights are usually accompanied by a flight physician and a flight nurse. Most air ambulance transports are 'bed-to-bed' transfers, and it the responsibility of the medical flight crew to ensure comprehensive handovers at the referring and the receiving facility.

Availability of spare seats for accompanying relatives on the flight will depend on the size of the aircraft.

Ground transport

It is important to remember that the transfer does not start or end at the airport. Arrangements for a ground ambulance must be in place at both sides prior to departure. Receiving hospitals occasionally send their own team to transport the patient to hospital but this has to be agreed before.

Immigration and other formalities

Even though immigration officers will normally come to the patient, they require the same travel documents as for anyone else. In special cases, alternative travel documentation can be generated, but this is often a complicated, lengthy process.

Professional standards

EURAMI (European Aero-medical Institute) and CAMTS (Commission on Accreditation of Medical Transport Systems) in the USA are the main international organisations providing professional standards and audit of air ambulance services. It is advisable to use air ambulance companies that are officially accredited by either to ensure quality.

Arranging international repatriation

Arrangements for international repatriation are often provided by Assistance Companies who offer services in medical situations during travel worldwide. Assistance companies sell their programmes in partnership with insurers, or direct to the consumer. Members can call the assistance company through a 24-hour call centre to receive help.

Assistance services can include:

- to arrange and pay for medical expenses away from home including cash advance
- to advise on medical service providers in unfamiliar places and organise treatment if required
- to communicate with the treating facility or medical service provider on behalf of the member, obtain medical reports and assist in appropriate health care decisions
- to plan and arrange international repatriation in conjunction with the local treating doctor and the receiving facility in the home country.

A variety of resources may be called upon to solve a medical challenge while the patient is in a foreign country.

Further reading

Conner R. Medevac from Luzon. Air & Space Magazine, July 2010.

IATA Medical Manual, 6th Edition, May 2013

Lam DM. Wings of life and hope: a history of aeromedical evacuation. Problems in Critical Care 4(4):477–94.

Martin T. Aeromedical Transportation: History of Medical Evacuation, Part 1 (1) 3-11, 2nd ed, 2006.

Neel H Jr., Medical considerations in helicopter evacuation. U.S. Armed Forces Medical Journal 1954;N2.

Neel H Jr., Medical evacuation in Korea. U.S. Armed Forces Medical Journal 1955;5.

McLaughlin RH. Criteria for medical repatriation and the context of inadequate access to care. American Journal of Bioethics 2012:12(9)

Page TN, Neel H Jr., Army Aeromedical Evacuation. U.S. Armed Forces Medical Journal, No. 8 (Aug 1957).

Veldman A, Diefenbach M. Air Med Journal, Mar-April (2) 2004.

CHAPTER 9

Critical Incidents

J.M. Droogh[1,2] and J.G. Zijlstra[2]

[1]Intensive Care Medicine; Mobile Intensive Care Unit, The Netherlands
[2]Department of Critical Care, University Medical Centre Groningen, University of Groningen, The Netherlands

---

OVERVIEW

- Transport related incidents are common
- Incidents can be divided into patient related, equipment related and team related
- Diagnosing and treating both physiological deteriorations and technical problems may be challenging due to the transport surroundings
- Most incidents are preventable by thorough preparation and technical knowledge of equipment used
- Critical incident training is highly recommended.

Introduction

'If anything can go wrong, it will' (Murphy's Law). This definitely has been proven for transport of the critically ill patient. Over the past decades several articles have been published detailing adverse events that occur during transfers. Adverse events rates reported varied from 3% to 75%. Incidents may be categorised as patient related, equipment related and team related.

Physiological deteriorations (Table 9.1)

Retrieval or transfer physicians are familiar with treating critically ill patients. Most of the medical problems faced en route are not different from those encountered in hospital, neither is the therapy. However, because of the transfer, some transport-related problems may arise. Furthermore, diagnosing and treating the problems can be challenging since one often has to work in a small compartment, on the move and with little back-up. Some examples are discussed below.

Respiratory events

Reported respiratory events are most often inadequate ventilation or oxygen desaturation, with incidences up to 15%. Hypoxaemia and sometimes high airway pressure may be the only initial sign of an unknown problem. Since auscultation may be difficult or

impossible due to a noisy environment, combining information of the patient's illness, findings gathered during the initial assessment prior to the transfer (e.g. tube position and fixation, wheeze on auscultation), ventilator readings (tidal volume, plateau and peak pressures), oxygen saturation, capnography and physical examination (symmetrical movement of the thorax), may all aid diagnosis.

Patient-related causes may be sputum mobilisation or endotracheal tube dislodgement. Both can occur on moving a patient or from vibration in an ambulance/helicopter/plane and therefore should be checked as a first priority. Other causes, like pneumothorax, are fortunately rare during transport, but emergency drainage should be considered when other causes are excluded.

Equipment-related causes include oxygen failure, ventilator failure, compression on or kinking of ventilation tubes.

Cardiovascular events

The most common cardiovascular events are hyper- and hypotension, brady- and tachycardias and arrhythmias (e.g. atrial fibrillation), with a reported incidence between 6% and 24%. These are most often provoked by the transfer process itself, i.e. patient-related causes like stress, inadequate analgesia or sedation, fluid shifts within the body and the use of vasopressors or inotropes. Therefore, first attention should be paid to patient comfort and the adequacy of intravenous drug delivery. If problems persist further evaluation should take place. Depending on the patient's illness, hemorrhage, pulmonary embolism, anaphylaxis or other less likely diagnoses should be considered.

Equipment-related causes may be infusions pump malfunction, kinking/displacement of intravenous lines and leakage of medication or infusion fluids at intravenous connection points (e.g. siphoning).

Primary equipment failure (Table 9.2)

Equipment failure or technical problems are common and may account for up to 46% of all incidents. Technical problems include power failure, gas supply problems (depletion or delivery problems) and missing or damaged equipment. Since there is no technical support available on the scene, the transfer team should have some technical knowledge of the equipment used, allowing

---

ABC of Transfer and Retrieval Medicine, First Edition.
Edited by Adam Low and Jonathan Hulme.

Table 9.1 Physiological deteriorations.

Signs	Differential diagnosis	Clues	Initial management
Hypoxaemia	Sputum mobilisation	Pneumonia/wheezes/rales	Suction
	Endotracheal tube dislodgement	Prior departure/x-ray changes	Repositioning tube/mask bag valve ventilation
	Failure of oxygen supply	Tube depth/capnography	Change cylinder
	Failure of ventilatory support	Check cylinders	Switch to bag valve
	Pneumothorax	Ventilator readings?	Decompression needle/chest drain
		High airway pressure/asymmetrical chest expansion	
High airway pressure	Sputum mobilisation	Pneumonia/wheezes/rales	Suction
	Stress/fighting the ventilator	Prior departure	Sedatives
	Tube obstruction	Look at the patient	Suction (change tube)
	Pneumothorax	Capnography?	Decompression needle/chest drain
	Bronchospasm	Hypoxaemia/asymmetrical chest expansion	ß2 agonists/magnesium sulphate
		History of asthma/allergy/wheeze	
Hypotension	Sedation	Responsiveness?	Decrease sedatives
	Hypovolaemia/SIRS/sepsis	Initial diagnosis, skin temperature, heart rate	Fluid challenges
	Haemorrhage	Initial diagnosis, heart rate, blood loss?	Blood (if available)/fluid , if severe: go to nearest hospital
	Cardiac tamponade	Initial diagnosis, jugular vein distension, cold skin	Sub-xiphoidal needle aspiration
	Anaphylaxis	History, quick deterioration, warm red skin, bronchospasm	Adrenaline (epinephrine), glucocorticoids, antihistamines
	Pulmonary embolism	Initial diagnosis, sudden onset of symptoms, hypoxaemia	Fluid, oxygen, thrombolytics
Hypertension	Stress/pain	Look at the patient, heart rate	Sedatives/analgesic
	Vasopressors/inotropes	Recent changed settings/syringe?	Decrease drip
	Intracranial embolism/haemorrhage	History, pupils	Antihypertensives
Cardiac arrhythmias	Atrial fibrillation/flutter		Magnesium/anti-arrhythmics
	Ventricle tachycardia/flutter/ fibrillation/arrest		ALS protocol

Table 9.2 Technical failure.

Some well known incidents	Signs	Initial management
Loss of airway control	Hypoxaemia/ capnography/ventilator alarms	Switch to mask bag valve ventilation. Make plans to resecure airway safely (360 access + follow SOP for RSI if available)
Failure of oxygen supply	Hypoxaemia	Check supplies/connections/tubing. If all else fails ventilate manually
Failure of ventilatory support	Hypoxaemia, ventilator alarms, capnography	Switch to bag valve ventilation/backup ventilator
Loss of vascular access	Depending on type of IV medication	New IV access peripheral/central or intraosseous
Failure of monitoring equipment		Regular non-invasive blood pressure measurement/clinical signs (pulse pressures/pallor, etc.)
Loss of electric power		Check battery status on all devices. Consider diversion to the nearest medical facility
Failure of infusion devices		Intravenous drip via a pressure bag

troubleshooting, reinforced by a lower incidence of technical problems reported by specialised retrieval teams. Some specific examples are discussed below.

Power loss

Unlike the in-hospital setting, during transfer there is not an unlimited power (or gas) supply. Familiarity with protocols regarding power supply and battery charging is essential. In case of a power loss minimum battery lifetime of equipment used should be known to calculate how much battery time is left.

Gas supplies

One should know how long gas supplies will last, taking into account not only the actual ventilator settings but also the volumes some ventilators use as a driving pressure (which might be as high as 3.5 litres per minute above the minute volume displayed by the ventilator). Other reported incidents involving gas supplies are caused by a lack of knowledge of capacity of different size gas cylinders and of how to connect them to ventilators. In cases of ventilator failure, the team should have a rehearsed plan B, i.e. is there a back-up ventilator available or should the patient be switched to bag valve ventilation?

Monitoring equipment

In case of a defective monitor one could switch to manual non-invasive blood pressure measurement. If a separate defibrillator is present, it can be used to monitor ECG and oxygen saturations.

Perfusor pump failure

In case of malfunction of an infusion device, the medication should be supplied by an intravenous drip. Preferably in a diluted solution administered via a pressure bag to provide a constant rate.

Road traffic collision

Ambulances are at high risk for involvement in a road traffic collision while driving under 'blue light' conditions, with potentially severe consequences. Protocols should be available for how to deal with such an event.

Furthermore, one has to take into account the necessity of caring for several patients on the scene of the accident, until additional ambulances arrive.

After a collision between our Mobile Intensive Care Unit (MICU) and passenger car, our MICU's steering gear was severely damaged (Figure 9.1). Fortunately, no personal injury occurred; however, our MICU could only drive very slowly. Since it was only another 300 meters to the destination hospital, we decided to pursue the trip.

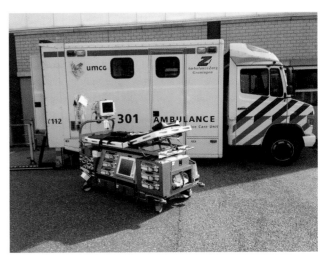

Figure 9.2 An example of a Mobile Intensive Care Unit with its sophisticated stretcher.

This time, we were lucky. However, we were fairly close to having to transfer our patient into another ambulance. This is rather difficult considering the use of the specialised retrieval ambulance and sophisticated stretcher with its necessary transfer equipment (Figure 9.2). This example emphasises the need for a back-up plan on how to evacuate the patient with the necessary equipment in case of a collision.

Prevention

Up to 31% of all transfer incidents are classified as significant, and up to 79% require an intervention. Strikingly, most may be preventable, (quoted as 52–91%). Good crew skills and teamwork, checking the equipment, using pre-departure checklists and re-evaluating the patient and monitors are thought to account for up to 82% of the incident outcome minimising factors.

One of the most important lessons regarding the safe transport of critically ill patients is to anticipate any problems that might occur during the transfer prior to the transfer. Preparation is therefore vital. Managing physiological aberrations during transfer is hampered by a lack of space, noise, movement and no immediate assistance. Even simple procedures may be extremely difficult. Therefore, equipment checks and maintenance and patient assessment and resuscitation prior to transfer are crucial. The team must be constantly vigilant of monitoring information and alarms. Anticipation of potential problems that might occur (e.g. when in doubt, intubate before departure) will help prevent critical incidents occurring mid transfer.

Debriefing and incident reporting

After every transfer, a debriefing should take place with all transfer team members. By asking each other simple questions, in an open atmosphere; for example, what went right and what could have been done differently, all aspects of the transfer can be evaluated. This is even more important when an incident has occurred during the transfer. Debriefings are therefore a vital tool for professionalising both the individuals and the team itself.

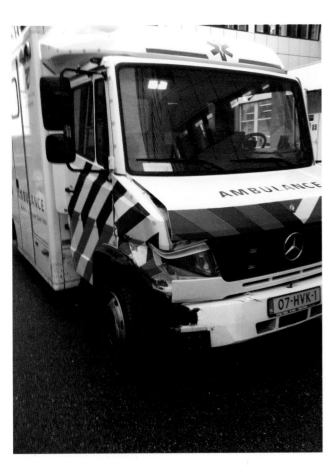

Figure 9.1 Road traffic collision.

The same can be said about incident reporting. Although most incidents are preventable, the nature of transfer work increases the chances of an incident occurring. To learn from these mishaps, and change predisposing organisational aspects, all incidents should be reported to at least the hospital's/retrieval organisation's incident reporting system and of course, where necessary, protocols should be adjusted.

Conclusion

Adverse events during transfer are common but potentially preventable. Transport of critically ill patients is like an expedition, participants have to be selected, preparation should be excellent, training extensive and surprises expected.

Further reading

Barry PW, Ralston C: Adverse events occurring during interhospital transfer of the critically ill. Arch Dis Child 1994;71:8–11.

Beckmann U, Gillies DM, Berenholtz SM, Wu AW, Pronovost P. Incidents relating to the intra-hospital transfer of critically ill patients. An analysis of the reports submitted to the Australian Incident Monitoring Study in Intensive Care. Intensive Care Med 2004;30:1579–85.

Droogh JM, Smit M, Hut J, de Vos R, Ligtenberg JJ, Zijlstra JG. Inter-hospital transport of critically ill patients; expect surprises. Crit Care 2012;16:R26.

Droogh JM, Kruger HL, Ligtenberg JJM, Zijlstra JG. Simulator-based crew resource management training for interhospital transfer of critically ill patients by a mobile ICU. Jt Comm J Qual Patient Saf 2012;38:554–9.

Flabouris A, Runciman WB, Levings B. Incidents during out-of-hospital patient transportation. Anaesth Intensive Care 2006;34:228–36.

Ligtenberg JJM, Arnold LG, Stienstra Y, et al. Quality of interhospital transport of critically ill patients: a prospective audit. Crit Care 2005;9:R446–51.

Wiegersma JS, Droogh JM, Zijlstra JG, et al. Quality of interhospital transport of the critically ill: impact of a Mobile Intensive Care Unit with a specialized retrieval team. Crit Care 2011;15:1122–5.

Waydhas C. Equipment review: Intrahospital transport of critically ill patients. Crit Care 1999, 3:R83.

Section 3

Transfer Equipment

CHAPTER 10

Electrical Supply and Batteries

G. Roberts[1] and J. Hulme[2,3,4,5,6,7]

[1]Department of Anaesthesia, University Hospital of Wales, UK
[2]Intensive Care Medicine and Anaesthesia, Sandwell and West Birmingham Hospitals NHS Trust, UK
[3]University of Birmingham, UK
[4]West Midlands Ambulance Service NHS Foundation Trust Medical Emergency Response Incident Team (MERIT), UK
[5]West Midlands Central Accident Resuscitation & Emergency (CARE) Team, UK
[6]Mercia Accident Rescue Service (MARS) BASICS, UK
[7]Midlands Air Ambulance, UK

OVERVIEW

- An efficient and reliable power supply is vital for retrieval work
- Many devices have rechargeable batteries: knowledge of battery life and factors influencing battery life are important
- Different transport modalities have internal power supplies that can be used for medical equipment.

Introduction

Having an efficient power supply in the pre-hospital environment is of upmost importance. The monitor/defibrillator unit, ventilator and syringe driver are the three important pieces of equipment that need a reliable power supply and are discussed in this chapter.

In the pre-hospital setting we do not have the luxury of mains current and therefore medical equipment must rely on a transportable power source. This can be in the form of an internal or external power supply.

Internal rechargeable batteries

Internal power supplies consist of removable rechargeable batteries. There are several available rechargeable battery types. The two commonest with relation to transfer medicine are lead acid and lithium ion.

Lead acid batteries are the oldest type and are found in automobiles, golf carts and emergency lighting systems.

Advantages: low cost, a large power-to-weight ratio and a high current output. Disadvantages: they are heavy, susceptible to erosion and carry a risk of explosion if over-heated or over-charged.

Lithium-ion batteries are common in consumer electronics such as mobile telephones and computers.

Advantages: lighter weight, safer and have a very low loss of charge when not in use.

Disadvantages: a potential risk of overheating and explosions; however in-built safety features tend to prevent this from happening.

ABC of Transfer and Retrieval Medicine, First Edition.
Edited by Adam Low and Jonathan Hulme.
© 2015 John Wiley & Sons, Ltd. Published 2015 by John Wiley & Sons, Ltd.

External power supply

External power supply can be either via a universal power supply (UPS) consisting of a collection of batteries, or can be run off a vehicle engine battery that is continually recharging via the engine alternator. These power sources all produce direct current (DC). Most medical equipment however requires alternating current (AC), and therefore an inverter is needed that converts DC to AC.

Power supply on board

Land ambulances

Land ambulances traditionally use the 12-V recharging engine battery as a power source. This relies on the engine to be ticking over to maintain charge. Land ambulances also use auxiliary lithium battery packs that can store charge. These can either be charged via the 12-V engine battery or in the ambulance stations, by plugging them into the external grid hook-up system. The charge time and battery duration of these auxiliary battery packs depends upon the electrical charge capacity (ampere hours). The charging time varies from 1 to 4 hours and the battery duration from 2 to 7 hours. Battery duration depends on the level of power consumption. Inverters are commonly built into the power supply of the ambulances

Ships

Power supply on ships is achieved via turbines and generators that produce current. A generator consists of a large electromagnet fixed to an axle. Copper cables surround the magnet and as the axle rotates via the movement of the ship a current is produced (Faraday's Law). This current is then stored as charge in a capacitor. If there is failure of this system then emergency power can be supplied by batteries or emergency generators. Emergency generators are separate from the turbines of the ship and traditionally run via a diesel engine in much the same way as the engine charges a car battery.

Helicopters and fixed-wing planes

Helicopters and fixed-wing planes generally do not have a power source that is compatible with medical equipment. They therefore rely on internal batteries or a UPS. All medical equipment on board must be CAA approved. Lead acid batteries with inverters as part of a UPS have been used within the military aeromedical field and can provide power for up to 6 hours. Their use however in the non-military setting is limited by flight safety regulations and weight. Alkaline battery based UPS are available for commercial use and their battery life can be up to four hours.

Monitor/defibrillator units

Zoll E-series

These monitors can use sealed lead acid or lithium ion battery packs. New and fully charged batteries can provide at least 2.5 hours of monitoring. This will be reduced with use of the defibrillator, strip chart recorder and pacemaker. The battery must be replaced and recharged when the 'low battery' message appears on the display in conjunction with two audible beeps.

The *Zoll E-series* batteries can be charged internally or externally. Internal charging requires an AC or DC mains input. The charger-on indicators at the bottom left of the monitor face will either show:

- *Orange-yellow*: device is off and charging or device is on with battery in situ.
- *Green*: device is off with fully charged battery.
- *Green/orange-yellow*: illuminate alternatively when no battery is installed or there is a battery charging fault.

External charging can be achieved via the Zoll Base Power Charger 4×4 or the Zoll Sure Power Charger. Testing of the batteries is automatic in both of these devices.

LifePak

These monitors have two rechargeable 11.1-V lithium ion batteries. They can only be charged by removing them from the monitor. Battery chargers can either be at the station or there is a mobile battery charger available. The batteries are not interchangeable with other LifePak models. The battery packs should be inspected routinely before insertion as the pins can become damaged. Each battery has a fuel gauge which indicates its approximate charge level.

Ventilators

The two transportable ventilators discussed are Dragers Oxylog®3000 and CareFusions ReVel™. SmithsMedicals ventiPAC and paraPAC are gas driven and therefore do not require an electrical power supply.

Oxylog3000

The Oxylog®3000 uses lithium-ion batteries that last up to 4 hours. These batteries have a built-in chip that provides the remaining battery capacity information. The batteries are easily exchangeable and can be charged using a battery charging station. Full charging takes 5 hours. External power can be supplied via a 24-V input cable.

ReVel™

This PTV series ventilator has lithium-ion easily exchangeable batteries that last up to four hours. Dual desktop battery chargers plus an external DC power supply are also available.

Syringe drivers

Syringe drivers commonly used in the pre-hospital setting are the Graseby, Alaris Asena GH and Braun Perfusor Space.

Graseby

Contains rechargeable 12-V DC nickel metal hydride (NiMH) batteries. Battery life is four hours based on an infusion rate of 5 mL/h.

Alaris Asena GH

Contains NiMH rechargeable batteries that take 2.5 hours to charge and last 6 hours when running at 5 mL/h at 20 degrees centigrade. An AC power cable is available.

Braun Perfusor Space

Contains rechargeable 12-V NiMH batteries with a temperature sensor to prevent overheating. Operating times vary according to infusion rates but can be up to 16 hours at 5 mL/h.

Further reading

Singh SK, Ingham R, Golding JP. Basics of electricity for anaesthetists. Contin Educ Anaesth Crit Care Pain 2011;11(6):224–8

CHAPTER 11

Transport Ventilators and Medical Gas Supply

J. Bingham[1,2,3,4,5]

[1]Department of Anaesthesia, University Hospital of North Staffordshire, UK
[2]Midlands Air Ambulance, UK
[3]West Midlands Ambulance Service Medical Emergency Response Incident Team (MERIT), UK
[4]North Staffordshire BASICs, UK
[5]West Midlands Central Accident Resuscitation & Emergency (CARE) Team, UK

OVERVIEW

- Ventilation during transfer should be no different to that prior to transfer
- Transfer ventilators have practical characteristics which facilitate portability
- A knowledge of physical gas law principles helps to anticipate and manage the problems of using compressed gases during transfer
- Gas cylinders come in a range of types, colours and capacities which, together with oxygen requirement calculations, allow necessary preparations for transfer.

Box 11.1 **The ideal characteristics of a transfer ventilator**

Practical

Lightweight
Robust
Easy to use
Minimal power requirement (gas or charge)

Clinical

Audible and visual alarms
Incorporate pressure and CO_2 monitoring
Provides all standard ventilatory modes including support for spontaneous ventilation

---

Introduction

Ventilation of a patient during the transfer process should follow the same basic principles as those used in hospital. In addition, the fundamental principle of transfer medicine stating that the level of care should not be less during the transfer than it was in the hospital environment is still observed. This means that ventilation of the patient should achieve adequate physiological variables of the level that would be targeted should the patient be in an intensive care environment. There should be no harm brought about by the use of a transport ventilator in place of a formal in-hospital one, including protection from volutrauma, atelectrauma and barotrauma. To facilitate this, monitoring of airway pressure and tidal volumes are necessary and capnography should be undertaken. Ideal characteristics of a ventilator are summarised in Box 11.1.

Before initiating ventilation, several things should be prepared. The ventilator should be checked (following manufacturer's instructions) prior to use and this would usually follow a process of ensuring basic operation, monitoring of pressures and setting of alarms where these exist.

The appropriate breathing circuit should likewise be checked and attached ensuring that, where fitted, pressure-monitoring lines are also connected. Many centres now advocate the use of single use

circuits but this is by no means universal and therefore care should be taken to check for wear and also that a filter device is fitted to protect multiple use equipment. Some manufacturers regard breathing circuit filters unnecessary but a filter with a humidifier is vital to retain airway moisture and preserve heat.

Selection of ventilation parameters may simply be a case of transfer of settings from in-hospital systems to those on the transfer ventilator but exceptions may have to be made where ventilator capabilities are different. As a general rule, for adults, a starting tidal volume based on 6–8 mL/kg of body weight and a frequency of 12 breaths per minute is adequate. Some ventilators will offer the option of positive end expiratory pressure (PEEP) that may reduce atelectrauma, improve oxygenation and lung compliance. Some may also allow setting of inspiration to expiration ratio. A maximum pressure limit should also be set (Box 11.2).

Box 11.2 **Suggested initial ventilator settings**

Suggested starting settings

Tidal volume: 6–8 mL/kg
Respiratory rate: 12 per minute
Pressure limit: 35–40 cmH_2O
positive end expiratory pressure dependent on clinical setting (at least 5 cmH_2O as a general rule)
Modify these settings before departure based on physiological parameters/ABG results

---

ABC of Transfer and Retrieval Medicine, First Edition.
Edited by Adam Low and Jonathan Hulme.
© 2015 John Wiley & Sons, Ltd. Published 2015 by John Wiley & Sons, Ltd.

Commence ventilation on the transport device for at least 15 minutes prior to departure, after which time assessment (clinical and blood gas analysis) is made regarding the effectiveness of the device and settings. Appropriate targets will depend on the clinical condition(s) being treated.

Types of portable ventilator

Portable ventilators are broadly divided into whether they are powered by compressed gas or by electrical energy (mains or battery). Gas-powered devices are often simpler in their mechanism and so may be smaller and lighter but require additional gas reserves to ensure their function. Electrically powered ventilators will operate with less gas but will require charging. Attention must be paid to the duration of battery power and options for charging.

Two of the commonest ventilators used for transfer of patients are of the Oxylog and Pneupac series (Table 11.1). Of course, others do exist but it would be impossible to list the specifics of each within this text.

Oxylog Series (Dräger)

The Oxylog 1000 ventilator provides a time cycled, volume-controlled and pressure-limited ventilation. It is completely gas driven with audible and visual alarms dependent on gas flow (or failing gas flow in the case of low pressure).

The Oxylog 3000 ventilator offers pressure-controlled and pressure-limited ventilation with pressure support. It is microprocessor controlled, driven by a high pressure gas supply. The Oxylog 3000 incorporates patient triggered modes that reduce the work of breathing during spontaneous ventilation.

The newer Oxylog 3000 plus model (Figure 11.1), in addition to the above, also features integrated capnography.

Pneupac series (Smiths Medical)

These ventilators are small portable gas-powered ventilators, requiring no electrical supply but with internal limited batteries to provide audible alarms. They are time-cycled, volume-preset, pressure-limited, flow generators (Figure 11.2).

Table 11.1 Characteristics of Pneupac and Oxylog portable ventilators.

Model and Weight	Power Source	Ventilation mode(s)	Driving gas consumption (in addition to O_2 to patient)	Controls and ranges	FiO$_2$ options	Notes
VentiPAC (3.1 kg)	Pneumatic Electrical alarm: batteries require change every year on average use Visual loss of O_2 display	Demand: allows spontaneous ventilation without support CMV/Demand – volume controlled, pressure limited ventilation, inhibited if patient breathes 450 mL tidal volume at a frequency set by the user	20 mL/cycle	Inspiratory and Expiratory times and inspiratory flow. Tidal volumes 50–1500 mL (controlled as a product of the flow rate and inspiratory time)	0.45 (air mix) or 1.0 (no air mix)	Optional PEEP valve 0–20 cmH$_2$O Pressure limit 20–80 cmH$_2$O MRI compatible
ParaPAC (2.5–3.1 kg)	Pneumatic Electrical alarm Visual loss of O_2 display	Demand and CMV/Demand modes (as above)	20 mL/cycle	Frequency (8–40/min) Tidal volume (50–1570 mL)	0.45 or 1.0	Optional PEEP valve 0–20 cmH$_2$O Pressure limit 20–80 cmH$_2$O MRI compatible
ParaPAC Plus (2.3 kg)	Pneumatic Electrical alarm Visual loss of O_2 display	Demand and CMV/Demand modes (as above) CPAP (310 model)	20 mL/cycle	Frequency (8–40/min) Tidal volume (70–1300 mL) Manual ventilation for CPR Optional CPAP and PEEP	0.5 or 1.0	PEEP 0–20 cmH$_2$O on 310 model Pressure limit 20–60 cmH^{2}O MRI compatible
Oxylog 1000 (3.15 kg)	Pneumatic Visual and audible alarm reliant on low gas pressures	IPPV/CMV	Approx 1 L/min	50–5000 mL (controlled by selection of minute volume and frequency)	0.6 (air mix) or 1.0 (no air mix)	Optional PEEP valve 0–20 cmH$_2$O Pressure limit 25–60 cmH$_2$
Oxylog 3000 (5.8 kg)	240-V AC main power Battery 4 hours approx	Volume controlled (CMV/AC/SIMV) Pressure controlled (BIPAP) SpnCPAP NIV	Average 0.5 L/min	Tidal volume (50–2000 mL) Frequency (2–60/min) A variety of mode options and flow and pressure variations via a menu system	0.4–1.0	PEEP of 0–20 cmH$_2$O Capnography (Oxylog 3000 plus) Pressure limit 20–60 cmH$_2$O

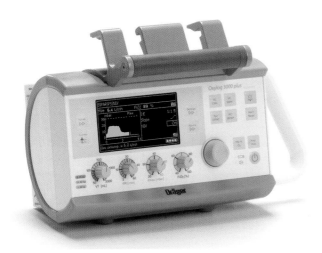

Figure 11.1 Oxylog 3000 plus transport ventilator. (Source: © Drägerwerk AG & Co. KGaA, Lübeck. Reproduced with permission of Drägerwerk AG & Co. KGaA, Lübeck).

They allow for a 'Demand' mode, which, if the patient attempts to breathe, opens up a valve to facilitate spontaneous ventilation without any pressure support.

The newest of the Pneupac series, the Parapac Plus, has options for CPAP and PEEP and is much lighter than the others at 2.3 kg.

Relevant physics

The way in which gases behave under a variety of physical conditions is important, as during transfer we are moving gas from the highly pressurised environment of a gas cylinder to that of atmospheric pressure. We may also be moving that gas through vastly different temperatures. The 'gas laws' are summarised in Chapter 3 and can be used to predict the behaviours and consequences of these changes.

How could these be relevant?

When considering oxygen cylinders, the high pressure of a cylinder allows it to contain a high mass of gas at a low volume. As it is released the pressure drops and so the volume increases giving a large volume of gas. Incidentally, additional gas laws now state that the reduction in pressure of the gas and increase in volume will mean that the temperature of the gas will drop and this may have implications for the patient. This may be seen in practice where Entonox® cylinders are used for prolonged periods, leading to build up of frost that can be seen on the outside.

Medical gases in practice

Gas cylinders come in a range of both size and type (Figure 11.3). Within Europe, gas cylinders have shoulders, which are coloured according to the contents, and this system is regulated and enforced (Table 11.2). Outside of Europe different systems exist and coding may not be controlled.

The most widely used medical gas for transport and retrieval is of course oxygen. However, depending on the transport system used, other medical gases may be available including medical air and nitrous oxide containing cylinders, e.g. Entonox®.

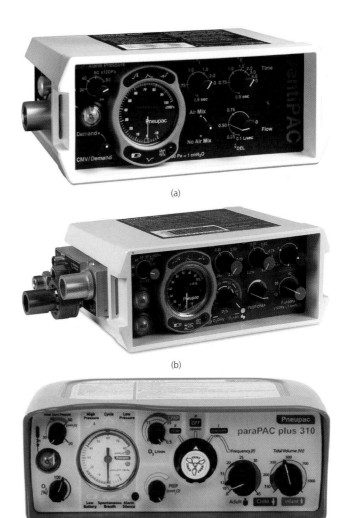

(a)

(b)

(c)

Figure 11.2 Examples of Parapac: (a) Ventipac (b) babyPAC (c) Parapac plus 310. (Source: Smiths International Ltd. Reproduced with permission of Smiths International Ltd).

Table 11.2 Colour coding for medical gases in Europe.

Contents	Shoulder colour
Oxygen	White
Air	White/black quarters
Carbon dioxide	Grey
Nitrous oxide	Blue
Entonox®	White/blue quarters

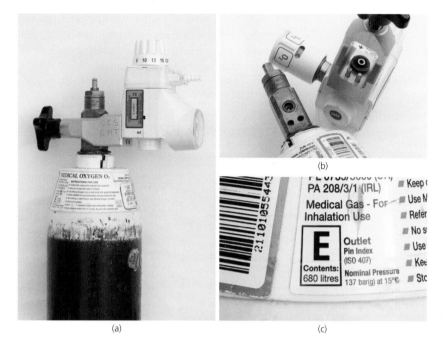

(a)

(b)

(c)

Figure 11.3 Medical oxygen cylinders. (a) Standard valve medical oxygen cylinder (b) Close up of pin index system on a standard valve cylinder (c) Integral valve CD sized cylinder. (Source: SWBH NHS Trust. Reproduced with permission of SWBH NHS Trust).

Table 11.3 Medical Gas cylinder characteristics and contents.

Cylinder type	Cylinder size code	Contents (L)	Notes
Integral valve	CD	460	Made of aluminium to reduce weight Flat base to help with storage.
Standard valve	C	170	Made of molybdenum steel
	D	340	Valve uses a pin index, which is gas
	E	680	type specific to prevent connection
	F	1360	of the wrong gas
	HX	2300	

Cylinder sizes must be appreciated to have an understanding of how much gas they will provide (Table 11.3). This is of particular importance with oxygen to allow calculation of supply volumes.

In addition, some transport and repatriation services, particularly whose which utilise fixed-wing aircraft for international transfers, may have more custom-made facilities (e.g. Lifeport) which provide greater quantities of oxygen (sometimes stored in its liquid state), in addition to compressed medical air and vacuum systems.

How much oxygen should I take?

One of the fundamental principles of good transfer practice is preparation and consequently ensuring the provision of sufficient oxygen, particularly in ventilated patients, is paramount. We need to know the amount of oxygen that needs to reach the patient, the amount of gas that the ventilator needs to drive the mechanism (if any) and the predicted transfer time. To ensure we have a good margin for error and to allow for unexpected delays, we allow for twice the time expected for the transfer. From these the following formula can be derived:

Oxygen required = 2 × (oxygen required to reach the patient
+ oxygen needed to operate the ventilator)
× transfer time

The amount of oxygen required simply to oxygenate the patient can be seen to be the product of the fractional inspired O_2 and the minute volume (MV). The minute volume may be displayed on the ventilator or calculated as the product of the frequency and tidal volume.

Therefore, putting these two statements together:

Oxygen required for transfer =
(FiO_2 × MV + driving gas) × (2 × expected transfer time)

Further reading

Fludger S, Klein A. Portable ventilators. Contin Educ Anaesth Crit Care Pain 2008;8(6):199–203.
www.draeger.com
www.smiths-medical.com
www.bochealthcare.co.uk

CHAPTER 12

Monitoring

A. Corfield[1,2] and S. Hearns[1,3]

[1]Emergency Medicine & Emergency Medical Retrieval Service, UK
[2]University of Glasgow, UK
[3]Emergency Medicine, Royal Alexandra Hospital, Scotland

OVERVIEW

- Equipment used in the transport environment must be designed and maintained for use in this setting
- Continuous ECG and SpO$_2$ monitoring are required for all patients
- End tidal CO$_2$ and invasive blood pressure are recommended for all ventilated patients
- Distracting factors in the transport environment mean that vigilance is required from attendants to detect changes in monitored parameters
- Underestimation of duration of transport is a frequent cause of equipment battery failure.

Monitoring of patients is a key part of ensuring a safe transfer. Patients being transferred are often critically ill or injured, in need of specialist medical attention and are being transferred for definitive care. Failure of monitoring equipment is a relatively common complication during retrievals that can have serious consequences.

Equipment

The transport environment places considerable additional strain on monitoring equipment beyond that normally encountered in the hospital environment (Box 12.1).

All monitoring equipment used in a transport setting must be capable of withstanding these additional challenges. Equipment should be compact and lightweight with bright displays that are visible in direct sunlight. Services procuring monitors should consider compatibility with disposable equipment used in referring sites.

Equipment used in the transport setting must also be secured appropriately during transport and tested to ensure it will remain secure in the event of a crash. In addition, any electrical equipment used in an aircraft must be certified for use in that particular aircraft.

ABC of Transfer and Retrieval Medicine, First Edition.
Edited by Adam Low and Jonathan Hulme.
© 2015 John Wiley & Sons, Ltd. Published 2015 by John Wiley & Sons, Ltd.

Box 12.1 Additional challenges for equipment in transport and retrieval environment

1. Physical hazards

Drop hazard
Handling of equipment
Acceleration and deceleration
Vibration

2. Environmental hazards

Exposure to moisture (rain or snow)
Exposure to extremes of temperature
Exposure to atmospheric pollution (dust)
Pressure changes due to altitude

In an emergency situation non-certified equipment may be brought on board and used, but this is entirely at the discretion of the aircraft commander.

Monitoring equipment used in the transport environment should have audio and visual alarms. The monitor display must be clearly visible to at least one transport team member at all times. During phases of increased activity such as patient movement into or out of aircraft or land ambulances, it is useful to have one team member assigned the role of watching the monitor. Audio alarms should be set at an appropriate volume to be heard above ambient noise. In aircraft this may be best achieved by plugging the audio output from the monitor directly into the aircraft communication circuit.

There is now a wide range of monitors (Figure 12.1) available for use in the transport and retrieval environment with the capability to deliver the monitoring outlined below.

How and when to monitor patients

Standards from various professional bodies outline the level of monitoring appropriate for patients in the transport and retrieval environment. A variety of modalities are available for monitoring of patients during transport and retrieval. Monitoring should always be used as an adjunct to the clinical assessment of a patient; however, during transport the ability to perform adequate clinical examination may be restricted.

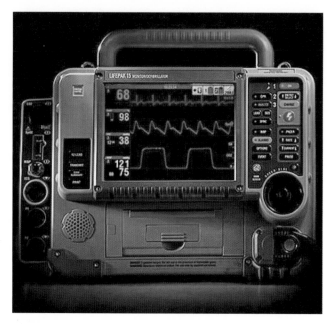

Figure 12.1 Example of a portable monitor used in transfer of critically ill patients used in transfers of critically ill patients. (Source: Harris T. (2013). Prehospital Monitoring. In: Nutbeam, T. and Boylan, M. (eds). ABC of Prehospital Emergency Medicine. John Wiley & Sons Ltd, Oxford, pp. 57. Reproduced with permission of John Wiley & Sons).

ECG

Continuous ECG monitoring is a standard of care for all unwell patients being transferred or retrieved. ECG traces are however prone to distortion due to vibration during transfer.

Many of the monitors available for patient transport also have the capability to deliver defibrillation and external cardiac pacing during transport.

Peripheral tissue oxygen saturation

Peripheral tissue oxygen saturation (SpO_2) monitoring is also required for all patients. Saturation monitoring is cheap and interpretation is straightforward. It is prone to interference from vibration and movement.

Non Invasive blood pressure

Non-invasive blood pressure (NIBP) is measured using an inflatable cuff around a limb, usually an upper limb. A sensor uses an oscillometric method to measure indirectly the arterial blood pressure by detecting changes in the pressure within the inflatable cuff. It is easy to use, is repeatable over a period of time and is non-invasive. NIBP is prone to interference from noise and vibration and is not necessarily an accurate reflection of the intra-arterial pressure in the transport environment. Patients also find repeated blood pressure measurements uncomfortable over prolonged periods. All patients should have an NIBP cuff in place, including those with invasive arterial monitoring in place, as an alternative in case of invasive pressure failure.

Invasive or intra-arterial blood pressure

The use of invasive blood pressure monitoring via intra-arterial catheters is increasingly common in hospital settings. Measurement of arterial pressure is through an indwelling intra-arterial catheter. This is connected via a continuous column of 0.9% saline, within plastic tubing to a transducer. The transducer measures the pressure and changes in pressure via a Wheatstone bridge. The changes in resistance are converted into a numerical value and visual representation of the arterial wave form on a suitable monitor.

Intra-arterial blood pressure monitoring is more accurate than non-invasive blood pressure monitoring in the transfer environment and gives information in real time. For patients being transferred and retrieved, invasive blood pressure monitoring is preferable to non-invasive for haemodynamically unstable patients, those on vasopressors and those being ventilated. It has the disadvantage of requiring a skilled operator to insert the cannula and the presence of an intra-arterial catheter is associated with an incidence of complications. It is essential that the catheter is adequately secured with sutures, dressing and tape during patient movement. Arterial lines also have the advantage of allowing arterial gas sampling during retrievals.

End tidal capnography

Electronic end tidal CO_2 ($ETCO_2$) monitoring has two main variants during patient movement. Arterial lines also have the advantage of allowing blood gas analysis to measure changes in CO_2 levels. In side stream monitoring, an adapter within the ventilation circuit allows a small amount of gas within the ventilation circuit to be continuously aspirated and analysed by a suitable monitor. This requires a motor within the monitoring unit and is more power intensive. Mainstream analysis relies on a device attached directly onto the ventilation circuit that measures via changes in the infrared spectroscopy of the gas within the ventilation circuit. Although this method uses less power, it is more sensitive to changes in moisture content within the ventilation circuit.

$ETCO_2$ monitoring is mandatory for a ventilated transport patient. $ETCO_2$ is a valid measure of arterial CO_2 in most patients and allows control of ventilation and gas exchange during transport. Sudden changes in $ETCO_2$ can indicate problems such as endotracheal tube displacement or ventilation/perfusion mismatch problems such as a drop in cardiac output. In a transport environment traditional assessment methods such as clinical examination may not be possible; therefore there is a higher reliance on monitoring to alert clinicians to potential problems.

Central venous pressure monitoring

Central venous pressure (CVP) has a limited role in resuscitation; however, many critically ill patients will have a central line sited prior to transfer or retrieval. The responsible transport clinician can then make a decision on whether CVP monitoring is required during transport.

Intracranial pressure monitoring

Intracranial pressure (ICP) can also be monitored during transport; however, it is unusual to do so outside of tertiary retrievals for specialised care. It would be unusual to institute ICP monitoring purely for transport; however, many neuro-critical care patients will have an ICP bolt *in situ* prior to the decision to transport. The decision on whether to continue ICP monitoring during transport will depend on many factors including cardiovascular stability, type of monitor, duration of transport and method of transport. stability, type of monitor available, duration of transport, method of transport.

Cardiac output monitoring

Invasive cardiac output monitoring is generally restricted to specialist retrieval work such as the movement of patients on extracorporeal life support. Improving technology has now made non-invasive devices such as oesophageal Doppler measurement a viable possibility in the transport environment. Consideration should be given to whether data from this type of device are likely to affect patient management during transport, before committing to carry and using it during transport.

Invasive temperature monitoring

Hypothermia is a recognised complication of transfer, especially in paralysed patients undergoing prolonged retrievals. Use of an invasive (oesophageal, rectal or bladder) temperature probe is essential for such patients to achieve accurate and real time temperature measurements.

Specific issues with monitoring in the transfer and retrieval environment

In addition to the physical and environmental hazards outlined above, other factors should be considered about monitoring equipment in the transport and retrieval environment by the transport team. One of the principal issues is power for any monitoring device. Monitoring devices, particularly when monitoring multiple channels such as invasive blood pressure and capnography, have a limited battery life. Battery types using nickel/cadmium-type technology generally have a shorter battery life than newer technologies such as lithium ion batteries. Often the duration of battery life will be shorter than the planned duration of patient transport. When planning for a patient transport, it is prudent to plan for a duration of transport that is twice that expected, as the multiple logistic challenges of patient transport lead to expected and unexpected delays.

If the battery life on a monitoring device is not sufficient to cover this period, then a contingency must be sought prior to departure. This can be AC or DC power from a transport platform; however, compatibility of connectors and external power supplies must be confirmed prior to departure. On secondary and tertiary retrievals, charging devices from a mains supply in the referring site may be an option to optimise battery power during transport.

Newer batteries can be 'hot swapped', so it may also be appropriate to carry a spare battery. Concern exists around the use of lithium ion batteries, particularly in an aeromedical environment because of the risk of fire.

Carrying spare consumables is prudent. This is especially the case with capnography sensors, arterial line equipment and disposable pulse oximeters.

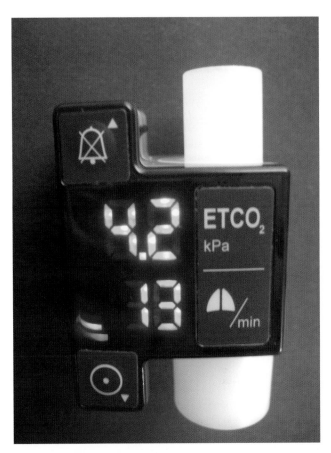

Figure 12.2 End tidal carbon dioxide monitoring.

Carrying back-up equipment is also advised. Stand-alone capnographs and pulse oximeters are small and relatively inexpensive. If these are carried, in the event of a monitor failure saturations, heart rate, respiratory rate and $ETCO_2$ can all still be measured (Figure 12.2).

Any patient monitoring used requires transport staff regularly to check the patient parameters and act if necessary. This can be challenging during patient transport because of multiple other distracting influences. This becomes especially true during longer distance transports and staff should alternate periods of being responsible for patient monitoring to combat fatigue.

Further reading

Association of Anaesthetists of Great Britain and Ireland. *Interhospital Transfer* 2009. http://www.aagbi.org/sites/default/files/interhospital09.pdf (accessed 9th February 2012).

Hearns S, Shirley PJ. Retrieval medicine: a review and guide for UK practitioners. Part 2: safety in patient retrieval systems. Emerg Med J 2006;23:943.

Intensive Care Society. *Guidelines for the transport of the critically ill adult.* 2012. http://www.ics.ac.uk/intensive_care_professional/guidance_transport_3_3_ (accessed 9th February 2012).

Lee SW, Hong YS, Han C, Kim SJ, Moon SW, Shin JH, Baek KJ. Concordance of end-tidal carbon dioxide and arterial carbon dioxide in severe traumatic brain injury. J Trauma 2009;67(3):526–30.

McMahon N, Hogg L, Corfield AR, Exton AD. Invasive versus non-invasive blood pressure measurement in flight. Anaesthesia 2012;67(12):1343–7.

CHAPTER 13

Drug Delivery

J. Cuell[1] and M. McCabe[2]

[1] West Midlands Deanery, Birmingham School of Anaesthesia, UK
[2] Anaesthetic Department, Worcester Royal Infirmary, UK

OVERVIEW

- The continuation or initiation of drug therapy while transferring patients is frequently required. Intravenous infusions are commonly used for fluids, sedative and vasoactive drugs
- Understanding the limitations of medical equipment and requirements for satisfactory functioning is paramount when working in isolated and adverse environments
- Numerous routes of drug administration are available to clinicians whilst transferring patients
- Oxygen is a drug with multiple modes of delivery providing both benefit and possibly harm
- The use of syringe pumps/drivers requires knowledge of the type of pump, associated equipment and contingency planning for inadvertent failure.

Introduction

In this chapter we will look at a few methods of drug delivery available, notably intravenous and oxygen delivery. Routes of drug administration are discussed elsewhere in this book.

Oxygen and inhaled delivery devices

A variety of delivery devices are available, all differing in their ability to provide a set fractional inspired oxygen concentration (FiO_2). Delivery systems can be classified as fixed- and variable-performance devices (Table 13.1).

Table 13.1 Classification of oxygen delivery systems.

Variable performance devices	Fixed performance devices
Hudson face masks and partial re-breathing masks	Venturi-operated devices
Nasal cannulae (prongs or spectacles)	Anaesthetic breathing systems with a suitably large reservoir
Nasal catheters	

Source: Al-Shaikh B, Stacey S. Essentials of Anaesthetic Equipment. Elsevier Ltd, 2007. Reproduced with permission of Elsevier.

ABC of Transfer and Retrieval Medicine, First Edition.
Edited by Adam Low and Jonathan Hulme.
© 2015 John Wiley & Sons, Ltd. Published 2015 by John Wiley & Sons, Ltd.

Variable performance devices

These deliver oxygen-enriched air to the patient. They entrain ambient air and the FiO_2 is dependent upon oxygen flow rates, the rate and pattern of ventilation, maximum inspiratory flow rate and a correctly sized and fitted mask to the patients face. Box 13.1 summarises their advantages.

Box 13.1 **Advantages of variable performance oxygen masks**

Patient comfort
Low cost
Simplicity
Ability to alter the FiO_2 without altering the appliance

These devices are utilised when a fixed oxygen delivery is not critical. Patients whose ventilation is not carbon dioxide dependent (i.e. chronic obstructive pulmonary disease) must be provided oxygen from a variable performance device with caution.

Fixed performance devices

These are sometimes known as *high air flow oxygen enrichment* (HAFOE) masks, but are more frequently referred to as a Venturi mask.

The Venturi mask uses the Bernoulli principle (Figure 13.1) in delivering a predetermined and fixed concentration of oxygen. As oxygen flows through a restricted orifice (Venturi device) a relative (compared to the surroundings) negative pressure is created, resulting in ambient air entrainment. The correct oxygen flow rate must be used for a predictable FiO_2 to be delivered. Less entrainment provides higher FiO_2 delivery. Total flows are often above peak inspiratory flow rates which assist in the flushing of expired gases from the mask, reducing rebreathing or an increase in dead space.

These devices are recommended for patients where the oxygen delivery content is known. Note that care should still be taken as the average FiO_2 delivered can be 5% more than expected.

Nebulisers

These create microdroplets ($1-20\,\mu m$) of solution in a gaseous medium. Microdroplet quantity is not dependent upon gas temperature. Smaller droplets are more stable and are deposited further down the respiratory tract. They deliver water and medications.

Bernoulli Principle

The total energy (kinetic & potential) of a system is constant. Flow through a constriction increases kinetic energy (velocity). Thus potential energy (pressure) falls.

The Venturi effect utilises the Bernoulli principle by using a constriction to accelerate the gas or fluid flow, reducing the surrounding pressure to the stream and allowing other gases or fluids to be drawn into the low pressure area.

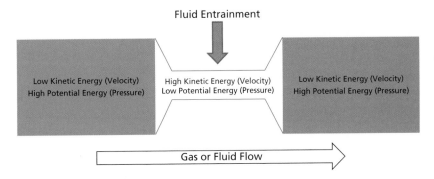

Figure 13.1 The Bernoulli principle.

There are three types of nebuliser:

1 Gas driven–employs a Venturi system entraining the liquid to be nebulised via a constriction and utilising the Bernoulli principle. Many designs incorporate a baffle or anvil that disperse the nebulised liquid into smaller droplets.
2 Spinning disc–motor driven, throwing out microdroplets via centrifugal force.
3 Ultrasonic–transducer produces ultrasonic frequency either in water or the solution is dropped onto it.

Intravenous delivery

Intravenous access

Intravenous access can be gained either peripherally or centrally. Central venous cannulae are commonly multi-lumen (quad/quin). The most important characteristic to note for all cannulae is the increase in flow rates as the diameter of the cannula increases (or gauge decreases). Peripheral cannulae have a standard colour attributed to each gauge.

The measurements in Table 13.2 are made using British Standards: distilled water at 22°C under 10 kPa pressure connected to 110 cm tubing with a diameter of 4 mm.

Intravenous administration

Fluid-giving sets are clear plastic tubing around 175 cm long with an internal diameter of 4 mm. Blood-giving sets have a filter mesh about 150–170 μm and a fluid chamber with a ball float (20 drops of clear fluid is 1 mL; 15 drops of blood is 1 mL). Sets without a

float or filter and with narrower lumen are unsuitable for blood administration.

Resistance and turbulent flow arises from extra tubing length, drip chambers and filters.

Lines used for drug delivery with syringe pumps should have low priming volumes limiting drug wastage, impact of free flow and significant delay in drug delivery.

Drug administration

Where multiple infusions are administered through a single lumen or cannula, backflow of drugs from the faster infusion rate-giving set up the slower infusion rate-giving set is a real possibility. Subsequently the correct doses of drug cannot be guaranteed and inadvertent drug bolus can occur with alterations in drug delivery rates.

To prevent this back flow, anti-reflux devices are recommended. These valves have a low opening pressure allowing fluid flow under gravity. Anti-syphon devices are also recommended to prevent free flow, especially when syringes are not correctly engaged in the pump mechanism or are located higher than the patient. Anti-syphon devices have a high opening pressure thus preventing free flow.

Syringe pumps/drivers

Infusion pumps or ck flow, anti-reflux devices are recommended. Infusion pumps or 'syringe drivers' are frequently used in numerous areas of medical practice to deliver drugs/ fluids to a patient via a number of routes including intravenous, enteral, subcutaneous and epidural. Infusion pumps can administer medications at rates as low as 0.1 mL per hour (too small for a drip), injections every minute, injections with repeated boluses requested by the patient (e.g. in patient-controlled analgesia) or fluids whose volumes vary by the time of day.

Types of infusion

Infusion pumps commonly request details on the type of infusion from the trained individual that sets them up:

- Continuous infusion: small pulses of infusion, between 500 nL and 10 mL depending on the programmed infusion speed.

Table 13.2 Cannula sizes, flow and colour.

Gauge	Flow rate (mL/min)	Colour code	Time to infuse 1000 mL
24G	13–24	Yellow	77–42 min
22G	23–42	Blue	43–24 min
20G	40–80	Pink	25–12.5 min
18G	75–120	Green	13.3–8.3 min
16G	130–220	Grey	7.7–4.5 min
14G	250–360	Orange	4–2.8 min

- Intermittent infusion: has a 'high' infusion rate, alternating with a low programmable infusion rate to flush the cannula. Often used to administer antibiotics, or other drugs that can irritate a blood vessel.
- Patient-controlled infusion: on-demand, usually with a pre-programmed ceiling to avoid intoxication. The rate is controlled by a pressure pad or button that can be activated by the patient. It is the method of choice for patient-controlled analgesia (PCA).
- Target-controlled infusion: mathematical models of body compartments determined by patient age, sex, weight and height deliver drugs to provide 'effector site' concentrations. Commonly used for anaesthetic and sedative drugs.

Types of pump

There are two basic classes of pumps. Large-volume pumps can pump nutrient or fluid solutions to feed a patient or administer intravenous crystalloid or colloid solutions. Small-volume pumps infuse hormones, such as insulin, or other medicines, such as opiates.

Large-volume pumps use some form of peristaltic pump. Classically, they use computer-controlled rollers compressing a silicone rubber tube through which the medicine flows. Another common form is a set of fingers that press on the tube in sequence. Small-volume pumps usually use a computer-controlled motor turning a screw that pushes the plunger on a syringe. Box 13.2 summarises the ideal features of an infusion pump.

Box 13.2 **The desirable features of an infusion pump**

- Portable
- Operates over a wide rate range
- Uses standard administration sets
- Easy to assemble and service
- Internal battery of good power for several hours
- Malfunction alarms
- Automatic keep-open device in alarm situations
- Accurate under a variety of situations (unaffected by altitude or motion)
- Resilient to temperature changes and inadvertent drop
- Easy to understand and operate.

Common infusion pump problems

These are frequently found problems worldwide:

- Software problems–causing the pump to be 'inoperable'. 'Key bounce', where a single keystroke is interpreted as multiple resulting in a 10 becoming 100.
- Alarm errors–the failure to generate an alarm when an occlusion or airlock is present. Generating an alarm in the absence of an occlusion. Inadequate alarm settings ensuring that an alarm is not detected.

- Broken components–resulting in over/under-infusing.
- Battery or electrical failure–from overheating, failure to recharge or not being replaced at the end of its life span.
- User interface (human factors)–confusing interface, poor design with power switches next to start buttons. Unclear units, warning messages and instructions. Unclear what infusion is running and to which venous access?

There are a wealth of troubleshooting tips for problems with infusion pumps but generally:

- ensure the right patient receives the right drug at the right dose via the right route at the right time
- plan ahead–contingency plan for failure of pump or tubing especially high risk infusions, i.e. sedation/inotropes
- label infusions and tubing at the port of entry
- use available drug library where appropriate
- check programmes and settings especially when changing them or syringes
- ensure the patient is appropriately monitored
- report problems encountered with equipment–to ensure equipment replaced, maintained and wider learning for others.

Vast numbers of infusion pumps are available (Figure 13.2); however, being familiar with their use, limitations and problems

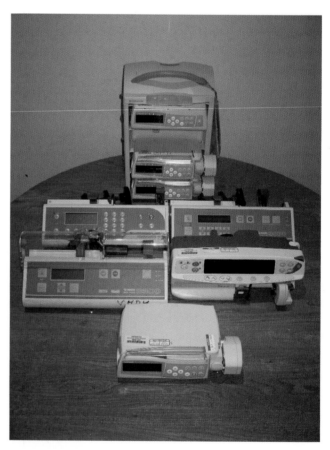

Figure 13.2 Examples of syringe drivers/pumps.

are paramount when working in isolation away from resources and notably a mains power supply.

Further reading

Al-Shaikh B, Stacey S. Essentials of Anaesthetic Equipment. Elsevier Ltd, 2007.

Keay S, Callander C. The safe use of infusion devices. CEACCP 2004; 4:81al.

MHRA. Device Bulletin: Infusion Systems, 2010.

Spoors C, Kiff K. Training in Anaesthesia. Oxford University Press, 2010.

U.S. FDA. White Paper: Infusion Pump Improvement Initiative, 2010.

CHAPTER 14

Near Patient Testing and Imaging

A. Low[1,2,3,4] *and T. Harris*[5]

[1] Anaesthetics, West Midlands Deanery, UK
[2] West Midlands Central Accident Resuscitation & Emergency (CARE) Team, UK
[3] West Midlands Ambulance Service NHS Foundation Trust Medical Emergency Response Incident Team (MERIT), UK
[4] AMREF Flying Doctors, Kenya
[5] Department of Emergency Medicine, QMUL and Barts Health NHS Trust London, UK

OVERVIEW

- Examples of near patient testing devices used in transfer and retrieval medicine
- Appreciation of some of the limitations of these devices
- Understanding of potential future developments
- Clinical indications and benefits of ultrasound in the retrieval setting.

Introduction

Point of care testing (POCT) refers to testing that is carried out in the proximity of the patient as opposed to in a dedicated laboratory. POCT has progressed rapidly in recent years. Over the next years it will be possible for around two-thirds of Emergency Department blood tests to be performed as POCT. This may or may not be cost-effective. This technology sees some POCT devices as suitable to use outside the hospital environment and will be discussed in this chapter. This chapter deals with POCT as applied to the retrieval environment. POCTs are usually blood or urine based and are all intermittent, as opposed to continuous readings (monitoring equipment discussed in Chapter 12). Table 14.1 provides a summary of different devices that may be utilised in retrieval medicine.

This technology enables early diagnosis of a wide range of conditions that may facilitate immediate care in the pre-hospital environment, such as hypoglycaemia or hypokalaemia, and allows a range of diagnoses that alters patient disposition and allows early institution of evidence-based practice. Examples of the latter include early diagnosis of acute myocardial necrosis by elevated troponin that allows immediate treatment with aspirin, clopidogrel and anticoagulation with heparin followed by transfer to an acute interventional cardiac facility; elevated lactate (>4 mmol/L) that mandates bolus fluid administration, broad-spectrum antibiotics and early referral to critical care specialist; early recognition of massive/submassive pulmonary embolism that may benefit from

thrombolysis, and early recognition of coagulopathy that may require correction with prothrombin concentrates.

The devices are usually small and simple to operate. However, they do require calibration and use along agreed guidelines and quality assurance measures.

Imaging POC devices are also now available in the form of ultrasound. Focused ultrasound is a term used to describe the use of ultrasound by non-imaging specialists to answer specific questions, as opposed to performing an organ-specific or regional study. Examples may include the focused assessment with sonography in trauma (FAST scan) to identify pericardial or intraperitoneal fluid, a focused biliary scan to identify gall stones or focused echo to identify the cause of a cardiac arrest. Specialist training schemes, notably in emergency medicine, now mandate a level of ultrasound competence as part of training. These skills translate readily into the retrieval and pre-hospital environments. Indeed a recent review identified seven studies in the use of trauma ultrasound in the pre-hospital arena.

POCT devices

Glucometers

Identification of hypoglycaemia allows immediate treatment. As such, glucose measurements are part of the skill base of most emergency medicine service (EMS) crews in the UK. A drop of blood is placed onto a test strip inserted into the meter. The test strip contains an enzyme (e.g. glucose oxidase) or chemical that reacts with the glucose in the blood generating a potential difference, which is read by the meter to provide a number on a calibrated scale (blood glucose level). The higher the electrical signal generated, the higher the number displayed.

Limitations

The glucose value displayed varies depending upon country of manufacture (mmol/L in UK, mg/dL in the USA and France). Above the calibrated scale, readings given will be 'Hi' or 'Lo'. All monitors must comply with international standards so that they are within 20% of a laboratory standard 95% of the time. However, meters can be affected by temperature, quality of blood sample, age of testing strip and contamination of the blood (e.g. glucose-containing substance on skin at sample site).

ABC of Transfer and Retrieval Medicine, First Edition.
Edited by Adam Low and Jonathan Hulme.

Table 14.1 Examples of clinical uses of POCT devices in the retrieval medicine setting.

Device	Example of clinical uses	Serial monitoring	Primary retrievals	Secondary/tertiary retrievals
Glucometers	Diagnosis of cause of collapse	In the management of DKA	Yes	Yes
I-Stat	Diagnosis of acute renal failure and acute coronary syndromes	CO_2 control in a ventilated patient with traumatic brain injury	?Yes	Yes
Hemocue	Decision to administer pre-hospital blood	Major haemorrhage	Yes	Yes
CoaguChek	Checking INR on patient with intracerebral bleed	No	?Yes – if you carry reversal agents	Yes
Hemochron Jr	Patients on intravenous heparin	Patients with IABP *in situ*	No	Yes
Urine Test strips	Diagnosis of pre-eclampsia	Ketones in DKA	Yes	Yes

I-Stat systems

This is a wireless, handheld blood analyser that provides rapid blood analysis. Of all current POCT systems it is the most readily applicable to pre-hospital care as the equipment is light, transportable, battery operated and well studied. It operates a wide range of diagnostic testing as defined in Box 14.1. It has a bar code scanner for patient identification purposes and serial tests. It can provide a variety of diagnostic tests based upon different cartridges inserted into the analyser.

Box 14.1 **Tests available with the I-Stat analyser. NB these are cartridge specific**

Arterial blood gases

pH
pO_2
pCO_2
Lactate
Base deficit

Total carbon dioxide

Haemocrit and haemoglobin
Renal function

- Electrolytes – Na, K, Ca, chloride and anion gap
- Urea
- Creatinine

Glucose
Cardiac enzymes

- Troponin
- Creatinine kinase
- B-type natriuretic peptide

Coagulation

- Prothrombin time/INR
- Kaolin ACT
- Celite ACT

The analyser goes through its own quality checks and results will not be given if these are not passed. Depending upon the test being processed, the cartridge will contain a reference electrode and a sensor for measuring the analytes (based upon a cascade of chemical reactions to produce electrons), and a buffered aqueous calibrant solution with known concentrations of the analyte and preservatives.

The I-Stat will not function outside temperature ranges of 18–30°C. If the software updates are not maintained (routinely sent out by the manufacturer), the analyser will shut down. The cartridges must be kept refrigerated (but not allowed to freeze) and used within 5 minutes of opening. Propofol/thiopentone infusions can interfere with certain cartridge analysis – check the cartridge you are using is compatible with these drugs. For samples other than tests of coagulation, sampling must be via heparinised syringes/capillary tubes. Air introduced into the sample in error may cause sampling to fail.

Hemocue

A portable photometer primarily used to measure haemoglobin. Blood is added to a microcuvette where the erythrocytes combine with reactants to release haemoglobin, the concentration of which is determined by the absorbance of light at 570 and 880 nm. The result is displayed in g/L. It is battery or mains operated. Microcuvettes can be stored at room temperature. There are other microcuvettes available that allow measurement of white cell count, and other analysers for glucose, HbA1C and albumin (urine sampling).

However, this device requires regular quality control and is inaccurate if used incorrectly. Contaminants (e.g. dirt) can cause inaccuracies.

CoaguChek

This system utilises reflectance photometry to derive the INR of a blood sample on a reagent strip compared to a control. Results correlate well with laboratory-based tests and are useful for testing patients on oral anticoagulants. This may facilitate pre-hospital notification of the requirement for prothrombin complex concentrates to reverse warfarin-related coagulopathy. This equipment is inaccurate if the finger is excessively squeezed (increases tissue factor level) or by contamination with alcohol/soap residue and if the patient is also on heparin. This may occur for inter-hospital transfers.

Hemochron Jr

This is a handheld device capable of deriving activated clotting time, activated partial thromboplastin time and prothrombin time. It is either battery operated or mains supply. Cuvettes are stored at room temperature. The device warms the testing cuvette to 37°C and a blood sample is added. This mixes with reagent (silica/kaolin/phospholipids) and moves back and forth within the measurement chamber. As coagulation occurs, the movement is impeded, detected by optical sensors, a timer is stopped to give a value. There are different cuvettes for each haemostatic test. This device is routinely used in cardiac theatres for monitoring heparin related coagulopathy. It may be of use in specialist retrieval settings in a similar manner to that described above.

Caution is required as results are provided as plasma equivalents. Poor quality samples and poor technique can influence results. Excessively low (<20%) or high (>55%) haematocrits will result in inaccuracies. Results are also affected by platelet dysfunction and fibrinogen level.

Non-blood-based tests

Urine dipstick

A quick and simple test. Test strips contain chemical reagents for up to 10 parameters (e.g. leucocytes, ketones, haemoglobin). The test strip is immersed in urine and left for 1–2 minutes before being read against a reference strip. The sensitivity of these strips may see positive tests for leucocytes in the presence of vaginal discharge or diarrhoea. Obtaining good-quality specimens may be a challenge in the pre-hospital environment and test results should always be interpreted in light of symptoms. Beta-hydroxybutyrate is the pre-dominant ketone in untreated diabetic ketoacidosis and may not be detected by urine dipsticks.

Pregnancy tests are simple to use, urine test strips that are a form of lateral flow test to detect the presence of the beta subunit of human chorionic gonadotrophin, confirming the presence of an implanted embryo. This, alongside an ultrasound scan, may be utilised in the diagnosis of ectopic pregnancy in the retrieval setting.

Pupillometry

One routinely monitors pupil size and reactivity as part of a neurological assessment. The Neuroptics Foresite Pupillometer uses rapid live photography coinciding with a light stimulus to record pupil sizes and reactivity (velocity). It is a small handheld, battery-powered device. Constriction velocity and pupil reactivity can be used to assess trends. Downwards trends potentially suggesting elevated intracranial pressure.

Limitations

This is a relatively novel technique and is yet to be validated for monitoring intracranial pressures. Inaccuracies may result from ocular pathology, intensity of retinal illumination, levels of alertness and time of day.

Future developments

Data from animal studies seem to suggest that samples from intra-osseous devices can be safely analysed through I-stat cartridges. Validation data from human studies are pending. There is an increasing amount of work being done to assess accuracy of monitoring parameters via infrared pulse oximetry (currently used to measure oxygen saturations) to encompass arterial blood gas parameters, haemoglobin and haematocrit. This would allow constant monitoring without blood based testing. Near infrared spectroscopy may allow resuscitation targeting microvascular flow as well as organ specific resuscitation. Studies are still awaited for both in-hospital use and extension into the retrieval setting.

Non-invasive means of monitoring ICP remain a priority in research and product development.

POCT devices exist for blood based diagnosis of infectious diseases such as HIV and hepatitis. Future developments include non-blood-based tests for diagnosis of HIV and TB, that may be of future use in the retrieval setting.

Imaging

Ultrasound in retrieval medicine

As ultrasound machines become smaller, lighter, battery powered and more robust, the ease with which they can be included in a retrieval services' equipment inventory increases. Skills in ultrasound are now required as part of the curriculum of emergency medicine training and are supported by the ICS and Royal College of Anaesthetists. The literature suggests that there is an evolving role for use of ultrasound in primary, as well as secondary and tertiary retrievals. Ultrasound is more sensitive than physical examination in identifying intra-abdominal and thoracic traumatic injuries.

Potential benefits include identifying sources of blood loss, warning the receiving hospital of injury complexes, identifying relevant specialities and suggesting the need for massive transfusion protocols. Thoracic scans may reduce the need for pleural drainage in patients transferred by air by identifying or excluding pneumothorax. Studies suggest that diagnosis of pneumothorax by clinical suspicion alone is associated with a very high false-positive rate leading to unnecessary procedures and risk.

Focused echocardiography may identify the cause of shock, and guide therapy. For example, massive pulmonary embolus with right ventricular failure may be diagnosed, so identifying the potential for thrombolysis; or pericardial effusion with tamponade may be diagnosed and treated by pericardiocentesis. Box 14.2 illustrates potential diagnostic uses of ultrasound. The physics of ultrasound and practicalities of performing scans are beyond the scope of this book, and require dedicated training programmes.

Pre-hospital-focused assessment (Figure 14.1) with sonography for trauma can have up to 93% specificity and 99% sensitivity in trained hands, as compared to in-hospital studies. Scans may be performed en route and so not delay transfer. While some aspects of patient immobilisation and packaging may limit useful 'windows' and views for ultrasound assessment, a protocol-based approach (e.g. Norwegian Air ambulance PHASE examination: combination

Box 14.2 **Diagnoses that can be made utilising point of care ultrasound**

CVS

Transthoracic echo to assess ventricular function
Diagnose RV failure due to suspected massive pulmonary pericardial effusion and cardiac tamponade
Abdominal aortic aneurysm
Severe hypovolaemic shock

RS

Assessment of a patient in respiratory distress to differentiate

- Pulmonary oedema
- Consolidation
- Pleural effusion and haemothorax
- Pneumothorax

GIT

Perforation
Free fluid in the abdomen suggestive of bleeding

Uterus

Foetal lie
Placental position/large abruptions (concealed haemorrhage)
Foetal viability (presence or absence of heart rate)

CNS

Diagnosis of middle cerebral artery occlusion
Increased intracranial pressure via transcranial Doppler or optic nerve sheath
… transcranial doppler or optic nerve sheath diameter

Musculoskeletal

Long bone fractures.

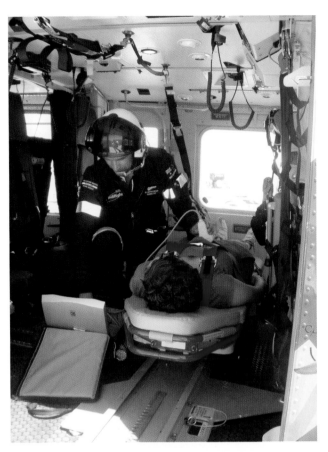

Figure 14.1 Use of ultrasound by a pre-hospital practitioner.

Box 14.3 **Factors that may impede the quality of ultrasound studies leading to inaccuracies.**

Environment

Bright sunlight

Patient factors

Obesity
Excessive movement

Patient packaging

Vacuum mattress
Limited space in HEMs missions

Technical failure

Battery failure
Machine malfunction

of heart, lung and peritoneal scanning, limited to 3 minutes) has been shown to have minimal extension of on-scene time in primary retrievals.

Experience to date suggests that ultrasound does not cause any electromagnetic interference with aircraft systems, and has been used in Scandinavian countries at low ambient temperatures. There does not appear to be interference with image quality from rotary-wing vibration or movement. Factors impeding ultrasound studies, particularly in primary retrievals are listed in Box 14.3. Feasibility studies have noted that manual dexterity is required from crews, with the ability to perform ambidextrous scans depending upon patient packaging in HEMs missions (Figures 14.2 and 14.3). In certain situations scanning may require the scanner to loosen their own, or the patients' restraints to gain access in flight. This requires close communication with aircrew to maintain crew and patient safety at all times.

In secondary and tertiary retrievals, ultrasound can help teams in diagnosis (Box 14.2) as well as undertaking therapeutic interventions and guiding resuscitation, as detailed in Box 14.4.

The main limitation associated with ultrasound relate to training and inter-user variability. This can be overcome by ensuring adequate skillset acquisition and maintenance through a service's clinical governance and internal training platforms. The ability for machines to capture and record data (several have USB ports as well), allows for peer review and quality assurance processes.

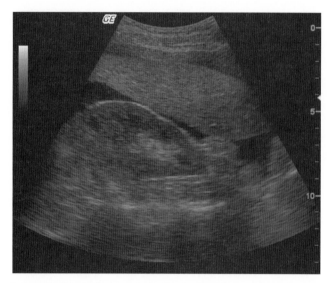

Figure 14.2 Diagnosis of ruptured ectopic pregnancy with ultrasound: free fluid in the abdomen.

Box 14.4 **Ultrasound guided therapeutic interventions and utilisation of serial studies to guide resuscitation**

Therapeutic interventions

Tracheal intubation (identifying oesophageal tracheal tube placement)
Aspiration of pleural effusion
Paracentesis
Lumbar puncture
Confirming cardiac pacing wire placement
Vascular access/central venous cannulation/intraosseus insertion

- delivery of inotropes
- monitoring central venous saturations and pressures

Peripheral nerve blockade

- introduction of nerve catheters for continuous infusion

Resuscitation

Fluid responsiveness: serial ECHO studies

- assessment of inferior vena cava collapsibility.

Further reading

Abbott Point of care testing. At: www.abottpointofcare.com

Busch M. Portable ultrasound in pre-hospital emergencies: a feasibility study. Acta Anaesthes Scand 2006;50(6):754–8.

Coagulation: The ins and outs – pointofcare.net. www.pointofcare.net/bayarea /coagulation_Ins_and_outs_062111.pdf

Curry and Pierce. Conventional and near-patient tests of coagulation. BJA CEACPP 2007;7(2):45–50.

Mazur SM, et al. The F.A.S.T.E.R trail. Focused assessment by sonography in trauma during emergency retrieval: a feasibility study. Injury 2008;39(5): 512–8.

Mazur SM et al. Use of point-of-care ultrasound by a critical care retrieval team. Emerg Med Austral 2007;19(6):547–52.

Pai NP et al. Point of care diagnostics for HIV and Tuberculosis: landscape, pipeline, and unmet needs. Discovery Med 2012;13(68):35–43.

Strandberg et al. Analysis of intraosseus samples using point of care technology – an experimental study in the anaesthetised pig. Resuscitation 2012;83(11):1381–5.

Taylor WR, et al. Quantitative pupillometry, a new technology: normative data and preliminary observations in patients with acute head injury. J Neurosurg 2003;98:205–13.

www.diagnosticpathology.org

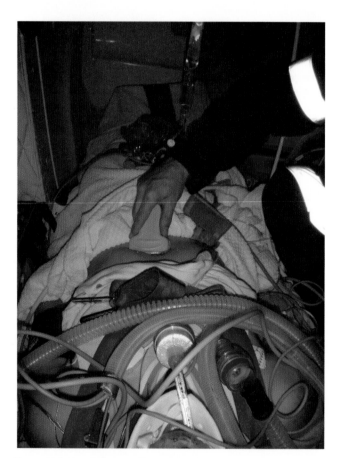

Figure 14.3 Use of ultrasound in a HEMs mission.

CHAPTER 15

Haemorrhage Control and Splinting

A. Hughes[1,2,3] and A. Weaver[4]

[1]Humanitarian and Conflict Response Institute, University of Manchester, UK
[2]Department of Emergency Medicine, Derriford Hospital, UK
[3]London's Air Ambulance, Barts and The Royal London NHS Trust, UK
[4]Emergency Medicine & Pre-Hospital Care, London's Air Ambulance, Royal London Hospital, UK

OVERVIEW

- More than one-third of trauma-related deaths are associated with uncontrolled bleeding
- Numerous steps taken in the pre-hospital environment can reduce these potentially preventable early deaths
- Interventions include recognising and minimising bleeding and reducing risk of trauma associated coagulopathy
- Adoption of a team based stepwise, systematic approach will help reduce time to definitive (often surgical) care for the injured patient.

Table 15.1 Active and passive interventions to reduce the risk of hypothermia.

Passive	Active
Remove wet clothing	Avoid infusing cold fluids or blood, use fluid warming devices e.g Buddy lite, Enflow
Shield from wind-chill	Warm air ventilation
Cover patient with blanket	Active core warming
Bubble wrap (naked skin next to wrap)	
Heating blanket	
Vehicle/Aircraft heating	

A stepwise approach to haemorrhage control is illustrated in Figure 15.1. With a team approach, these can often happen concurrently. The other important aspects of haemorrhage control as part of the stabilisation process are considered in this chapter.

Temperature control

Hypothermia (core body temperature less than 35°C) in trauma patients represents an independent risk factor for increased bleeding and mortality. Patients lose heat through a number of mechanisms, illustrated in Figure 15.2.

Hypothermia has an adverse effect on coagulation and is associated with an increased risk of severe bleeding. When body temperature drops, hypothermia-induced coagulopathy occurs secondary to a combination of platelet dysfunction, enhanced fibrinolytic activity and alteration of temperature-dependent enzyme function, thus risking ongoing haemorrhage. This effect is in addition to the intrinsic coagulopathy of severe injury, known as acute traumatic coagulopathy (ATC). In individuals with ATC, hypothermia will exacerbate coagulopathy and should be avoided.

Hypothermia is also associated with an acidosis. Synergistically these can impair coagulation in human whole blood, a combination commonly referred to as the 'lethal triad', significantly reducing the chances of recovery from critical injury (Figure 15.3).

Prevention of hypothermia and implementation of simple thermoregulatory interventions to maintain normothermia (Table 15.1)

are important steps in a damage control approach to the bleeding patient.

Minimising movement

Whole blood clotting time in a normothermic patient is approximately 10 minutes. A patient sustaining a traumatic injury will begin to form a clot using their own clotting factors. Disrupting this 'first' clot can contribute to ongoing bleeding, thus gentle handling and minimal movement from first point of contact, particularly in patients with suspected pelvic fracture, is important. Traditional 'log-rolling' onto an extrication or long board should be avoided. Excessive rotational movement of the patient can be prevented by using alternative devices such as an orthopaedic scoop stretcher. Limited 'log roll' techniques utilise a minimal 10° 'buttock off the ground' roll to place the device between the patient's skin and their clothes on each side of the patient (Figure 15.4). This allows simultaneous application of a carefully placed pelvic splint. The scoop stretcher can be lifted onto a vacuum mattress for packaging or equivalent device for loading into the vehicle. On arrival at the ED, counter-traction to allow removal of the scoop incurs minimal patient movement, i.e. no rotation (Table 15.2).

External haemorrhage control

Compressible haemorrhage

Effective wound compression will reduce external evidence of bleeding, but coagulopathy may still occur. Thus, despite achieving

ABC of Transfer and Retrieval Medicine, First Edition.
Edited by Adam Low and Jonathan Hulme.
© 2015 John Wiley & Sons, Ltd. Published 2015 by John Wiley & Sons, Ltd.

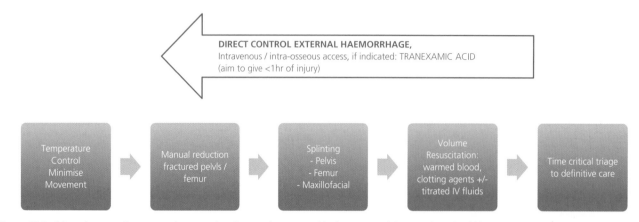

DIRECT CONTROL EXTERNAL HAEMORRHAGE,
Intravenous / intra-osseous access, if indicated: TRANEXAMIC ACID
(aim to give <1hr of injury)

| Temperature Control Minimise Movement | ⇒ | Manual reduction fractured pelvls / femur | ⇒ | Splinting - Pelvis - Femur - Maxillofacial | ⇒ | Volume Resuscitation: warmed blood, clotting agents +/- titrated IV fluids | ⇒ | Time critical triage to definitive care |

Figure 15.1 Although a stepwise systematic approach to haemorrhage control is demonstrated, interventions should be undertaken concurrently by the team.

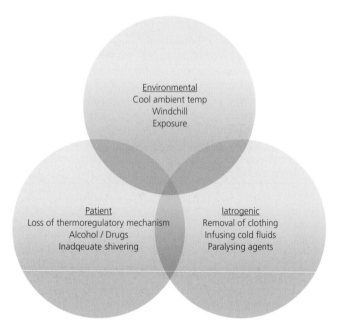

Environmental
Cool ambient temp
Windchill
Exposure

Patient
Loss of thermoregulatory mechanism
Alcohol / Drugs
Inadqeuate shivering

Iatrogenic
Removal of clothing
Infusing cold fluids
Paralysing agents

Figure 15.2 Risk factors for hypothermia in retrieval medicine.

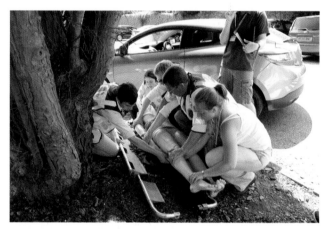

Figure 15.4 Minimal roll onto a scoop stretcher. 10° roll allows placement of the scoop and application of a pelvic splint if necessary, minimising risk of clot disruption. (photography by Brian Aldrich).

Table 15.2 Rotational movements incurred during log roll versus limited log roll.

	Semi-prone patient: total rotational movement	Supine patient: total rotational movement
Log roll and long board	510°	360°
10° Roll and scoop	170°	90°

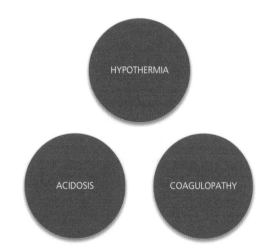

HYPOTHERMIA

ACIDOSIS

COAGULOPATHY

Figure 15.3 The lethal triad.

haemorrhage control using direct manual pressure, damage control interventions must also be implemented (see earlier) (Table 15.3).

Non-compressible haemorrhage

Commonly used in military practice, the combat application tourniquet (CAT) can be applied single or double handed by/to a patient suffering from limb trauma with major haemorrhage. Effective tourniquet use can provides temporary haemorrhage control and has been associated with increased survival. However, concern

Table 15.3 Equipment for management of external haemorrhage.

	Composition and design	Use	Benefits and limitations
Emergency compression bandage	Sterile, elastic wrap with non adherent pad. Direct pressure applicator integrated	Multiple sites for compressible haemorrhage. Provides high downward pressure over dressing area but not throughout wider bandage thus preventing tourniquet effect	Prevents slippage of applied bandage, direct compression effect over wound
Blast bandage 20 × 20 inch	Sterile elasticated wrap with large non-adherent wound pad. Removable occlusive layer 19 × 19 inch – can cover abdominal contents reducing heat and moisture loss. Slippage of dressing prevented by composition of wrap	Traumatic amputations, burns and large wounds. Eviscerated abdominal contents	Large coverage – whole back or chest, multiple points of adhesion preventing slippage of elastic during wrapping process
Suturing	Size 0/1/0 non-absorbable large sutures	Scalp wounds - closed with sutures with additional direct pressure can achieve good haemostasis	Easy, removable, quick and effective if combined with compression
May loosen and wound ooze
Staples	Surgical staples	Scalp wounds	Easy, quick, effective along with compression
Can loosen, haematoma can form underneath
Tourniquet	Small lightweight one handed tourniquet allowing complete occlusion of blood flow in extremity; self-adhering band and friction adaptor buckle. Windlass system for circumferential pressure	Limb trauma with haemorrhage, difficult to use at junctional points	Application before onset of shock associated with increased survival; self applied, simple, effective, lightweight
Complications such as tissue damage, compartment syndrome and nerve palsy reported after prolonged use; time of application must be noted

remains regarding tissue damage associated with prolonged use. Clinicians should be alert to this complication particularly during primary and secondary retrieval missions. Non-compressible haemorrhage in junctional zones, e.g. neck, may be cautiously managed with insertion and inflation of a Foley catheter or Epistat balloon.

Haemostatic agents

Topical haemostatic agents can be used as adjuncts, in combination with other methods described. Correct use and application is important. In particular, direct pressure is still required once a haemostatic agent has been applied. Agents may be categorized by the active ingredients: kaolin, chitosan and poly-*N*-acetyl glucosamine. All have differing mechanisms of action (Table 15.4). They are particularly useful for bleeding sites which are difficult to access, e.g. cavities.

Non-topical haemostatic agents

Direct targeting of altered clotting factors in bleeding patients has been shown to be beneficial. Tranexamic acid is an antifibrinolytic agent acting as a competitive inhibitor of plasminogen. It has been shown to reduce mortality in bleeding trauma patients or those at risk of significant haemorrhage. Current evidence suggests administration within 3 hours (ideally <1 hour) after injury, delivered intravenously at a dose of 1 g (adult) over 10 minutes, followed by a 1-g infusion over 8 hours.

Splinting

Splinting aims to achieve effective anatomical reduction. This promotes:

- reduction in haemorrhage (apposition of the fracture site and reduced movement of bone ends which may disrupt a formed clot)
- tamponade effect (in some cases)
- analgesia (secondary to reduction to anatomical alignment)
- reduction in swelling, haematoma formation and reduced risk of neurovascular compromise.

Pelvis

Unstable pelvic fractures (Figure 15.5) are associated with massive haemorrhage and high mortality, and often correlate with significant intra-abdominal injury. The application of a simple circumferential non-invasive splintage device, in conjunction with temperature control and careful patient handling, can reduce blood loss and improve pelvic stability by controlling vascular and bone bleeding through 'closing' of the pelvis. Simple effective splinting can be achieved using a correctly positioned formal pelvic splint but also, in less resourced environments, improvised techniques using a bed sheet, clothing, or triangular bandage can be effective.

Application of pelvic splint

Traditional teaching encouraged the practice of 'springing the pelvis' as part of the primary survey – this action results in

Table 15.4 Summary of the characteristics of haemostatic dressings.

Haemostatic agent	Composition	Mechanism of action	Use and benefits	Limitations
Hemcon Chitoflex (gauze)	Chitosan	Naturally occurring polysaccharide and antimicrobe, metabolised by the liver into glucosamine. Chitsosan induces platelet adhesion and aggregation, promoting sealing of the wound. Must be placed directly onto bleeding wound.	Open wounds, difficult access, more compliant than earlier versions, dual sided chitosan roll	Risk of rebleeding, correct application important as if not fully unrolled prior to application may 'glue' together when in contact with blood; folded multiple times to treat difficult access wound
HemCon chitogauze (gauze roll)	Chitosan		Open wounds, difficult access wounds, quick time to haemostasis; controls rate of blood flow through dressing;	
Celox gauze (Gauze roll and granular form)	Chitosan		Works independently of patient clotting mechanism. Open wounds, junctional zone; quick, highly effective and easy to use. Simple to use; cheap; small and robust; Non allergenic, non exothermic, functions in cold environments; high performance and effective – outperforms other dressings, second longest wound packing time; period of compression immediately after application recommended	Powder can be difficult to apply in field, especially in wind. Syringe application available
Quickclot combat gauze (gauze)	Kaolin	Kaolin is a potent activator of the intrinsic clotting pathway. Pro-coagulant. Clot is formed within and around Quickclot gauze	Open wounds, external haemorrhage not amenable to tourniquet use, proper wound packing and pressure very important in its use	Longer time to achieve clotting; potentially greater blood loss as a result; dependent on functional clotting cascade to achieve haemostasis
Quickclot Advanced clotting sponge (granules)	Modified zeolite	Initial generation contained zeolite, which created an exothermic reaction after absorbing water in blood, concentrating cells and clotting factors and resulting in haemostasis. Concerns regarding the exothermic reaction thus second generation dressing was developed with modified zeolite.	Open wounds, external haemorrhage	Reduced exothermic reaction; Longer time to achieve clotting; difficult to place in small incisions; requires functioning clotting cascade to achieve haemostasis, granules may stick to wounds making removal harder and may promote risk of thrombo-emboli formation
Modified rapid deployment haemostat (dressing)	Poly-N-acetyl glucosamine	Activation of platelets and coagulation cascade, local vasoconstriction and agglutination of red blood cells	Effective for controlling bleeding in hospital setting	Rebleeding may occur at dressing removal; modified version more effective at controlling sever bleeding, expensive

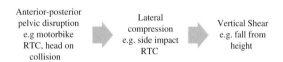

Figure 15.5 Examples of "unstable" pelvic fractures. Accurate interpretation and understanding of the underlying mechanism of injury is important when determining presence of a likely pelvic fracture. Approximate rotational movements of the pelvis, comparison of traditional log-roll with limited log-roll.

compression and distraction of the fracture site and promotes clot disruption and further haemorrhage and so must be avoided. Pelvic injuries should be managed based on suspicion of injury following examination and interpretation of the mechanism of injury. Accurate early placement of the splint (Table 15.5) directly onto skin at the level of the greater trochanter is crucial to restore some structural integrity and compression to the pelvis. The splint

can be applied simultaneously with a scoop stretcher thus reducing unnecessary additional movement. The pelvic splint must not be removed until radiological imaging to exclude unstable injury is completed (Figures 15.6 and 15.7).

Femur

Femoral fractures are often secondary to high-energy trauma and associated injuries must be excluded. The femur has a good vascular supply and injury can result in significant blood loss. Clinical features include pain, shortening and rotation of the leg, swelling and fullness to the thigh. Splintage with traction is the management of choice for shortened mid-shaft femur fractures (open or closed). Wound irrigation may be performed in open fractures with gross contamination. Irrigation and application of 0.9% saline soaked dressing should occur prior to splint application. Irrigation is particularly important if there is significant delay

Table 15.5 Examples of pelvic splints.

	Composition and design	Use	Benefits	Limitations
SAM pelvic sling II	Material compression. Velcro strap to allow tension	Pelvic fractures	Controlled and consistent stabilisation with an auto stop buckle to reduce risk of over compression. Radiolucent so can be left in situ for imaging. Safe and quick to apply	Can be applied in wrong position negating compression and stabilization effect. Access to groin and femoral vessels limited, soft tissue damage
Other pelvic binders:	Geneva belt – first described in 1999 Stuart splint London splint Dallas pelvic binder Trauma pelvic orthotic binder T-POD splint			Trauma Pelvic Orthotic Binder: I x case of bilateral peroneal nerve palsy after sheet (direct pressure to fibula head secondary to binding around knees). T-POD: application of forces? in excess of that necessary for splinting; wide device
Pneumatic anti-shock garment	In the 1970s Medical Anti Shock Trousers (MAST) and G suits were introduced	Pelvic fracture		Difficult to apply; cumbersome, Compression of lower extremities and abdomen especially if prolonged use; altitude effect on volume; does not allow for controlled pelvic reduction; restricts access to abdominal and pelvic area, abdominal compartment syndrome
Sheet or material	Successful realignment of open book fracture in 1997	Pelvic facture	Simple, good improvisation if resources not available, especially humanitarian environments	No control on how tightly the sheet is applied. Difficult to secure; further damage to skin wounds over area

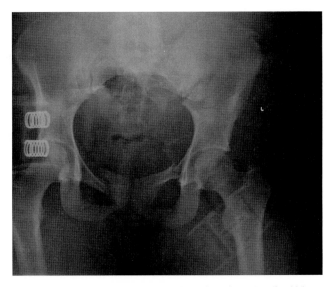

Figure 15.6 Incorrectly applied SAM II pelvic splint. The springs (buckle) visible on the X-ray represent almost the top of the commonly used SAM II pelvic sling. The buckle of the splint should be place at the level of the greater trochanters.

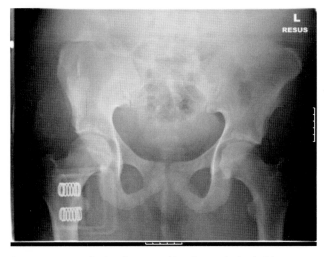

Figure 15.7 Correctly placed SAM II pelvic splint, at the level of the greater trochanter.

prior to operative management. Following analgesia, immediate manual in-line traction can be applied (Figure 15.8). Manual traction can be continued until a traction splint (Table 15.6) is ready to be placed and can continue whilst a pelvic splint is positioned in patients with concurrent pelvic fractures. Ideally, the pelvic splint should be positioned and secured prior to the femoral splint. Following reduction, distal pulses and perfusion should be assessed and recorded. Examples of other splintage devices are given in Table 15.8.

Fluid resuscitation and permissive hypotension

Recent studies demonstrated that aggressive fluid resuscitation methods initiated pre-hospitally may be detrimental to trauma patients. Early aggressive fluid resuscitation can promote dilution of coagulation factors, increase the incidence of coagulopathy, disrupt clots and therefore increase blood loss from bleeding points. Considered low-volume resuscitation with crystalloids in the non-traumatic brain and/or non-spinal injured patient, especially in the absence of blood and blood products, is recommended. Ideally, volume resuscitation with high ratios of fresh frozen plasma

Table 15.6 Examples of femur splint.

	Composition and design	Use	Benefits	Limitations
Kendrick traction device	Lightweight, robust and versatile. Weight 0.5 kg	Femoral fracture particularly mid-shaft	Simple, portable and compact, lightweight, can be used with pelvic splint, no pressure on perineum, multiple uses (humerus).	Protrudes beyond end of stretcher; difficult to use in associated ankle or foot fractures; pressure sores prolonged use
Sager traction device	Splint and ischial perineal cushion	Femur fractures – proximal third and mid-shaft. Placed on inner side of leg with padded cross piece that presses against the ischial tuberosity for counter traction	Provides quantifiable dynamic traction padded cross piece so safe traction applied with limited possibility of overtraction, dynamic traction force, movement and lifting without loss of traction, can be applied in any patient position, bilateral traction can occur	Large, non compactible, generally contraindicated in pelvic fractures, contraindicated in supracondylar fractures of distal end of femur as traction can cause anterior rotation of distal bone fragment, CI in fractures ankle or foot; pressure sores from prolonged use
Thomas splint	Adjustable, stainless steel,	Femur fractures	More suitable for hospital environment, Durable and universal, good traction	Pressure sores from prolonged use, difficult to apply in pre hospital environment, protrudes beyond patients foot
Improvised femur splints	Tape or equivalent, waking poles	Femoral fractures	Good for improvisation when resources or kit not available	Appropriate traction difficult to determine, aim for 10% body weight, may loosen

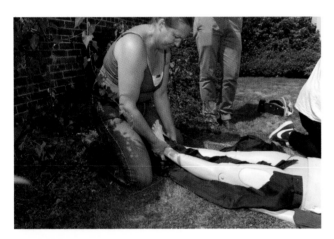

Figure 15.8 Manual traction on the femur. (Source: Brian Aldrich. Reproduced with permission).

and red blood cells (FFP:RBCs), in conjunction with haemorrhage control interventions, is best.

Permissive hypotension (systolic 80–90 mmHg) maintains a level of tissue perfusion that is adequate for short periods of time but it is important to weigh effects of this against transport time and patient comorbidities.

Blood and clotting agents

Pre-hospital blood transfusion

Internationally, pre-hospital and retrieval teams have access to packed red blood cells (PRBCs) for specific purposes and many retrieval services have blood storage facilities at their bases or pre packed boxes ready to be taken out for appropriate missions. In 2012, London's air ambulance became the first pre-hospital service in the UK to carry routinely 4 units (O negative) PRBCs on every

mission and this practice is replicated by some of the other UK air ambulances for immediate resuscitation, although the evidence base for improved patient outcome is unclear.

Increased distances to hospital may warrant the availability of blood for pre-hospital/retrieval teams. In remote settings and amongst some military teams, whole blood transfusion has been found to be an efficient way of delivering blood in extreme circumstances. Pre-screened donors can donate at the scene of the incident in a short time, negating the requirement to carry multiple components in austere environments.

Blood transportation and storage

Several options exist but the pre-hospital environment presents some unique challenges (Box 15.1). The Minnesota Thermal Science 'Golden Hour Box' has passed both military and civilian validation tests (Figure 15.9). It maintains steady state temperature (2–6°C) for 48–72 hours with no battery or power supply requirement.

Box 15.1 **Challenges and issues with pre-hospital blood administration**

RISKS OF TRANSFUSION

Emergency blood supplies must not be wasted. Compliance with regulations ensures that products are kept in optimal condition and can be redistributed when they are not used.

Blood transfusion may exacerbate hypothermia and hence coagulopathy. Every effort should be made to deliver warmed blood.

Hypocalcaemia and hyperkalaemia may occur during/after transfusion and electrolyte monitoring can help to detect these imbalances and allow early treatment.

Transfusion reactions are infrequent using universal donor group emergency blood but clinicians should monitor patients during transfusion for adverse reactions.

Table 15.7 Considerations for carrying blood products with a retrieval service.

Temperature control	Storage and protection of unit	Traceability	Quality assurance	Aircraft damage
Ability to maintain steady state temperature at 4°C > 18 h to avoid wastage and allow circulation and resupply Data loggers for continuous temperature recording, downloadable data to demonstrate compliance Method for detecting unusable units	Capacity to store 4 units PRBCs/blood products Robust portable container and packing Portable and small Lightweight and waterproof Resilient Easy to access contents	Supply and delivery Data recording Patient linked to unit Avoiding wastage	Team training SOPs Governance	Leakage onto floor of aircraft affecting electronics, avionics and airframe.

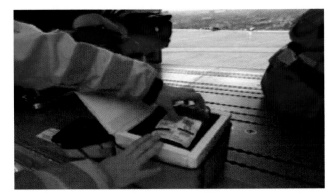

Figure 15.9 The Minnesota Thermal Science box.

Table 15.8 Examples of other splintage devices.

	Splintage	Benefits	Limitations
Humerus Ulna/radius Tibia/fibula Ankle Hand	SAM splints, vacuum splints, box splints, moulded splints (e.g. Benecast), air splints, improvised splints	Lightweight, simple to use, can be cleaned and reusable, versatile, minimal training required	Vacuum and air splints may be affected by altitude; pressure sores, no traction applied; may "hide" external haemorrhage
Maxillofacial	Definitive airway (intubation), dental blocks, collar then epistats	Good haemorrhage control when used in combination, gives structural integrity to facial skeleton; easy to use	Risk of further anatomical distortion if epistats are overinflated

Compliance with regulations and legislation

SOPs encourage compliance with hospital standards. Key points for transfusion in the pre-hospital/retrieval environment include:

- clear indications for transfusion
- obtaining pre-transfusion blood sample
- checking of blood type and expiry date prior to transfusion
- warming of blood (Buddy Lite/Enflow)
- documentation and paperwork to ensure 100% traceability
- communication with laboratory.

The future

The ability to transfuse PRBCs is a significant step forwards in the pre-hospital management of the severely injured bleeding patient. Provision of supporting blood products such as thawed fresh frozen plasma (FFP)/freeze dried components to administer in high ratios (current recommendations 1:2 (plasma:RBCs)) with PRBCs and helping to target the acute traumatic coagulopathy (Table 15.7). Freeze dried FFP and concentrated factors are likely to become more readily available in the near future and will provide additional options for pre-hospital teams. Research continues as to the most effective ratio of blood products for patients with acute traumatic coagulopathy.

Further reading

Brodie S, Hodgetts TJ, Ollerton J, et al. Tourniquet use in combat trauma: UK military experience. J R Army Med Corps 2007;153:310–3.

Brohi K, Singh J, Heron M, Coats T. Acute traumatic coagulopathy. Journal Trauma 2003;54,1127–30.

Hewitt Smith A, Laird C, Porter K, Bloch M. Haemostatic dressings in pre hospital care. Emerg Med J 2012;0.1–6.

Lee C, Porter K. The pre hospital management of pelvic fractures. Emerg Med J 2007;24:130–3.

Lockey DJ, Weaver AE, Davies GE. Practical translations of hemorrhage control techniques to the civilian trauma scene. Transfusion 2013;53;17S–22S.

Kragh J, Walters T, Baer D, Fox C, Wade C, Salinas J, Holcomb J. Survival with emergency tourniquet use to stop bleeding in major limb trauma. Ann Surg 2009;249:1.

Shakur H, Roberts I, Bautista R, Caballero J, Coats T, Dewan Y, et al. CRASH-2 Trial Collaborators. Effects of tranexamic acid on death, vascular occlusive events and blood transfusion trauma patients with significant haemorrhage (CRASH-2): a randomised, placebo-controlled trial. Lancet 2010;376(9734):23–32.

Spahn D, Cemy V, Coats T, et al. Management of bleeding and coagulopathy following major trauma: an updated European Guideline. Critical Care 2013;11:R17. Online at http://ccforum.com/content/11/1/R17.

CHAPTER 16

Stretchers, Incubators and Vacuum Mattresses

H. Bawdon[1,2,3] and M. Ward[4]

[1]West Midlands Deanery, UK
[2]West Midlands Central Accident Resuscitation & Emergency (CARE) Team, UK
[3]West Midlands Ambulance Service NHS Foundation Trust Medical Emergency Response Incident Team (MERIT), UK
[4]West Midlands Ambulance Service, UK

OVERVIEW

Stretchers have a number of strengths and weaknesses:

- know your stretcher's capabilities
- request specialist stretchers where required
- consider maximum weight limits
- Mattresses should be appropriate to the type of transfer being undertaken
- Scoop stretchers are useful in minimizing patient movement during transfer
- Vacuum mattresses are especially useful for prolonged transfers and reduce the risk of pressure sores
- Incubators provide an optimum environment for the care of neonatal and infant patients.

Stretchers utilised in transfer

Stretchers in common use within ambulance services can be categorised into two distinct loading designs:

1 The stretcher is placed into a loading system located at the rear of the vehicle; the legs then fold into the body of the stretcher while the stretcher is either manually pushed or automatically loaded into the vehicle using a motorised system.
2 The stretcher is either wheeled up a ramp or onto a lift, and then loaded into the vehicle.

There are also an increasing number of both types of stretcher that can be adapted to convey bariatric patients. Careful attention should be given to the maximum working load of the stretcher.

The ideal properties of a stretcher are summarised in Table 16.1.

All movements of the patient should be undertaken using the TILE mnemonic as described in Table 16.2.

There are a number of devices available to assist with the transfer of patients to and from the stretcher. These include slide sheets, transfer mattresses and hoists. Follow the manufacturers' guidelines when securing the patient to the stretcher, ensuring you only utilise appropriate restraint straps.

ABC of Transfer and Retrieval Medicine, First Edition.
Edited by Adam Low and Jonathan Hulme.
© 2015 John Wiley & Sons, Ltd. Published 2015 by John Wiley & Sons, Ltd.

Table 16.1 The ideal properties of a stretcher.

Properties of the ideal stretcher	
Adaptable	Able to carry various sizes, shapes and weights of patients
Adjustable	Able to be easily re-positioned so that the patient can be transferred in any position and also allow for resuscitation to be commenced rapidly
Height adjustable	Has a variety of lifting, loading and lowering mechanisms; these can be manual, hydraulic, electric, or a combination of any of the three
Capable	Able to carry equipment to enable the administration of drugs and fluids, i.e. syringe pumps, oxygen and fluid bags Able to carry equipment to allow continuous monitoring of the patient
Secure	Fitted with a restraint system to secure the stretcher within the transfer vehicle
Transferable	Allows easy and comfortable transfer between the vehicle and the unit.

Table 16.2 TILE pneumonic.

Risk assessment for patient transfers	
Task	Manufacturers' guidelines should be available for each item of equipment and the instructions followed. *Remember*: using equipment outside of these guidelines is hazardous and may risk patient and clinician safety
Individual	All members of the transfer team should be trained in safe manual handling techniques and the use of each item of equipment *Remember*: effective communication and teamwork will ensure safety for all
Load	Safe Working Loads (SWL) should be clearly labelled on each piece of lifting or load bearing equipment *Remember*: take into account both the weight of the patient and any equipment when considering the maximum SWL
Environment	Consideration should be given to access and egress; most ambulance trolleys are designed to be used on flat surfaces. *Remember*: small wheels do not cope well with uneven or loose surfaces

The adaptation of standard ambulance stretchers to carry additional equipment should always be pre-planned and in line with manufacturer's guidelines. There are legal implications to the provider of the ambulance and also individual implications for the driver of the vehicle. They should refuse to transport patients if the equipment being utilised could cause injury to the patient or transfer team.

Mattresses

The stretchers commonly in use come with a fitted mattress; this may be a single formed design or made up of a number of elements. The mattress must be firm enough to enable CPR to be delivered, but compliant enough to be comfortable for the conscious patient. The mattress should be checked every day for:

- integrity of the covering
- attachment to the stretcher
- cleanliness.

Damage or deformity to the mattress may lead to the patient sustaining pressure sores.

Pressure sores

Pressure sores are breaks in the skin caused by compression of the tissues. They form when points of the body are in prolonged contact with a hard surface. Force concentrated over a small area causes high pressure in the area; if that pressure exceeds the pressure of blood supplying the tissues, necrosis and tissue breakdown may ensue. Areas most at risk therefore include bony prominences (e.g. hips, heels and shoulder blades) and parts with little body fat covering (e.g. the small of the back).

Risk factors for development of pressure sores can be divided into three categories (Table 16.3): patient comorbidities, presenting illness and iatrogenic causes.

Risk is minimised by limiting time spent immobilised (aided by minimising on scene time) and using optimum equipment. Scoops are thought to be lower risk than long boards; vacuum mattresses provide the best care.

Scoops

The orthopaedic stretcher, commonly known as the scoop stretcher, is a lifting device which can also be used for the short-term

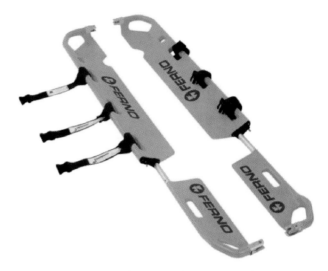

Figure 16.1 The scoop stretcher separated into two parts. (Source: Ferno. Reproduced with permission of Ferno).

immobilisation of a patient during transfer. The scoop is especially useful for patients that need to be maintained supine and where a full log roll is not appropriate. Prior to application it is separated into two halves, facilitating minimal patient movement (Figure 16.1).

The scoop is not a carrying device; therefore it should always be used in combination with another device when carrying patients over a distance.

Patients should not remain on a scoop for longer than 45 minutes. It can be used to transfer onto a vacuum mattress.

Vacuum mattress and splints

Vacuum mattresses are commonly made of a polyurethane material filled with polystyrene balls. The device is sealed and has valves fitted that allow for the air within to be extracted. This forces the balls together causing the device to become rigid. This maintains the patient in the position in which the device has been applied, making it the perfect device for the transfer of patients with spinal injuries.

A correctly applied vacuum mattress distributes pressure evenly across the body and therefore reduces the chances of a pressure sore developing, minimises patient movement and therefore improves patient comfort during transportation.

Vacuum splints use the same principles but come in a range of sizes allowing for the immobilisation of limbs. They can be moulded to fit any deformity and are therefore very versatile.

Devices fail if punctured; care should be taken during use when sharp objects such as broken glass are present.

Incubators

An incubator is a box-shaped device which optimises the environment in which neonatal and infant patients can be cared for. The transfer of neonatal patients between care facilities is undertaken using a portable incubator. Incubators can either be attached to

Table 16.3 Risk factors for the development of pressure sores.

Patient comorbidities	e.g. diabetes, chronic steroid use, malnutrition, incontinence.
Presenting illness	e.g. sensory impairment, reduced level of consciousness.
Iatrogenic	Spinal boards are no longer recommended for prolonged transfers, as their hard inflexible flat structure increases the risk of pressure sores developing. Excessive time spent immobile on any piece of equipment will also lead to pressure sores.

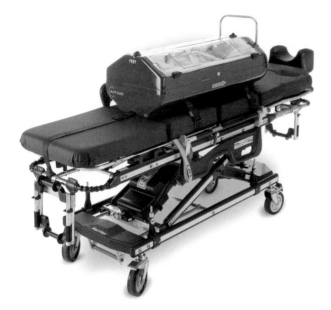

Figure 16.2 An incubator securely fastened to an ambulance trolley. (Source: Ferno. Reproduced with permission of Ferno).

stretcher bases or are an integral unit incorporating the stretcher (Figure 16.2).

The incubator allows the environment within to be maintained; this prevents inappropriate cooling, maintains humidity levels and protects the patient during transfer.

Incubators used in transfers often have the monitoring, oxygen, ventilator and power supply built into the unit. The internal batteries have variable operational capability ranging from 45 minutes to >6 hours; it is strongly recommended that the charging cable remains with the incubator at all times.

Remember that when undertaking a transfer ensure that the power adaptors and restraint system for the incubator are compatible with the transfer vehicle.

The authors have reviewed the technical specifications for a number of transfer incubators: weight ranges of between 1 and 6 kg are quoted in these. However, the specific guidance for the product must be followed.

Further reading

Lovell ME, Evans JH. A comparison of the spinal board and the vacuum stretcher, spinal stability and interface pressure. Injury 1994;25: 179–80.

Luscombe M, Williams J. Comparison of a long spinal board and vacuum mattress for spinal immobilisation. Emerg Med J 2003;20:476–8.

CHAPTER 17

Personal Protective Equipment

C. Bosanko[1,2] *and S. Hepburn*[3]

[1]Emergency Medicine, University Hospital North Staffordshire, UK
[2]West Midlands Ambulance Service NHS Foundation Trust Medical Emergency Response Incident Team (MERIT), UK
[3]Emergency Medicine and EMRS, Department of Emergency Medicine, Western Infirmary, UK

> **OVERVIEW**
>
> By the end of the chapter you should know
>
> - The principles of risk assessment and hazard mitigation
> - The process for risk assessment
> - Risk assessment in the out of hospital environment
> - How to select appropriate personal protective equipment for your role.

Introduction

Ensuring the safety of individuals in the course of their work is not only desirable, but is also a legal responsibility of the employer. The hazards and risks to a team member when working in the retrieval environment are equal and at times greater than when working in hospital, and can be unpredictable and dynamic. This is especially so for aeromedical retrieval.

An organisation must be able to demonstrate a robust mechanism for identifying hazards and the actions taken to minimise risk to their team members, or they may be criticised in the event of any adverse incident. An organisation which invests appropriate time and resource to provide safe and effective personal protective equipment (PPE) will both meet its legal duty and be viewed as a professional, responsible service. Most items of PPE can include service logos where appropriate to display corporate branding; this is particularly important to services that rely on charitable donations for funding, and allows rapid identification to other out of hospital agencies.

Legislation

The legal responsibility for provision of PPE in the UK is mandated under the Personal Protective Equipment Regulations (2002), which in turn fall under the Health and Safety at Work Act 1974 and its various revisions/amendments. The Health and Safety Executive (HSE) is the independent regulator that acts in the public interest to reduce work-related death and serious injury.

ABC of Transfer and Retrieval Medicine, First Edition.
Edited by Adam Low and Jonathan Hulme.
© 2015 John Wiley & Sons, Ltd. Published 2015 by John Wiley & Sons, Ltd.

The HSE provides robust guidance about requirements for different industries. The regulations also govern assessment of suitability, maintenance, storage, instruction in, and use of, PPE. In the USA, the Occupational Health and Safety Administration has published similar guidelines. The CAA, and its umbrella European organisation the Joint Aviation Authorities, produces specific guidance about aviation-related risk management, that is pertinent to the field of retrieval and transfer medicine.

Identifying risks

Risks and hazards can exist from a variety of sources in the out of hospital environment, some that may be controlled, others not. Some are inherent from the nature of the mission, for example infection transmission from patient to medic. Some may be predictable from the logistics of the mission, particularly method of transport and route implications.

It is not the purpose of this chapter to describe every risk, but to outline a process of evaluation and implementation of control measures. Generally, the process for managing risks should be kept simple, and follow a simple staged assessment of recognising hazards, identifying who could be harmed, evaluating the risks, recording the outcomes and ensuring there is a process of review (Box 17.1).

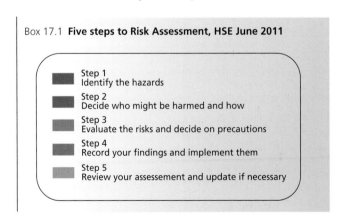

Box 17.1 **Five steps to Risk Assessment, HSE June 2011**

Step 1
Identify the hazards

Step 2
Decide who might be harmed and how

Step 3
Evaluate the risks and decide on precautions

Step 4
Record your findings and implement them

Step 5
Review your assessement and update if necessary

Even using a structured approach, assessing the risks to team members, for example, undertaking a protracted aeromedical transfer from a remote environment, can quickly become a daunting task. For this reason, potential risk assessors should aim to forge links with other services and share risk assessments wherever possible. Many assessments are generic and can be readily exchanged between services. Some are more service specific and relate to unique working conditions, and will require a more bespoke approach.

Box 17.2 outlines the potential risks to personnel and patients during a land transfer. Fixed wing or rotary transport will present different hazards

---

Box 17.2 The hazards associated with road transport

Driving at speed – increased collision risk

Unrestrained clinicians delivering care – likelihood of injury in the event of a collision increased

Driver is also a caregiver – distraction

Equipment failure – both vehicular, encompassing lights/sirens, and patient care devices

Oxygen carriage

Controlled drug security

Lifting patients – manual handling

Exposure to bodily fluids and generation of clinical waste.

It is crucial to emphasise that the assessment process is dynamic in nature, and over time new risks will manifest themselves. Risks will need to be reviewed periodically to ensure the controls put in place are still appropriate or required. Close links to an organisation's adverse event reporting mechanisms, a key part of any service clinical governance system, are vital. Team members should be proactively encouraged to report occasions when, for example, they felt PPE was not adequate. This should then trigger a risk analysis using the five-step process in Box 17.1.

Managing risks

Once a risk has been identified, some form of control or response is required. As mentioned above, the risks to the out of hospital team and their patients will vary from one setting to another, and therefore the controls need to be appropriate. Protracted low-level helicopter transfers across water will require a plan for the event of ditching into water, whereas a land-based unit should not need to consider this risk! The risk mitigation plan will include ensuring the helicopter is suitably equipped for an emergency over water, training the crew for this eventuality and the PPE requirements will include life jackets (Table 17.1).

Patients and the healthcare workers transferring them present potential hazards to one another (see Chapter 40 for more detail). Routine precautions aimed at infection control such as hand washing and safe sharps disposal are essential. Single patient use equipment should be used when available. If equipment is reused, appropriate sterilisation must be performed between patients. Ventilated patients are a potential source of transmission of respiratory tract infection, and filters which remove bacteria and viruses with closed circuits are required. PPE will also be worn to reduce infection transmission (Table 17.2).

PPE

PPE encompasses any item of clothing/device carried by the rescuer to reduce their risk of harm, when a hazard cannot be removed or avoided. Table 17.2 outlines some examples of hazards encountered in the out of hospital setting and PPE that may be used to mitigate the risk.

Table 17.1 Example of risk assessment and control.

Nature of mission	Risk/hazard	Who is at risk?	Controls already in place	Solution	Relevant UK legislation
Primary response to RTC	Visibility at roadside	All crew Present flight suit does not meet visibility standards for roadside work	Scene safety SOP Scene control by Police and Fire and Rescue Service Vehicle extrication training with Fire & Rescue Service	High visibility jackets (Class 3) to be worn over flight suits on HEMS missions	BS EN ISO 20471:2013
	Debris and broken glass – risk to eyes, hands and feet	All crew Flight helmet impractical as limits communication if worn on the ground		Protective hard hat helmet with integral visor Fire-retardant and sharp resistant gloves Footwear with ankle support and reinforced toe cap	BS EN 397:2012+ A1:2012 BS EN 443:2008 BS EN 388: 2003 BS EN ISO 20345:2011
	Exposure to blood and body fluids	All clinical crew	Safe sharps management	Medical procedure gloves Eye protection	BS EN 455-2:2009 +A2:2013 BS EN 166: 2002
Helicopter transport	Fire	All crew	Emergency exit procedures Passenger briefing Fire Training Fire extinguisher on board and at helipads	Flight suit with flame retardant properties	BS EN ISO 11612:2008
Helicopter transport over water	Emergency over water	All crew	Helicopter Underwater Escape Training course (HUET) Team fitness and CRM	Immersion Suit for prolonged "over-water" missions Lifevests with STAS breathing apparatus Personal Locator Beacons	EASA Regulations

Table 17.2 Hazards and PPE in the out of hospital environment.

Hazard category	PPE	Notes
Patient-borne hazards Blood Body fluids Respiratory infections	Gloves	Worn when risk of exposure to blood or body fluids, mucous membranes or when handling contaminated equipment. Latex, nitrile or vinyl. Sterile for invasive procedures.
	Aprons Sleeve protectors Eye protection Face masks	To protect healthcare workers clothing, and thereby reduce contamination transferred between patients. Worn when there is a risk of splashing body fluids or blood onto face. Face masks may reduce transmission of airborne pathogens. Should be changed if they become damp.
	Filtering facepiece masks FFP3	Recommended for aerosol generating procedures in recent episodes of influenza pandemic.
Environmental hazards RTC wreckage including broken glass, distorted metal Fire Service heavy rescue machinery Low light and roadside incidents CBRN contamination	RTC helmet Eye protection Boots	A hard hat, increasingly produced to meet firefighter standard. May include an integrated visor. The toe cap should be able to withstand an impact up to 200 joules. OSHA and ANSI guidance recommends minimum height 4 inches, cut/puncture and abrasion resistance, barrier protection to chemicals, and safety toe.
	High visibility clothing	Class 3 garments incorporate a minimum of 0.8 m^2 of fluorescent background material and 0.2 m^2 of retroreflective material. See Figure 17.1.
	Escape hoods	Provides a sealed system which filters harmful particles and gases preventing inhalation. Temporary device, worn when an individual suspects a risk to themself from a CBRN hazard, allowing them to withdraw from the hazardous area.
	Specialist, e.g. CBRN, water rescue, working at height, breathing apparatus	As the risk of a CBRN incident increases, specialist emergency service personnel are training to work with casualties in the hot zone or who have become contaminated. These individuals often have additional skills in water and working at height, e.g. HART paramedics
Transport hazards Fire Collision Ditch into water	Flight suit Helmet	Flight suits with flame retardant fabric, reflective strips, and knee and elbow pads. Helmets have a role in both protection of the head and communication between crew members, and are deemed compulsory for HEMS activities by the CAA.
	Lifejackets Immersion suit	The CAA requires that survival suits and life jackets shall be worn by crew and passengers when operating beyond autorotational distance from land in accordance with JAR-OPS 3.827
	Specialist e.g. Personal Locator Beacons	May be carried to assist in location of casualties following a ditch into water.

OSHA, Occupational Health and Safety Administration; ANSI, American National Standards Institute; EN, European standard.

It should be emphasised that PPE should be considered the final control measure to prevent injury, when all attempts at reducing or removing risks have been made. It should not be used as a first-line or sole risk reduction strategy. See Figure 17.1 for an example of the items of PPE required for an individual responding to primary out of hospital missions. Since clinicians undertaking transfer and retrieval medicine work in a variety of settings, the full kit may need to be adapted.

The protection offered by an item of PPE may be identified by the BS (British Standard Mark) or the CE label, which references the quality of the equipment or materials used (Figure 17.2). It should be noted that on occasion, the BS mark may refer to a component of the PPE, for example the material used to manufacture a jacket, rather than the entire garment.

Use, storage and checking of PPE

Equipment checks including PPE ought to be part of a scheduled review process which is incorporated into a service policy, or SOP.

This document should include clear unequivocal guidance about what equipment is worn and carried, which checks should be performed, frequency and actions to be taken in the event of faults found. All checks should be recorded and audited. The equipment lifespan should be monitored against manufacturer's recommendations, taking into account its frequency of use, which may in some cases reduce its lifespan.

Beyond scheduled checks, the importance of daily checks on items of PPE cannot be overemphasised. It is clearly in the interests of the individual using the equipment to check that the equipment is in good functioning order, and is appropriate for the missions they will be undertaking. Arriving for a shift a few minutes early will allow time to perform a visual and functional check of necessary equipment as per manufacturer's recommendations. It is good practice to perform these checks personally.

PPE can often be bulky and requires areas for safe/protective storage when not in use. Ideally this should be an area specifically designated for PPE use to reduce unnecessary damage, wear and tear.

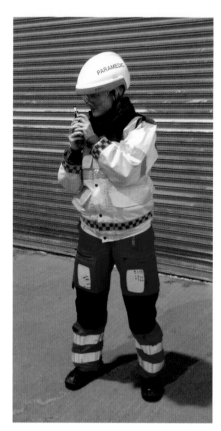

Figure 17.1 Personal protective equipment suitable for primary response. Helmet including markings to indicate job role and eye protection, high visibility jacket, with identifying markings, work trousers, with pockets and knee protection, steel toe cap boots.

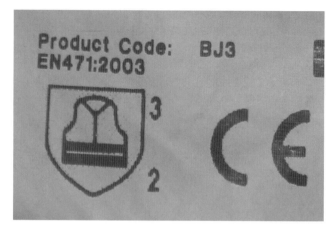

Figure 17.2 Example of the labelling that might be used to indicate personal protective equipment quality standard.

nature of an organisations workload and its adverse event reporting mechanism.

Although there is an onus on any organisation to ensure its members are appropriately equipped for the work they perform, there is also a responsibility, and an inherent interest, for the individual using the PPE to ensure it is looked after, and is in good working order.

Conclusion

The provision of PPE requires a process of risk identification, analysis and implementation of controls, with regular review and maintenance schedules. This process is dynamic, and integrates with the

Further reading

Association of Anaesthetists of Great Britain and Ireland. Safety Guideline: Infection Control in Anaesthesia. Anaesthesia 2008; 63:1027–36.

CE Marking http://www.bsigroup.com/en-GB/our-services/product -certification/ce-mark/

Five steps to risk assessment, HSE June 2011, accessed at http://www.hse .gov.uk/pubns/indg163.pdf May 2013

Health and Safety Executive (HSE) www.hse.gov.uk

The Personal Protective Equipment Regulations 2002. Accessed at http:// www.legislation.gov.uk/uksi/2002/1144/pdfs/uksi_20021144_en.pdf

CHAPTER 18

Communication and Navigation

I. Locke

West Midland Ambulance Service, NHS Trust, Midlands Air Ambulance, UK

OVERVIEW

- The benefit of a formal voice procedure in telecommunications
- The advantages of conference calls in the transfer planning stage
- Communication equipment available to transfer teams
- Interagency cooperability and the communication issues that are presented
- Navigation equipment utilised by differing transfer modalities
- Understanding the role of the co-driver in emergency driving situations.

Communication

The importance of communication starts at the decision to transfer. The AAGBI highlight that the decision to transfer should not be taken lightly: it puts the patient at an increased risk of morbidity and creates extra pressure on hospitals to organise and *potentially* provide staff to effect the transfer. Mitigating the increased risk is balanced by providing adequately qualified and experienced staff to handle the transfer and equipment that is fit for purpose.

Once the request for transfer has been made, interrogation by the transfer team should take the form of a formal voice interrogation with the sending unit. This should use a set format such as the Safe Transfer and Retrieval (STaRs) ACCEPT model (Box 18.1).

Box 18.1 **The ACCEPT model for transfers**

A: Assessment
C: Control
C: Communication
E: Evaluation
P: Preparation/Packaging
T: Transport

The UK trauma network has been active since 2012. The networks are centred on a MTC which is supported by a network of smaller trauma units (TUs). Within the West Midlands Trauma Network in the UK, the Ambulance Service has a Regional Trauma Desk (RTD) staffed by an experienced Critical Care Paramedic (CCP). When a transfer has been identified the RTD will initiate a conference call between the sending unit/receiving unit and transfer team. The conference call and use of a formal planning template allows for a systematic, methodical assessment of the need for transfer including:

- ascertaining the referrer, the receiving unit and named responsible clinician, including relevant unit/individual phone numbers
- discussing patient condition, risk of en route complications, resuscitation needs, equipment and drug needs, plus transport modality
- reduced need for multiple phone calls
- allowing imaging or the need for imaging to be discussed and if necessary completed and linked to receiving unit pre-transfer
- enabling the transfer team to plan transport modality, arrange timings for these resources to be available, ensure requisite skill level and required speed of transfer.

If a blue light transfer is required, it might be necessary for both of the ambulance crew to remain in the front of the vehicle. The role of the co-driver is to operate the radio, check the navigation system, liaise with control as required and help identify hazards. If a long-distance transfer is required under emergency conditions, it may be necessary for the crew to swap drivers. This may affect the transfer team if they had expected an extra pair of hands or are not used to operating in the back of an ambulance with unfamiliar equipment.

If tasked to a primary transfer from a remote location, or a long distance transfer at night or in poor weather, it is useful to consider the military Search and Rescue (SAR) team/Coastguard. Requested through the Aeronautical Rescue Coordination Centre (ARCC) at RAF Kinloss, the ARCC can dispatch Military and Coastguard aircraft depending upon the tasking. Advantages and disadvantages to consider:

- aircraft is operated outside of weather/daylight limits set upon civilian/HEMS operators.
- confirmed winch capability to reach primary remote locations (e.g. mountains, coast)
- most aircraft will be at coastal station and have a longer journey if used for an interhospital transfer

ABC of Transfer and Retrieval Medicine, First Edition.
Edited by Adam Low and Jonathan Hulme.
© 2015 John Wiley & Sons, Ltd. Published 2015 by John Wiley & Sons, Ltd.

- airframes are generally larger and may not be suitable for some hospital helipads
- ARCC resources and mountain rescue teams are currently not using the new ambulance/emergency service digital communications system. Relying upon VHF radios/mobile phone systems, direct communications may have to be relayed through ARCC.

Equipment

Terrestrial trunked radio (TETRA) is the digital, secure network utilised by all UK emergency services. Unlike conventional analogue radio, it boasts complete coverage utilising multiple networks and allows for interoperability between services. It has the ability to be used as a radio, broadcasting to a group channel, individual to individual or as a mobile phone. It is secure, will source signal even when in enclosed spaces and has the benefit of being flight tested and used by HEMS units. It is battery powered, and spare batteries are carried on many, if not all, emergency service vehicles. Transfer teams should ensure the availability of spares/extra batteries especially on long transfers. Handset distribution is limited, if operating in a private vehicle/aircraft only the transfer team will have the handsets.

While transfer teams should have a specific phone, many individual members will have personal mobile phones. These add an extra level of resilience when planning and during transfers if there is a problem with the primary communication source. Invariably they are small, easily stowed, can be used internationally and can be charged easily if a 12-V adaptor is available.

Limiting factors include network coverage dependent upon individual providers, geographic areas with differing levels of coverage and remote areas that have no signal. It is an unsecure device and not suitable for aero medical usage.

Satellite phones, if they have line of sight access to the sky, will receive full signal and the ability to communicate no matter how remote the user's location. They can be used to transfer data, and provide an extra level of safety in the event of a transfer/retrieval from a remote location or an aircraft systems failure or other emergency. Coverage is affected adversely by cloudy/inclement weather and being inside or close to tall buildings. Individual unit costs are higher than a conventional cell/mobile phone and call charges even higher.

VHF radios have been phased out of most front line ambulance services but are still used by HEMS units as aircraft utilise radio systems for communication between the helicopter and air traffic control. They can also communicate aircraft to aircraft via 123.1 MHz VHF or the Emergency Communications channel 156.125 MHZ. This can be very useful if the transfer team are on a HEMS aircraft and need to communicate/operate in conjunction with UKSAR force or Mountain Rescue teams.

Navigation

Depending upon the transfer modality, team involvement in active navigation will vary. The ambulance crew will usually perform all necessary navigation required, leaving the critical care team (CCT) to focus on clinical tasks. If part of the HEMS or emergency care team, some or all of the team will be involved both in the planning and navigation en route.

Land ambulance

Most UK ambulances utilise satellite navigation systems that are usually linked to ambulance control. As a case is assigned to an ambulance (crew) the location is automatically plotted with the Satellite system. A–Z map books, usually limited to the geographical location the service covers, are provided as an adjunct. Local knowledge should not be overlooked as they can often reduce unnecessary delays:

- ambulance crew knowing the quickest, most efficient route allowing for local traffic and local road conditions
- CCT teams understanding the layout of receiving units better than the Ambulance crew.
- knowledge of simple but crucial information such as the right entrance for specific wards/units.

Helicopter services

Rotary services all have a GPS system. Using a six-figure grid Ordnance Survey reference with the correct prefix will enable the aircraft to fly to any specific location. In the UK, all hospital helipads and landing sites have to be pre-surveyed by the Civil Aviation Authority and classified according to aircraft type and landing profiles. As a result hospital helipads (or their nearest landing sites) with grid references and landing profiles are kept in a database that units can access either electronically or as a hard paper copy.

Many hospitals will not have a primary helipad and will require a secondary transfer from the landing site. Essential information will be the grid reference for the landing site, the A–Z reference for the transfer vehicle and an estimated time of arrival to minimise delays on landing.

Many UK HEMS units are physician led. These teams enable transfers as an independent unit. The majority of HEMS teams are single pilot operators; meaning the pilot is qualified and experienced to fly with no assistance from the crew. In the planning phase the role of the HEMS crew is to:

- aid with navigation
- operate GPS coordinates
- utilize aeronautical charts, OS maps and A–Z maps to track flight plans and identify hazards en route to the pilot.

If GPS system fail, adverse weather occurs or operating in areas unknown, the pilot may request assistance from the HEMS crew member.

Fixed wing

Fixed-wing aircraft, preferably pressurised, should be used for transfer distances over 150 miles (240 km). Fixed wing aircraft involve a separate flight crew who will handle all matters of aviation including navigation to the designated airfield. However, close liaison with local ambulance services is required to ensure associated land ambulance is ready and in place.

Further reading

AAGBI. (2009) *Interhospital Transfer*. AAGBI. London

AAGBI. (2006) *Recommendations for the safe transfer of patients with brain injury*. AAGBI. London.

Association of Ambulance Chief Executives. (2012) *Driver Training Advisory Group, UK Ambulance Services Emergency Response Drivers Handbook*. Class Professional. Bristol.

Bledsoe B, Benner R. (2006) *Critical Care Paramedic*. Pearson. New Jersey.

Bond Air Services. (2005) *HEMS Crew Member Training Course*. Staverton.

Brooks A, Mahoney P, Hodgetts T. (2007) *Major Trauma*. Churchill Livingston. London.

Gentleman D, Dearden M, et al. Dundee Royal Infirmary, Dundee UK. Guidelines for resuscitation and transfer of patients with serious head injury. BMJ 1993;307:547–52.

Greaves, I., Porter, K., Hodgetts, T., Woollard, M. 2nd ed. *Emergency Care A Textbook for Paramedics*. Saunders. Edinburgh, 2006.

JRCALC. (2004) *Clinical Practice Guidelines For use in U.K. Ambulance Services*. ASA. London.

NICE. (2007) Clinical Guideline 56. *Head Injury. Triage, assessment, investigation and early management of head injury in infants, children and adults*. NICE. London.

STaR (2006) *Safe Transfer and Retrieval: The Practical Approach/Advanced Life Support Group* (2nd Edition). Oxford. Blackwell Publishing.

Section 4

Pharmacology of Transfer Medicine

CHAPTER 19

Routes of Administration

T. Nutbeam[1,2] and R. Fenwick[3]

[1] Department of Emergency Medicine, Derriford Hospital, Plymouth Hospitals NHS Trust, UK
[2] West Midlands Ambulance Service NHS Foundation Trust Medical Emergency Response Incident Team (MERIT), UK
[3] Emergency Department, Shrewsbury and Telford Hospitals NHS Trust, UK

OVERVIEW

- The pros and cons of the various routes of administration with which the retrieval and transfer practitioner needs to be familiar
- The principles of safe drug storage and transport
- The principles of prescribing, preparing and delivering drugs safely and effectively
- How to use and trouble shoot central venous catheters, mucosal atomisation devices and intraosseous devices.

Routes of administration

The principle routes of administration of drugs/medications are outlined below.

Oral

This is the most commonly used route of administration in general medicine. If the patient is fully conscious, clinically well and has an intact swallow/ gag then this may be an appropriate route to choose. The bioavailability of medications administered will vary widely; not only from person to person but also in relation to other factors (Box 19.1) at the time of administration. This inherent unreliability, coupled with the limitations related to administration, limits the usefulness of this route in the unwell patient. It is however an excellent, well tolerated route for administration of antiemetics to transfer team members!

Box 19.1 **Factors which affect bioavailability of orally administered medications**

Medication characteristics (e.g. lipid solubility)
Gastrointestinal mobility
Gastric pH
Reaction between medication and other gastrointestinal contents (foods, other medications etc.)
Gastrointestinal blood flow (decreased in shocked states).

ABC of Transfer and Retrieval Medicine, First Edition.
Edited by Adam Low and Jonathan Hulme.
© 2015 John Wiley & Sons, Ltd. Published 2015 by John Wiley & Sons, Ltd.

Sublingual/buccal

Drug absorption is rapid and avoids first pass metabolism. Glyceryl trinitrate for angina/congestive cardiac failure (CCF) is the medication most commonly administered by this route. Other examples are listed in Box 19.2.

Box 19.2 **Medications commonly administered via the sublingual or buccal route**

Glycerytrinitrate
Opiates (e.g. buccal fentanyl)
ACE inhibitors in acute CCF
Dextrose gel for hypoglycaemia

Rectal

Drugs via this route are rapidly absorbed. Indications and examples can be found in Box 19.3.

Box 19.3 **Indications for use of rectal route of administration**

Drug is particularly effective by this route/ other forms not readily available, e.g. indomethacin for renal colic
Drug cannot be taken orally due to vomiting/aspiration risk, e.g. aspirin in acute embolic stroke
Intravenous access unavailable, e.g. diazepam in a fitting child

---

Nasal

This is an ideal route for the infrequent administration of potent, low volume drugs, which require rapid onset, bypassing first pass metabolism. Antimigraine and anti-allergy medications are commonly administered via this route. The retrieval and transfer practitioner is more likely to use them in the context of analgesia and sedation (see 'Mucosal atomisation device', MAD).

Inhalation

Oxygen delivery, the use of nebulisers and other inhaled anaesthetic agents are covered elsewhere in this text.

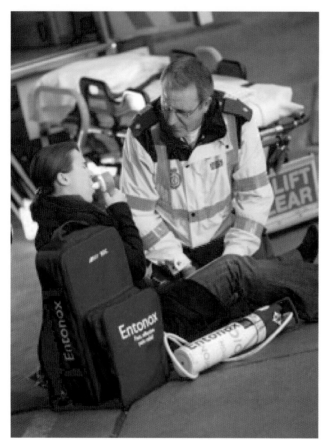

Figure 19.1 An Entonox cylinder: note the blue and white shoulders. (Source: Hulme, J. (2013). Prehospital Analgesia and Sedation. In: Nutbeam, T. and Boylan, M. (eds). ABC of Prehospital Emergency Medicine. John Wiley & Sons Ltd, Oxford, p. 53. Reproduced with permission of John Wiley & Sons).

Nitrous oxide and oxygen

This 50:50 mixture of nitrous oxide and oxygen is commonly known as Entonox (Figure 19.1) or 'gas and air'. It is used commonly in the pre-hospital environment and in labour suites. It benefits from extremely rapid onset/offset and can be used with most conscious patients (see Chapter 20).

Methoxyflurane

Penthrox or 'the green whistle' is widely used in pre-hospital care in Australia. It is usually available in an inhaler format which can be self-administered by those over the age of 5 years. It is commonly used as an analgesic agent in the setting of trauma. It provides analgesia following six to eight breaths that lasts for several minutes. Owing to the risk of kidney injury it is relatively contraindicated in the context of diabetes mellitus and pre-existing renal disease.

Topical/cutaneous

Drugs commonly administered by this route include; local anaesthetic agents used prior to cannulation in children (EMLA, Amitop), opiates in chronic pain (fentanyl patches) and topical hormone use. This route (including ophthalmic administration) will have limited utility to the retrieval and transfer practitioner.

Q	Flow rate
P	Pressure
r	Radius
η	Fluid viscosity
l	Length of tubing

$$Q = \frac{\pi P r^4}{8 \eta l}$$

Figure 19.2 Poiseuille's Law dictates maximal flow rates through a cannuale.

Subcutaneous and intramuscular

Absorption by this route is unreliable and extremely variable. Rate-limiting factors include those related to the drug itself, and local blood flow at the site (difficult to predict or monitor). Commonly administered subcutaneous agents include anti-thrombosis medications and insulin. Intramuscular injection of 1:1000 adrenaline (epinephrine) is used in the initial treatment of anaphylaxis.

Intravenous

The intravenous route provides the fastest (alongside intraosseous) and predictable route of administration. Intravenous 'push' will result in a high peak concentration of the drug (e.g. in rapid sequence induction) with this variability being avoided using a continuous infusion. The closer the delivery device is (usually the end of the catheter) to the point of action (heart/ brain, etc.) the quicker the onset. Maximum volume of drug delivered is dictated by Poiseuille's law (Figure 19.2).

Intraosseous

The intraosseous route is used in the setting of difficult or delayed intravenous access. Drugs, blood and other agents can be delivered via this route. Time to onset and flow rates are similar to that achieved via a central line. See 'Intraosseous' section for more details.

Others
Intrathecal

Rarely initiated by the retrieval and transfer practitioner. A detailed explanation of monitoring and trouble shooting an intrathecal infusion is beyond the scope of this text.

Via endotracheal tube

Rarely used except in extremis. Intratracheal adrenaline (epinephrine) may have a role in the treatment of life-threatening asthma.

Safe medication

Safe storage

The storage of controlled drugs is strictly regulated in law. All medicinal products should be stored in accordance with their product information leaflet. This will normally require a secure,

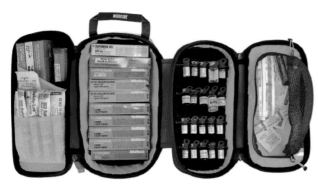

Figure 19.3 StatPack medication storage device. (Source: StatPack. Reproduced with permission of StatPack).

dark, temperature controlled environment. Certain medications (e.g. muscle relaxants) may require refrigeration for long-term storage. The use and storage of all medications should be subject to mandatory audit. Regular stock checks should be performed alongside drug rotation.

Safe transport

The transport of controlled drugs, both in terms of storage device used and maximal quantities permissible to be held by different healthcare professionals is controlled by law. Many retrieval and transfer practitioners will choose to carry their medications in a purpose designed carry case: normally with padding or elastic loops to restrict the movement of ampoules (Figure 19.3). Consideration should be given to the use of plastic ampoules when available: this can prevent breakages though not all medications are available in this format. The use of prefilled syringes for time critical medications (e.g. cardiac arrest medications) may be warranted as well as the drawing up of emergency drugs (e.g. for RSI) at the beginning of a shift/tasking.

Safe prescribing and documentation

All medications delivered to a patient should be both prescribed and the administration recorded. Care should be taken when working out complex drug doses/calculations and these should ideally be

Table 19.1 Medications according to weight.

Ideal body weight (IBW)	Corrected body weight	Total body weight (TBW)
Calculations		
Broca formula:	(CBW)	
IBW in Kg =	(CBW = IBW + 40%	
Men: Height in cm minus 100	of excess weight)	
Women Height in cm minus 105		
Examples		
Propofol	Fentanyl	Suxamethonium
Thiopentone	Sugammadex	Midazolam bolus
Ketamine	Local anaesthetics	Atracurium
Rocuronium	Antibiotics	
Vecuronium		
Morphine		

double-checked. Prescriptions should be written in accordance with the guidance in Box 19.4.

When calculating medication doses, care should be taken to ensure the appropriate dose is calculated according to patient's ideal weight, corrected body weight or total body weight (see Table 19.1).

Safe preparation

Assemble the required materials in ideally a clean location designated for the task. Where possible, this area should be uncluttered and free from interruption and distraction.

Calculate the volume of medication required to give the prescribed dose then prepare the label for the medication.

Wash hands and apply disposable gloves in accordance with local policy. When preparing the medication be sure to use a non-touch technique to avoid bacterial contamination. Immediately label the syringe or infusion once prepared.

Record any reasons for deviation from clinical guidelines on the prescription and in the patient's notes.

Safe delivery

Medication should ideally be checked by two practitioners prior to delivery – this process should be clearly documented – particular care should be taken when titrating medication to effect (see Box 19.5. Details on use of intranasal, central line and intraosseous delivery can be found later in the chapter.

Box 19.5 **The 'Six Rights' of medication administration**

1 Right patient – is the medication indicated for this patient; no contraindications; no allergies
2 Right drug – the correct name (trade name vs. generic name); correct concentration
3 Right dose
4 Right route
5 Right time – slow or rapid administration
6 Right documentation

Central venous catheters

Use of central venous catheter lines

Whenever accessing the line, a strict aseptic technique must be used as Central venous catheters (CVC) are frequently associated with bacteraemia. Always check that blood can be drawn back from a lumen prior to use to ensure patency of the selected port. If a transducer set is to be used ideally it should be attached to the distal lumen (largest gauge); however, if this is not possible then proximal or medial ports are acceptable. The lumen with the transducer set 'flush line' can be used to give boluses or short infusions such as antibiotics or fluid boluses. Under no circumstances should potent drugs such as potassium or inotropes be attached to the flush line for risk of bolusing if the line were to be flushed. All other ports should have either a bionector (bung with a one way valve) or a double lumen extension set, therefore allowing multiple therapies to be used. An overview of port designation can be found in Table 19.2.

Each lumen can be treated as separate with regards to combining drugs, however only those that are compatible should be attached to a double lumen extension.

If an infusion is stopped it should be disconnected and blood drawn back on the lumen, then flushed, to ensure continued patency.

Common problems

- Occluded lumens – there may be a clot in the lumen, occasionally they rest against the vessel so making it difficult to draw back blood. Attempt to draw back with patient in a head down position. Do not flush if you suspect a clot or you do not know what drug has last been used in that lumen.
- Inconsistent measurements – this can be due to incorrect positioning of transducer, secure it to the patients arm if possible to ensure consistent pressure readings.
- Difficulty calibrating – check all connections, if more than one transducer set in-situ (ABP monitoring) check the correct modules and transducer sets are being used.
- Infusions on transducer line – certain infusions can be given via this port (IV antibiotics, fluid boluses), ensure they are turned off at the tap in order to take a CVP reading.

Mucosal atomisation device (MAD)

The intranasal route offers a non-invasive alternative for medication administration. The MAD creates 30-μm particles that offer rapid absorption across mucosal membranes to the blood stream and into the brain/cerebrospinal fluid via the olfactory mucosa, avoiding first pass metabolism. Absorption can be affected by

Table 19.2 Central line lumens.

Distal (largest gauge) – brown	Medial – blue/grey	Proximal – white
Blood administration	TPN	Blood sampling
High volume fluids	Drug administration	Drug administration
Drug administration		
CVP monitoring		

Table 19.3 Commonly used Intranasal medications.

Indication	Medication	Dose
Analgesia	Diamorphine	0.1 mg/kg
	Ketamine	0.5–1.0 mg/kg
	Fentanyl	2.0 µg/kg
Sedation	Midazolam	0.5 mg/kg
	Ketamine	3 mg/kg
	Fentanyl	1.5–3.0 µg/kg
Seizures	Midazolam	0.2–0.3 mg/kg (10 mg adult dose)
Opiate overdose	Naloxone	2 mg

the presence of blood or mucous discharge (which may require suction), however atomization offers superior effects compared with drops or sprays (quicker bioavailability and more reliable administration) (Table 19.3).

The ideal volume for intranasal administration is 0.2–0.3 mL and the maximum is 1 mL per nostril (for volumes above 0.3 mL it is recommended that half should be administered in each nostril to increase the available mucosal surface area). Therefore, the administered medication is required to be both high concentration and low volume. When preparing the device and calculating medication, it must be remembered that the MAD has a dead space of 0.1 mL, which must be accounted for to prevent underdosing. Commonly administered IN drugs can be found in Table 19.3.

Intraosseous

Indication

The immediate requirement for vascular access when IV cannulation is unsuccessful or delayed.

Contraindications

The only widely acknowledged contraindication is a proximal fracture of the targeted bone.

There are a number of relative contraindications:

- previous intraosseous attempts at the proposed bone (extravasation)
- previous orthopaedic surgery at the proposed site e.g. total knee replacement (needle unable to penetrate metalwork)
- infection of the overlying soft tissues (increased theoretical risk of osteomyelitis)
- inability to identify landmarks, e.g. due to obesity (misplacement)
- bone disease, e.g. osteoporosis/ osteogenesis imperfecta

Insertion sites (see Figure 19.4)
Humerus – greater tubercle

Adduct the patients arm, flex the elbow and place their hand onto their umbilicus. Palpate the anterior mid-shaft humerus. Continue palpating proximally up the anterior surface of the humerus until the greater tubercle is met. Palpate coracoid and acromion. Imagine a line between them and drop a line approximately 2 cm from its midpoint to the insertion site (adults).

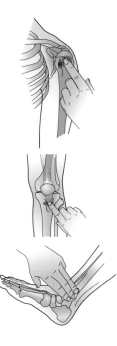

Humeral head
- Abduct arm to body and flex slow to 90°
- Internally rotate arm so hand over umbilicus
- Greater tubercle now lies arrierior on shoulder
- Insert needle perpendicular to bone
- Splint limb to side to prevent dislodgement

Proximal tibia

Adult
- One finger breadth medial to tibial tuberosity

Child
- One finger breadth below and medial to tibial tuberosity
- Two finger breadth below patella and one finger medial

Distal tibia

Adult
- Three finger-breadths above tip of medial malleolus

Child
- Two finger-breadths above tip of medial malleolus

Figure 19.4 Intraosseus insertion sites. (Source: Dawes, R.J. (2013). Circulation Assessment and Management. In: Nutbeam, T. and Boylan, M. (eds). BC of Prehospital Emergency Medicine. John Wiley & Sons Ltd, Oxford, pp. 35–43. Reproduced with permission of John Wiley & Sons).

Proximal tibia – anteromedial surface

Two fingerbreadths below and medial to the tibial tuberosity in adults. Most commonly utilised as it is easily accessible with good flow rates and can be secured.

Distal tibia – medial surface

Two fingerbreadths proximal to the tip of the medial malleolus in adults.

Pain during insertion is reported to be similar to that of a wide-bore cannula; therefore, subcutaneous infiltration of lignocaine should be considered in the conscious patient. Consent should be sought wherever possible although this is not required in the obtunded patient.

An initial flush of at least 10 mL of 0.9% sodium chloride is required to create a lacuna to receive the fluid on administration. Without this flush, flow rates will be considerably reduced. In the conscious patient, this flush creates a diffuse visceral pain and slow lignocaine administration (40 mg to 4 mL of 1% or 2 mL of 2%) should be utilised if time allows.

Always give fluids or drugs via the connect tube in the EZ-IO set, as directly attaching the syringe to the intraosseus needle can cause the syringe to break, rendering the device unserviceable. To achieve maximal flow rates it is recommended to use a syringe and three-way tap (50-mL syringe, draw fluid from bag then manually push fluid).

The use of stabilisation dressings specifically designed for use with each device may reduce the incidence of displacement and extravasation. Other complications, e.g. osteomyelitis, are negligible if aseptic insertion techniques are utilised and the device is removed within 24 hours of insertion.

Fluid warming devices

The use of warmed fluids has not been demonstrated to actively rewarm patients but rather stop their temperature falling further with large transfusions or infusions.

Considerable focus on the prevention of hypothermia has led to a number of commercial devices being available on the market. There is currently no evidence directly comparing the devices efficacy in either the retrieval or pre-hospital environments. These devices are designed to be rugged and portable while providing the ability to warm all fluids and blood products prior to both high and low volume infusions.

Further reading

Dougherty L, Lister S. *Royal Marsden Hospital Manual of Clinical Nursing Procedures* (Professional Edition). London: Wiley Blackwell 2011.

Nutbeam T, Daniels D (eds). *ABC of Practical Procedures*. London: BMJ Publishing Group; 2009.

UCL Pharmacy. *UCL Hospitals Injectable Medicines Administration Guide*. London: John Wiley and Sons; 2010.

CHAPTER 20

Pre-hospital Sedation and Analgesia

J. Hulme[1,2,3,4,5,6]

[1]Intensive Care Medicine and Anaesthesia, Sandwell and West Birmingham Hospitals NHS Trust, UK
[2]University of Birmingham, UK
[3]West Midlands Ambulance Service NHS Foundation Trust Medical Emergency Response, UK
[4]Incident Team (MERIT), UK
[5]West Midlands Central Accident Resuscitation & Emergency (CARE) Team, UK
[6]Mercia Accident Rescue Service (MARS) BASICS, UK

OVERVIEW

- Pain is subjective, influenced by culture, previous pain events, beliefs, mood and ability to cope and should be managed accordingly in a stepwise manner
- Analgesia is the relief of pain through administration of drugs or other methods
- Sedation is a continuum from alert anxiolysis through procedural sedation to complete unresponsiveness
- Increasing depth of sedation increases the risk of:
  - over-sedation = anaesthesia
  - agitation or confusion
  - hypotension
  - apnoea
  - death

Practitioners should follow predefined standard operating procedures for sedation and advanced analgesia.

Introduction

In this chapter we will consider agents and techniques for analgesia and sedation. Adherence to standard operating procedures (SOPs) and minimum monitoring standards are recommended.

Analgesia

Pain is common. Effective analgesia is important: it improves early and late physiological and psychological parameters and facilitates easier transfer. It improves patient assessment by reducing distress and enables treatment otherwise not possible without increased pain.

Principles of management of acute pain

1 Mandatory assessment of presence and severity using reliable tools.
2 Appropriate use of non-pharmacological and pharmacological interventions.

3 Supported by adequate documentation within a service using a quality assurance system.

The World Health Organization (WHO) has described an 'analgesic ladder'. Step onto the ladder at the best height for your patient; it should not always be climbed from the bottom rung! Healthcare providers underestimate analgesic needs due to psychological and educational barriers. Reliable tools to score pain and titrate treatment exist; use them.

Non-pharmacological interventions

Non-pharmacological techniques are potent; a calm, professional manner ('therapeutic communication') helps your patient and team. Anxiety is a modulator of pain (Box 20.1).

Box 20.1 **Techniques that reduce pain**

Treat the cause: relocate dislocated limb/digit
Immobilise fractures: reduces pain/bleeding
Treat muscle spasm: it is extremely painful (e.g. following femoral fracture) and counteracted by traction
Cooling and shielding burns from touch/airflow reduces pain. Consider cooling duration vs. risk of hypothermia

---

Pharmacological interventions

Use synergistic agents rather than a larger dose of one drug if the timeframe allows, e.g. paracetamol (acetaminophen), codeine and non-steroidal anti-inflammatory drugs (NSAIDs) reduce opioid requirements (Box 20.2). For urgent transfers, the immediate benefit may not be seen but the principle remains, although the number of co-administered drugs is likely to be smaller.

Some agents cause analgesia and sedation, e.g. opioids, ketamine. This can be useful, e.g. procedural sedation. Remember, most

---

Box 20.2 **Classes of analgesic agents used during retrievals**

Non-opioids
Opioids
Inhalational agents
Local anaesthesia

ABC of Transfer and Retrieval Medicine, First Edition.
Edited by Adam Low and Jonathan Hulme.
© 2015 John Wiley & Sons, Ltd. Published 2015 by John Wiley & Sons, Ltd.

sedatives are not analgesic – depressed consciousness does not equal pain relief.

Non-opioids

Paracetamol

There are few reasons why paracetamol should not be part of every analgesic prescription. For patients with reduced gut function, intravenous paracetamol (1 g QDS IV) has an effect in 5–10 minutes, peaking at 1 hour and is available in 100-mL plastic bottles.

NSAIDs and COX-2 selective inhibitors

For acute mild to moderate pain, e.g. acute back pain. Numerous drugs and administration routes exist.

Side effects include gastrointestinal intolerance and bronchospasm (only in a minority of asthmatics). Death due to thrombotic episodes increases with ischaemic heart disease for some NSAIDs.

COX-2 selective inhibitors offer theoretical freedom from adverse effects associated with NSAIDs but can cause other serious harm.

Ketamine

An anaesthetic agent used at lower doses as sedative, and analgesic for moderate and severe pain (Figure 20.1). It has a large therapeutic index: the difference between effective dose and amount in overdose causing significant harm is large (Box 20.3).

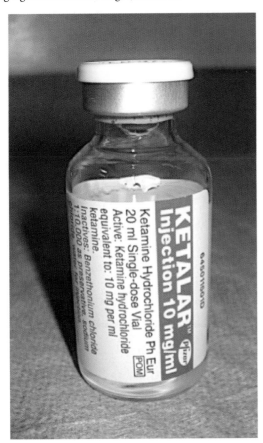

Figure 20.1 Ketamine is a widely used agent for analgesia, procedural sedation and anaesthesia of the critically ill or injured patient.

Box 20.3 **Suggested dosing regimes for ketamine**

Analgesia:	0.25 mg/kg incrementally
Sedation:	0.5 mg/kg
Anaesthesia:	1–2 mg/kg (reduced if severe cardiovascular compromise)

Rapid onset (1 minute) and offset (longer lasting anterograde amnesia) requiring repeat doses to maintain analgesia but making ketamine valuable to allow short, painful procedures (chest drain insertion, fracture manipulation).

Patients describe hallucinations and nightmares after ketamine, sometimes long term. Up to 20% experience emergence phenomenon: acute agitation/psychological distress as the ketamine wears off. It is reduced by benzodiazepines or morphine.

Ketamine solutions contain structurally different molecules (enantiomers). Preparations omitting psychoactive versions are not yet widely used.

Ketamine suppresses breathing less than most anaesthetics; apnoea is unusual unless the IV/IO dose has been administered too rapidly. Airway patency and reflexes are often (not always) usefully preserved. Increased muscular tone following ketamine can make extrication difficult (limbs difficult to flex/hands clasped onto steering wheel) and dislocations more difficult to treat. Ketamine can cause nausea and vomiting.

Opioids

Opioids are widely used for severe pain, especially morphine, fentanyl and diamorphine. Morphine is considered a 'gold standard' for severe pain treatment, although has several shortcomings.

Significant inter-patient dose requirements necessitate dose titration. However, the onset of analgesic effect is 20 minutes, meaning titration is impractically lengthy. Opioids fail to provide dynamic analgesia (i.e. during movement). Respiratory depression is uncommon with careful titration. Antiemetics are typically co-administered.

Fentanyl and diamorphine are faster acting, shorter lasting and more lipid soluble than morphine. This last property enables delivery via alternative routes while longer lasting analgesia is arranged. The 'fentanyl lollipop' is not licensed for acute pain although it is used for this purpose by many.

Inhalational agents

Inhalational agents have rapid onset/offset if the patient is cooperative while longer lasting analgesia is established, or they can be used as adjunctive analgesia during painful episodes, e.g. splinting. No common significant side effects except sedation and nausea.

Nitrous oxide:oxygen (50/50 mix): Entonox®

This is contraindicated in patients with air-containing closed spaces (pneumothorax, intracranial air after head injury, decompression sickness) as N_2O diffuses in increasing pressure.

Entonox® separates into its component gases at −6°C, risking delivery of a hypoxic mixture. Repeated inversion of the cylinder before use at low temperatures is recommended to mix gases.

The cylinder and delivery system are heavy and can mean that a useful analgesic is left behind if other equipment needs to be carried.

Methoxyflurane: Penthrox™

A volatile anaesthetic agent that at low concentrations produces analgesia equivalent to 10 mg of morphine. Pain relief may be superior to Entonox®, which may achieve its effect due to inattention secondary to euphoria. It can be safely administered to patients in shock.

The Penthrox™ Inhaler (Medical Developments International, Melbourne, Victoria, Australia) is a lightweight, single patient use, handheld device like a large whistle. Oxygen can be administered via an inlet port. One 3-mL bottle of methoxyflurane provides 25 minutes of analgesia. Maximum dosage is 6-mL per day. A hole near the mouthpiece when covered by a patient's finger causes a higher concentration to be inhaled, increasing analgesia if required.

Easy to use and well tolerated, it is used extensively in Australia and by remote teams, e.g. military, expeditions. Coughing and respiratory symptoms have been reported by staff in enclosed environments, e.g. ambulance. An optional scavenger attachment is available that reduces this problem and is recommended to reduce regular, longer-term exposure of health workers.

Local anaesthesia

Topical application: venepuncture in non-time critical situations, for children and needle phobic adults.

Peripheral nerve blocks

Profound analgesia without sedation, e.g. femoral nerve blocks. Accurate injection may be problematic in a primary setting; splinting and ketamine/morphine obviate need for (suboptimal) regional anaesthesia performed in difficult practical circumstances. Excellent for long-lasting safe analgesia during secondary transfer. The use of nerve stimulation and ultrasound guidance is commonplace within hospital facilities to increase the success of a number of nerve blocks, including femoral.

Sedation

Sedation is a continuum although discrete definitions are proposed (Table 20.1). Deeper levels are indistinguishable from general anaesthesia. This is reflected in multi-speciality recommendations describing staff competencies and equipment (see further reading).

The dissociative state produced by ketamine is considered akin to general anaesthesia by the Royal College of Anaesthetists and the College of Emergency Medicine in the United Kingdom and should be treated accordingly by those considering its use (Figure 20.2).

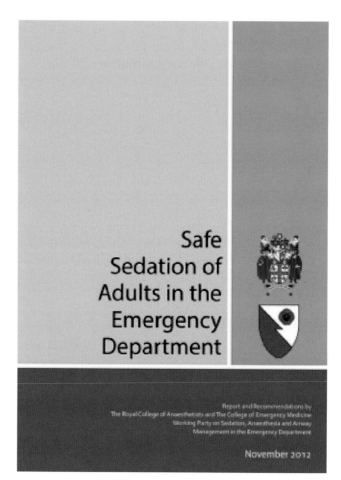

Figure 20.2 There are many examples of recommendations for the safe practice of sedation that highlight the need for training, monitoring and teamwork. Those pertinent to the country of practice should be familiar to clinicians using these skills. (Source: Royal College of Anaesthetists and the College of Emergency Medicine. Reproduced with permission of the Royal College of Anaesthetists and the College of Emergency Medicine).

Table 20.1 Continuum of depth of sedation.

	Minimal sedation/anxiolysis	Procedural sedation (formerly 'conscious sedation')	Deep sedation	General anaesthesia
Responsiveness	Normal response to verbal stimulation	Purposeful* response to verbal or tactile stimulation	Purposeful* response following repeated or painful stimulation	Unable to be roused even with painful station
Airway	Unaffected	No intervention required	Intervention may be required	Intervention often required
Spontaneously ventilation	Unaffected	Adequate	May be inadequate	Frequently inadequate
Cardiovascular function	Unaffected	Usually maintained	Usually maintained	May be impaired

*Reflex withdrawal from a painful stimulus is NOT considered a purposeful response. Excerpted from Continuum of Depth of Sedation. Definition of General Anesthesia and Levels of Sedation/ Analgesia of the American Society of Anesthesiology. From the ASA, 520N, Northwest Highway, Park Ridge, Illinois, 60068-2573, USA.

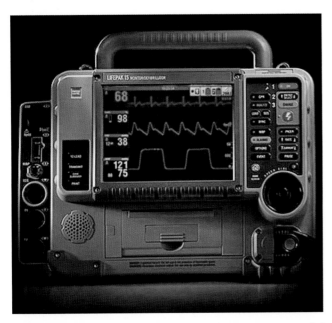

Figure 20.3 Multimodal monitoring of the sedated patient is recommended. (Source: Harris T. (2013). Prehospital monitoring. In: Nutbeam, T. and Boylan, M. (eds). ABC of Prehospital Emergency Medicine. John Wiley & Sons Ltd, Oxford, pp. 57. Reproduced with permission of John Wiley & Sons).

Sedation during retrieval and transfer takes one of two forms:

1 Procedural sedation: administration of short-acting sedatives and analgesics to facilitate distressing/painful interventions, e.g. extricating the injured, trapped patient, insertion of intercostal drain. Patient maintains purposeful response to verbal commands, alone ± light tactile stimulation (reflex withdrawal from painful stimulus is NOT considered purposeful). Airway, breathing and cardiovascular function are maintained without interventions.
2 Deep sedation/general anaesthesia: ongoing administration of sedatives and analgesics, often as infusions, to facilitate mechanical ventilation. Neuromuscular blockade often co-administered.

Monitoring

In accordance with minimum standards used during anaesthesia (Figure 20.3). Capnography in non-intubated sedated patients gives a regular respiratory trace and is likely to become routine (see Further reading) (Box 20.4).

Box 20.4 **Minimum mandatory monitoring standards**

ECG (three lead)
Pulse oximetry
Blood pressure (NIBP auto-cycle every 3–5 minutes/arterial line)
Capnography
Visual monitoring (respiratory rate, alertness, response to stimuli)

Equipment

Kit and drugs to manage cardiovascular collapse and emergency anaesthesia.

Training

Procedural sedation can, without intention, become general anaesthesia and precipitate physiological decompensation (airway loss, respiratory compromise, cardiovascular collapse). Illness and injury increase likelihood of adverse events even with small amounts of sedation.

In-hospital sedation by non-anaesthetists has been cause for concern. Recommendations endorsed internationally and in the UK by all major bodies involved in prehospital care are that procedural sedation should only be undertaken by 'practitioners … competent to undertake RSI and tracheal intubation'. Transfer of anaesthetised patients requires a skill set beyond this.

Drugs

Administer supplemental oxygen to all sedated patients.

Procedural sedation

Numerous drug combinations have been used; avoid unnecessary polypharmacy. Successful analgesia and sedation are readily achieved for most patients using one or two drugs, e.g. opioid and benzodiazepine/ketamine. In difficult situations what is usually needed is more patience to titrate correctly the therapeutic agent, additional non-pharmacological methods (e.g. splinting) and better teamwork: not an extra drug.

Maintenance of general anaesthesia

A sedative (propofol/midazolam) plus opioid (fentanyl/morphine) are most commonly used.

Further reading

Safe Sedation Practice for Healthcare Procedures. Standards and Guidance. Academy of Medical Royal Colleges. October 2013.

Safe sedation of adults in the emergency department. The Royal College of Anaesthetists and The College of Emergency Medicine Working Party on Sedation, Anaesthesia and Airway Management in the Emergency Department. November 2012.

Prehospital anaesthesia: safety guideline. Association of anaesthetists of Great Britain and Ireland (AAGBI) (endorsed by the Royal College of anaesthetists, Joint Royal Ambulances Liaison Committee, College of Emergency Medicine, the British Association for Immediate Care, Faculty of Prehospital Care of the Royal College of Surgeons of Edinburgh, Royal Centre for Defence Medicine). February 2009.

Recommendation for standards of monitoring during anaesthesia and recovery. AAGBI. March 2007. (www.aagbi.org/sites/default/files/standardsofmonitoring07.pdf)

The use of capnography outside the operating theatre. AAGBI, London. 2011 (www.aagbi.org/sites/default/files/Capnographyaagbi090711AJH%5B1%5D_0.pdf)

CHAPTER 21

Sedation and Neuromuscular Blockers

E. Joynes[1] and B. Munford[1,2,3]

[1]Careflight Darwin, Australia
[2]Anaesthetist, Liverpool Hospital, Australia
[3]UNWS Medical School, Australia

OVERVIEW

- Intubated patients require sedation ± muscle relaxation to facilitate ventilation
- There is a choice of agent, with differing characteristics
- Choice of drug should take account of drug and patient characteristics.

Emergency anaesthesia (rapid sequence induction (RSI)) is undertaken in a range of environments, from the controlled environment for elective anaesthesia to remote sites (in and out of hospital) with limited support. It is indicated in a very small proportion of the cases attended by pre-hospital healthcare professionals; most often for trauma patients (Box 21.1).

Box 21.1 **Indications for RSI prior to transfer**

Multiple trauma
Head injury
Unconsciousness
Anticipated deterioration in clinical course
Humanitarian
Respiratory failure
Failure of airway patency/protection
Flight/pre-hospital safety (agitated/unmanageable patient)

Drug choice is multifactorial and will depend upon the patient, clinician training and clinical context. Standard operating procedures help to standardise interventions such as emergency anaesthesia including drug choices.

Induction agents

Potential induction agents in all these settings include ketamine, propofol, thiopentone and etomidate (Table 21.1 and Figure 21.1).

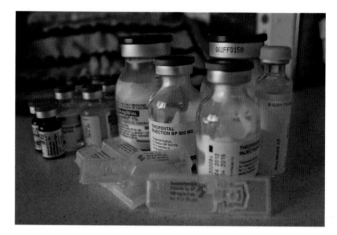

Figure 21.1 Thiopentone, propofol and etomidate are examples of induction agents.

Ketamine can be used for induction and maintenance of anaesthesia and is the drug of choice in most critically ill patients due to a better haemodynamic stability profile. Etomidate is an alternative as it also causes less cardiovascular compromise than thiopentone and propofol, but even a single dose may inhibit the adrenal axis (can block adrenal cortisol production for up to 8 hours in healthy individuals and up to 24 hours in the critically ill).

Ketamine's cardiovascular effects commonly include tachycardia, hypertension and increased cardiac output. These effects may make it detrimental if there is shock due to myocardial ischaemia, but beneficial in most critically ill or injured patients. There has been controversy over its use in brain injury following descriptions of increased cerebral blood flow and raised intracranial pressure. This concept, although still often quoted, is now largely discredited. The effects do not occur if hypoventilation and hypercapnia are avoided and the maintenance of blood pressure is likely to outweigh effects on intracranial pressure. There is some evidence to suggest that in brain injuries, ketamine may have protective effects via N-methyl-D-aspartate (NMDA) receptors.

Neuromuscular blockers

Neuromuscular blocking drugs (NMBDs) for emergency RSI include suxamethonium and rocuronium. Alternative intermediate

ABC of Transfer and Retrieval Medicine, First Edition.
Edited by Adam Low and Jonathan Hulme.
© 2015 John Wiley & Sons, Ltd. Published 2015 by John Wiley & Sons, Ltd.

Table 21.1 Drugs for induction/sedation.

Drug	Thiopentone	Ketamine	Propofol	Etomidate	Midazolam
Use	Induction agent Status epilepticus Brain protection	Analgesia/sedation/induction (dissociative anaesthesia) Hypotension/shock, Asthma	Induction/maintenance of anaesthesia Status epilepticus/sedation	Induction agent	Induction/sedation/pre-medication
Chemical	Thio-barbiturate	Phencyclidine derivative	Phenol derivative	Imidazole ester	Benzodiazepine
Presentation	500 mg sodium thiopental yellow powder, reconstitute with water	Clear/colourless solution 10/50/100 mg/mL	Aqueous emulsion 1% or 2%	Lipid emulsion or clear colourless solution containing propylene glycol, at concentration of 2 mg/mL	Clear/colourless solution 1/2/5 mg/mL
Induction dose	IV 2–7 mg/kg Onset 30 seconds Duration 5–15 minutes	IV 1.5–2 mg/kg Onset 1–2 minutes Duration 5–10 minutes IM 10 mg/kg Onset 2–8 minutes, duration 10–20 minutes	IV 2–3 mg/kg (increase 50% children) Onset 30 seconds Duration 10 minutes Infusion 1–4 mg/kg/hour	IV 0.3 mg/kg	Sedation dose 0.05–0.1 mg/kg IV/0.07–0.08 mg/kg IM rapid onset short duration
Pharmacokinetics Absorption Distribution Metabolism Excretion	Highly protein bound Rapid onset/offset (re-distribution) Liver Renal	Well absorbed IM Offset mainly due to redistribution (brain to peripheral tissues) Liver Renal	Highly protein bound Rapid offset (redistribution) Liver Renal	Rapid offset (redistribution) Liver/plasma esterases Renal	Well absorbed IM Highly protein bound Liver Renal
Pharmacodynamics Caution	CVS/RS depression, Laryngospasm Decrease cerebral blood flow/ICP Anticonvulsant Incompatible with many drugs	Increase BP, use in shocked patients, Bronchodilation, Preserves airway reflexes Dissociative anaesthesia ?effect on CBF (may be safe in head injury if normocarbia maintained) Nausea/Vomiting salivation Emergence phenomena Avoid in cardiac ischaemia	CVS depression, care in shocked patients Suppresses laryngeal reflexes Decrease cerebral oxygen consumption Epileptiform movements Anti-emetic, anti-convulsant Pain on injection, egg allergy	Small reduction CO/BP – use in shock Apnoea – transient, less than other agents/cough/hiccup Nausea/Vomiting Inhibits adrenal steroid production – care in elderly/critically ill.	CVS/RS depression Antrograde amnesia, sedation, anxiolysis, anticonvulsant Effects reversed with flumazenil

to long acting muscle relaxants include vecuronium, pancuronium, atracurium and cisatracurium (Table 21.2).

Suxamethonium, the only depolarising muscle relaxant in use, has a rapid onset and short duration. Its numerous side effects include raised intraocular pressure and hyperkalaemia. For these reasons it is not recommended in penetrating eye injury, crush injury or burn injury after the first 24 hours. The major reason for its continued use is its short duration of action so that if primary airway management fails, the patient will not remain paralysed and can be woken up.

Rocuronium is an alternative to suxamethonium and at high doses (1.2 mg/kg) time to intubating conditions are comparable. It is safe in neuromuscular disorders, hyperkalaemia and penetrating eye injuries.

Higher doses of rocoronium last more than an hour although rapid reversal with sugammadex is possible. In many patients treated within the pre-hospital or emergency department setting, waking the patient if initial airway management plans are unsuccessful is not a truly viable option as the effects of injury will still be present plus the additive effect of anaesthetic agents (Box 21.2). The need for ongoing resuscitation and emergency transfer (e.g. to hospital or to the operating room) remains and as securing the airway is a priority the long duration of rocuronium may be helpful during supraglottic airway use or surgical airway access.

Box 21.2 **Primary transfer RSI case study**

A 22-year-old male is ejected from a vehicle traveling at a speed of 70 km/hr. The nearest trauma centre is 30 minutes away.

Upon arrival your initial assessment is as follows:

A. moaning, no blood or foreign material

B. RR 14, good air entry bilaterally, sats 98% breathing air, trachea midline

C. cool peripheries, capillary refill 4 seconds, radial pulse steady, 120 regular, SBP 88 mmHg, no obvious abdominal or pelvic injury, deformed right femur

D. GCS 7 (E1, V2, M4), PEARL 2 mm

Think about which drugs you would use for the RSI and ongoing sedation and analgesia in this case.

Ketamine combined with rocuronium or suxamethonium are commonly used RSI agents in trauma. In an isolated head injury you may consider a thiopentone induction. Etomidate is less likely to cause hypotension; however, adrenal suppression may increase morbidity and mortality in critically ill patients. Given the patient's haemodynamic instability, ketamine would be many experienced clinicians first choice of anaesthetic agent. Ongoing paralysis is advisable in head injury to prevent coughing and straining on the ET tube as this caused surges in ICP. Rocuronium given as a bolus would be practical given the proximity of the trauma centre.

Table 21.2 Muscle relaxants.

Drug	Depolarising: suxamethonium	Non-depolarising: rocuronium	Non-depolarising: vecuronium	Non-depolarising: pancuronium	Non-depolarising: atracurium	Non-depolarising: cis-atracurium
Use	RSI Muscle relaxation to facilitate intubation for RSI	RSI Facilitate intubation/use in crush injury/extrication	Muscle relaxation to facilitate intubation/ventilation	Muscle relaxation to facilitate intubation/ventilation	Muscle relaxation to facilitate intubation/ventilation	Muscle relaxation to facilitate intubation/ventilation
Chemical	dicholine ester of succinic acid	Amino-steroid Intermediate action	Amino-steroid Intermediate action	Amino-steroid Long action	Benzyl isoquinolinium ester	Benzyl isoquinolinium ester isomer of atracurium, 4 × potency
Presentation	Clear solution 50 mg/mL store at 4°C	Clear solution 10 mg/mL, store <30°C for 3 months	Powder, dissolved in water to make a clear solution 2 mg/mL Store 21°C	Clear solution 2 mg/mL pancuronium bromide	Clear solution 10 mg/mL 4–10°C	Clear solution 2 mg/mL 4–10°C
Dose for induction/intubation	IV 1–2 mg/kg, IM 3 mg/kg Rapid onset 30–60 seconds, duration 5–10 minutes	IV 0.9–1.2 mg/kg Rapid onset ~60 seconds, duration 60 minutes	0.1 mg/kg Slow onset 3 minutes, lasts 30 minutes	0.05–0.1 mg/kg Onset 90–150 seconds, lasts 45–60 minutes	IV 0.6 mg/kg Slow onset ~90 seconds Used for infusion as recovery is 10–16 minutes independent of length of infusion	IV 0.05–0.1 mg/kg Slow onset –150 seconds Used for infusion as recovery independent of length of infusion
Pharmacokinetics	Metabolised by plasma cholinesterase. Some patients abnormal enzyme – prolonged metabolism	Metabolised by liver, excreted by hepatobilary and renal systems (clearance > GFR)	Metabolised by liver excretion hepatic/renal	Metabolised by liver Excretion renal	Breakdown mainly spontaneous via Hofmann degradation, remainder is via plasma esterases	Breakdown mainly spontaneous via Hofmann degradation, rest renal excretion unchanged
Pharmacodynamics	Bradycardia, especially on second dose and in children Raises serum potassium 0.4 mmol/L (more in muscle injury) Fasciculation's	Minimal CVS/RS effects Action prolonged by dehydration, acidosis	Minimal CVS effects, RS apnoea, bronchospasm extremely uncommon CNS no effect on ICP	Increase HR, BP, CO secondary to vagolytic action, RS apnoea, bronchospasm extremely uncommon	CVS stable, may cause bronchospasm	CVS stable, no histamine release
Caution	Raised potassium (crush injury), muscle trauma, burns (over 24 hours), penetrating eye injury, risk anaphylaxis/malignant hyperpyrexia	Risk anaphylaxis	Anaphylaxis rare	Anaphylaxis rare	histamine release – can cause hypotension	Renal failure – decreased clearance. This does not prolong its action.

Sedation in the pre-hospital setting

Interventions performed in the resuscitation and stabilisation of patients may require analgesia and/or sedation (Box 21.3). Choice of drug will depend upon the clinical status of the patient and the skillset of the retrieval team. Common classes of drugs used include opiates, benzodiazepines and ketamine.

Box 21.3 **Indications for analgesia/sedation in the retrieval setting**

To provide patient comfort for inter-hospital or prolonged pre-hospital transfer
To tolerate mechanical ventilation
To reduce blood loss and cerebral oxygen demand
To facilitate procedures/extrication
To relieve agitation/aggression (i.e. in acute psychosis)
To facilitate pre-oxygenation in the agitated patient.

Maintenance of sedation

Following intubation, patients require sedation, analgesia and in the acute setting, ongoing paralysis to tolerate mechanical ventilation. Common drug regimens include midazolam, propofol or ketamine for maintenance of sedation in combination with an opioid analgesic such as morphine or fentanyl (Boxes 21.4 and 21.5). Drugs are preferably administered intravenously (or intraosseously) as this route is fast acting and reliable. Intramuscular administration in these circumstances is avoided due to unpredictable absorption and onset.

Box 21.4 **Drug regimens for analgesia and sedation**

Morphine and midazolam

Analgesia and sedation. Commonly used combination, often as a 1:1 ratio mixed as compound infusion for a syringe driver or infusion pump. This decreases number of pumps. Side effects: hypotension, respiratory depression.

Propofol (± opioid for analgesia)

Indications include sedation of ventilated and occasionally spontaneously breathing (e.g. psychiatric) patients, especially short term when rapid awakening is planned; status epilepticus. Side effects: profound hypotension – caution in shocked patients, pain on injection.

Ketamine

Analgesic properties used with midazolam for short procedural sedation, use in agitated patients or difficult access scenarios. Usually maintains cardiovascular stability, respiration and airway reflexes. Side effects: hallucinations, may still cause hypotension in shocked patients.

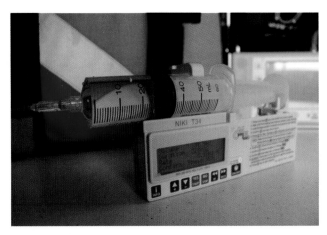

Figure 21.2 Sedative agents are commonly administered as infusions via syringe driver in the retrieval setting.

Infusions are commonly used for on-going analgesia/sedation (Figure 21.2) although small intermittent boluses can be an alternative for some transfers (e.g. short primary transfer) as these involve less preparation and avoid the complexity and bulkiness of infusion pumps.

Box 21.5 **General considerations when sedating patients**

Maintain minimum monitoring standards: BP, ECG, SpO_2, $ETCO_2$ plus presence of appropriately trained clinician. In intubated and paralysed patients monitor for potential awareness (hypertension, sweating, tachycardia, pupil dilation)
Complications of sedation include airway obstruction, hypoventilation, aspiration and hypotension. There may be an emergency requirement for advanced airway management
Mechanical ventilation: usually requires paralysis with neuromuscular blocking agents to be tolerated
Dose variation: shocked trauma patients require decreased doses of anaesthetic / sedative agents. Stable hospitalised patient on sedation may require increased dose to tolerate transport
Drug safety: Draw up and label syringes carefully/consider pre-filled syringes.
Controlled drugs: Follow local policy to ensure accountability/security. Consider anti-tampering seals.

Further reading

Ankam JA, Hunter JM. Pharmacology of neuromuscular blocking drugs. Cont Educat Anaesthe Crit Care Pain 2004;4(1):2–7.

Ellis D, Hooper M. *Cases in Pre-hospital and Retrieval Medicine.* Churchill and Livingstone, New South Wales, Australia 2010.

Lupton T, Pratt O. Intravenous drugs used for the induction of anaesthesia. Anaesthesia UK 2006. At: http://www.frca.co.uk/article.aspx?articleid=100634.

Sasada M, Smith S. Drugs in Anaesthesia and Intensive Care. Third Edition. Oxford University Press, New York 2003.

Stevenson C. Ketamine: A review. Update Anaesthes 2005;20:25–9.

CHAPTER 22

Inotropes and Vasopressors

A. Fergusson[1] and R. Tipping[2,3]

[1]Peninsula Deanery, South West School of Anaesthesia, UK
[2]Queen Elizabeth Hospital, UK
[3]West Midlands Ambulance Service NHS Foundation Trust Medical Emergency Response Incident Team (MERIT), UK

OVERVIEW

- Positive inotropes increase the force of contraction of the heart; vasopressors cause arteriolar vasoconstriction
- Both positive inotropes and vasopressors are used to treat shock, aiming to maintain end organ perfusion
- They have various mechanisms of action, the commonest of which is as agonists at adrenoreceptors throughout the cardiovascular system
- The majority are given as infusions via a central venous line
- Adequate preparation of drugs and equipment is essential prior to transfer.

Introduction

Shock is a common pathology in patients requiring transfer or retrieval. It is characterised by inadequate tissue and organ perfusion. It can be classified according to aetiology as summarised in Box 22.1. Treatment often includes the use of inotropes and vasopressors to maintain tissue perfusion and minimise end organ damage.

Box 22.1 **Classification of shock**

Hypovolaemic shock: blood loss, dehydration
Distributive shock: anaphylaxis, septic shock, neurogenic shock
Obstructive shock: cardiac tamponade, pulmonary embolus
Cardiogenic shock: myocardial infarction, arrhythmias, heart failure

---

Box 22.2 **Key terminology**

Positive inotropes are agents which increase the force of contraction of the heart, thereby increasing the cardiac output
Vasopressors are agents which cause arteriolar vasoconstriction, thereby increasing SVR and blood pressure

---

ABC of Transfer and Retrieval Medicine, First Edition.
Edited by Adam Low and Jonathan Hulme.
© 2015 John Wiley & Sons, Ltd. Published 2015 by John Wiley & Sons, Ltd.

The terms defined in Box 22.2 are often incorrectly used interchangeably. Collectively, they can be termed vasoactive agents. Both positive inotropes and vasopressors can be endogenous or synthetic agents.

Cardiovascular physiology

A basic understanding of the physiology will enable the clinician to understand how the manipulation of different variables can increase cardiac output or oxygen delivery.

$$\text{Cardiac output (CO, L/min)} = \text{stroke volume (SV, L)} \times \text{heart rate (HR, bpm)}$$

Cardiac stroke volume is determined by:

- pre-load (cardiac filling pressure)
- myocardial contractility
- afterload SVR.

$$\text{Cardiac output} = \text{MAP} - \text{CVP (mmHg)}/\text{SVR (dyne s/cm}^5\text{)}$$
$$\text{Oxygen delivery (DO}_2, \text{L/min)} = \text{CO (L/min)} \times \text{CaO}_2$$
$$\text{CaO}_2 \text{(mL O}_2\text{/dL)} = (\text{Hb (g/dL)} \times \text{SaO}_2 \times 1.34) + (10 \times \text{PaO}_2\text{(kPa)} \times 0.0225)$$

CaO_2 is the O_2 content of arterial blood; SaO_2 is the oxygen saturation in arterial blood; 1.34 mL is Hüfners constant, the volume of oxygen carried by 1 g of haemoglobin.

Classification of vasoactive drugs

These are summarised in Table 22.1.

Mechanism of action

Catecholamines and direct-acting sympathomimetic agents act as agonists at adrenoceptors, a family of G-protein-coupled receptors which span the extracellular membrane. $\alpha 1$ adrenoceptors are found in vascular smooth muscle. Stimulation causes vasoconstriction, increasing systemic vascular resistance (SVR) and blood pressure. $\alpha 1$ adrenoceptor agonists are therefore vasopressors.

$\beta 1$ adrenoceptors are found in the heart. They are Gs receptors; stimulation causes activation of adenylate cyclase, leading to an

Table 22.1 Classification of catecholamines.

Catecholamines	Naturally occurring: Adrenaline (epinephrine) Noradrenaline (norepinephrine) Dopamine Synthetic: Dobutamine Isoprenaline
Non-catecholamine sympathomimetic amines	Metaraminol Ephedrine Phenylephrine
Phosphodiesterase (PDE) Inhibitors	Milrinone Enoximone Aminophylline
Others	Calcium gluconate/calcium chloride Levosimendan Glucagon Vasopressin

increased level of cAMP and resultant increase in intracellular Ca flux and Ca concentration. The result is an increase in contractility, increasing CO. β1 adrenoceptor agonists are therefore positive inotropic agents (Figure 22.1).

The majority of other positive inotropes share a similar final pathway, increasing cAMP levels and subsequently increasing intracellular Ca concentration. Phosphodiesterase inhibitors prevent the enzymatic breakdown of cAMP. Glucagon increases cAMP levels by activating adenylate cyclase. Calcium chloride or gluconate increases intracellular Ca levels. Finally levosimendan increases the sensitivity to calcium.

Commonly used drugs

These are summarised in Tables 22.2 and 22.3.

Practicalities

Prior to the initiation or escalation of vasoactive drugs, care must be taken to ensure an adequate circulating volume. Factors which guide decisions on whether or not fluid is required will include BP, HR, CO monitoring, fluid losses and clinical condition.

An in depth discussion of the choice of fluid is outside of the remit of this book and the choice of fluid will be situation and clinician dependent (see Box 22.3).

Box 22.3 **Classes of intravenous fluids available**

The colloid/crystalloid debate has been ongoing for many years
The choice of resuscitation fluid may affect morbidity and mortality in critically ill patients.
Crystalloids are cheaper and less likely to cause anaphylaxis
Hydroxyethyl starches (HES) have been shown to contribute to acute kidney injury and have adverse mortality effects in certain subgroups of patients; these concerns have led to their recent withdrawal by manufacturers.

An adequate supply of fluid should be available, including blood and blood products where appropriate. Any blood products used during transfer must have the relevant documentation returned to the issuing blood bank.

Vasoactive drugs tend to be very potent and have short half lives, often 1–2 minutes. They are therefore usually given as an infusion. The majority must be given via a central line, with the exception of metaraminol, ephedrine, dobutamine and adrenaline (when used in cardiac arrest or anaphylaxis). Extravasation of vasoactive drugs can cause significant tissue necrosis and morbidity, so correct placement of lines should be ensured. Invasive arterial blood pressure monitoring should be used where possible; in addition to providing a beat

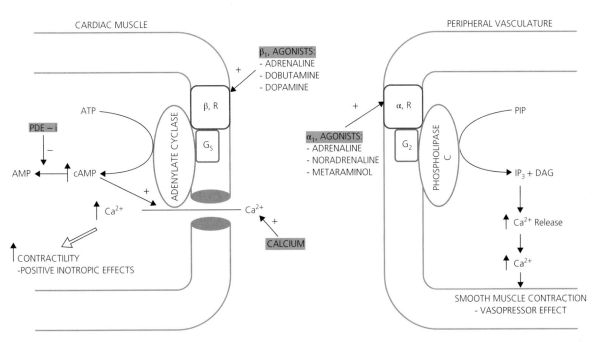

Figure 22.1 Mechanism of action of positive inotropes and vasopressors.

Table 22.2 Vasopressors.

Drug	Mechanism of action	Uses	Dose	Notes
Noradrenaline	Predominantly an α1 agonist, causing peripheral vasoconstriction. It also has some effects at β1 adrenoceptors, causing some positive inotropic effects	Refractory hypotension, low SVR states	Solution containing noradrenaline base 40 μg/mL, initial rate 0.16–0.33 mL/minute, adjusted as necessary. NB 1 mg of noradrenaline base is equivalent to 2 mg of noradrenaline citrate acid	A reflex bradycardia may be seen when BP is restored
Metaraminol	Pure α1 agonist	Hypotension where central IV access is unnecessary or unavailable.	0.5–5-mg bolus, can also be given as an infusion	Can be given peripherally
Ephedrine	Direct B1 and 2 agonist and also acts indirectly on α1 adrenoecptors by causing noradrenaline release	Hypotension where central IV access is unnecessary or unavailable	3–9 mg bolus	Can be given peripherally. May demonstrate tachyphylaxis
Vasopressin	Acts on V1 receptors in vascular smooth muscle, resulting in vasoconstriction	Refractory hypotension. Also used as vasopressor in brainstem-dead donors	0.01–0.04 units/min	

Table 22.3 Positive inotropes.

Drug	Mechanism of action	Uses	Dose	Notes
Adrenaline	Agonist at α1, β1 and β2 adrenoceptors	Low cardiac output states, anaphylaxis, cardiac arrest, bronchospasm, with local anaesthetic agents, in croup. etc.	Inotrope: infusion of 0.01–0.15 μg/kg/min Anaphylaxis: 500 μg (0.5 mL of 1 in 1000) IM or 50 μg (0.5 mL of 1 in 10000) IV, repeated as necessary Cardiac arrest: 1 mg (10 mL of 1 in 10,000), repeated every 3–5 minutes as necessary	At low doses, β effects predominate, causing positive inotropy, chronotropy and bronchodilation. At higher doses, α1 effects predominate, causing peripheral vasoconstriction, increasing SVR and BP
Dobutamine	Potent agonist at β1 and β2 adrenoceptors	Low cardiac output states, especially when secondary to myocardial infarction, cardiomyopathy and cardiac surgery. Also used in septic shock to improve oxygen transport to tissues.	Infusion of 2.5–10 μg/kg/minute	Often causes tachycardia. Tachyphylaxis can occur with prolonged use
Dopamine	Agonist at α1, β1 and δ1 (dopamine) adrenoceptors	Low cardiac output states	Infusion of 2–5 μg/kg/min	β1 effects predominate at lower levels, α1 effects predominate at higher levels No evidence of a reno-protective role. More dysrhythmogenic than other intropes
Isoprenaline	β1 and β2 adrenoceptor agonist	Bradyarrhythmias	Infusion of 0.02–0.2 μg/kg/min	Chronotropic effect more pronounced than inotropy
Enoximone	PDE type 3 inhibitor, preventing breakdown of cAMP	Low cardiac output states	Initially 90 μg/kg/min over 10–30 minutes, then infusion of 5–20 μg/kg/min	It has both positive inotropic and vasodilatory properties, and is therefore known as an 'inodilator'

by beat measurement of blood pressure, it uses less monitor battery life than regular non-invasive blood pressure measurements. Cardiac output monitoring may also be appropriate.

Infusions of vasoactive drugs should ideally be well established prior to commencing a transfer. The lowest dose, which achieves the required response, should normally be targeted; however, a transfer may not be an appropriate time for constant fine tuning. Care must be taken with choosing an appropriate port of the central line and preventing flushing of an inotrope line, which can result in an inadvertent bolus.

Sufficient amounts of drugs should be prepared, with back-up syringes or bags available, checked and ready to go. Given the short half lives, interruption of delivery during syringe changes will be poorly tolerated. This can be overcome by 'double pumping' – running both syringes via a three-way tap and weaning down the rate of the old syringe whilst the rate of the new syringe is increased.

Conclusion

Vasoactive drugs will be commonly used during retrieval and transfer of critically unwell patients. Knowledge of their mechanism of action and basic pharmacodynamic and pharmacokinetic properties, along with an understanding of basic physiological principles, will allow these drugs to be used safely and effectively.

Further reading

Peck TE, Hill S. *Pharmacology for Anaesthesia and Intensive Care*, 3rd ed. Cambridge, Cambridge University Press, 2008.

Rang HP, Dale MM, Ritter JM et al. *Rang and Dale's Pharmacology*, 7th ed. London, Churchill Livingstone, 2011.

Smith S, Scarth E, Sasada M. *Drugs in Anaesthesia and Intensive Care*, 4th ed. Oxford, Oxford University Press, 2011.

CHAPTER 23

Specialist Pharmacology: Haemostatics and Uterotonics

P. Morgan[1] and D. Lockey[1,2,3]

[1]North Bristol NHS Trust, UK
[2]London's Air Ambulance, UK
[3]University of Bristol, UK

OVERVIEW

- Haemostatic dressings are a useful adjunct to the management of traumatic haemorrhage
- Early administration of tranexamic acid significantly reduces mortality in traumatic haemorrhage
- Oxytocics used in the third stage of labour significantly reduce the risk of post-partum haemorrhage
- Tocolytics in preterm labour should only be considered if they facilitate transfer to an appropriate facility or for drug therapies to be completed before delivery
- Hypertonic saline is more effective than mannitol in reducing intracranial pressure in severe head injury.

Specialist haemostatic dressings for pre-hospital use

Haemostatic dressings are used in severe haemorrhage and are particularly useful in junctional areas, for example neck, axilla where tourniquets are unsuitable. They are impregnated gauzes or granules within a bag.

Zeolite (Quick Clot Advanced Clotting Sponge®) and kaolin (QuickClot Combat Gauze®) accelerate the clotting cascade. Chitosan (Celox Gauze® and HemCon ChitoFlex®) attract blood components to the dressing (electromagnetic charge) and do not rely exclusively on the clotting cascade; hence still effective in coagulopathy. It is derived from shellfish, but not considered a problem in patients with allergy.

Directions

Remove other dressings. Remove pooled blood. Identify bleeding point and pack the wound maintaining pressure. After 3–5 minutes of pressure apply a bandage over the dressing to hold it in place. Proximal tourniquets can be slowly released; re-apply if haemorrhage occurs (Figure 23.1).

ABC of Transfer and Retrieval Medicine, First Edition.
Edited by Adam Low and Jonathan Hulme.
© 2015 John Wiley & Sons, Ltd. Published 2015 by John Wiley & Sons, Ltd.

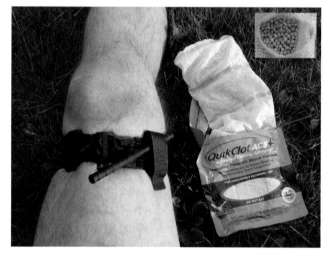

Figure 23.1 A combat application tourniquet applied to the lower limb and example of haemostatic agents.

Tranexamic acid

Tranexamic acid inhibits fibrinolysis and is used to prevent/reduce haemorrhage associated with excessive fibrinolysis. If administered within 3 hours (greatest effect in first hour) of significant traumatic haemorrhage all cause mortality is significantly reduced (CRASH-2 trial). There is conflicting evidence in major obstetric haemorrhages: Royal College of Obstetricians and Gynaecologists consensus is that it is rarely indicated.

- Cautions: increased risk of thrombosis in embolic disease or oral contraceptive pill use (Not demonstrated in trauma in CRASH-2). Rapid infusion may cause hypotension. Avoid co-administration of penicillins or blood products through the same intravenous cannula.
- Contraindications: history of convulsions (lowers the seizure threshold and increases cerebral oedema); isolated head injuries (currently under investigation in CRASH-3 trial).
- Side-effects: nausea, vomiting, diarrhoea, dizziness, convulsions. Rare: thromboembolic events, visual disturbance.
- Dose: trauma – 1 g IV over 10 minutes, further 1 g IV over 8 hours. In severe renal failure maintenance 1 g should be given over 16 hours following the 1-g bolus.

Mannitol and hypertonic saline

Both are osmotically active and will lower intracranial pressure (ICP), indicated in severe head injury. Hypertonic saline increases intravascular volume, increasing the mean arterial pressure and thus cerebral perfusion pressure. A recent meta-analysis showed it to be more effective at reducing ICP compared to mannitol; however, it increases serum sodium and chloride levels.

- Cautions: mannitol crystallizes in cold conditions.
- Contraindications: dehydration, severe cardiac failure/ pulmonary oedema.
- Side-effects: thrombophlebitis, pulmonary oedema, cardiac failure. Mannitol: significant diuresis, dehydration and renal toxicity.
- Dose: mannitol bolus 0.5 g/kg (max 1 g/kg) 20% solution over 30–60 minutes. Hypertonic Saline 100 mL (5%) over 10 minutes.

Uterotonics

Routine oxytocic use in the third stage of labour is associated with a 60% reduction in the risk of postpartum haemorrhage (PPH). The synthetic analogue (Syntocinon®) causes uterine (smooth) muscle contraction and is used in vaginal deliveries with low risk of PPH (5–10 iu IM). Following Caesarean section it should be administered slowly IV (5–10 iu). In the atonic uterus, (e.g. prolonged second stage or twin delivery) an infusion of 40 iu in 500 mL 0.9% Saline or Hartmanns solution over 4 hours will reduce the risk of delayed PPH; 500 μg of ergometrine (IM/slow IV) should also be considered (Figure 23.2).

Ergometrine stimulates uterine contraction. Oxytocin 5 iu/mL combined with ergometrine 500 μg/mL (Syntometrine®) is effective for incomplete miscarriage and managed third stage of labour

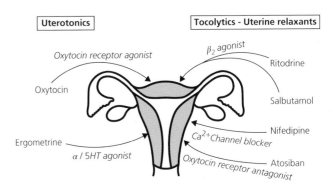

Figure 23.2 Uterotonics and tocolytic agents.

(IM/slow IV). Oxytocin in lower doses is used for induction of labour (0.001 iu/min, increased at 10 minute intervals -to a maximum of 0.02 iu/min, until three to four contractions per 10 minutes). Foetal monitoring is essential.

- Cautions
  - ergometrine: significant nausea, vomiting and hypertension due to vasoconstriction
- Contraindications
  - ergometrine: known hypertension/pre-eclampsia, cardiac disease, or severe renal impairment
  - oxytocin: enhances sympathomimetics; antidiuretic effects may complicate fluid resuscitation and coagulation disorders
- Side-effects:
  - ergometrine: palpitations, pulmonary oedema and abdominal pain
  - oxytocin: headache, vomiting, hyponatraemia, hypotension if rapidly bolused. In excess: disseminated intravascular coagulation and uterine rupture.

Table 23.1 Anti-emetics.

Drug	Indication	Mechanism	Dose	Side Effects/ Contraindications
Prochlorperazine	Vertigo, GI tract associated causes, e.g. opiates, gastric irritation	Dopamine antagonist	20 mg orally, further 10 mg after 2 hours if required. IM 12.5 mg 6 hourly	*Contraindications*: Neuroleptic malignant syndrome *Side effects*: Hypotension with rapid IV injection Tardive dyskinesia, extrapyramidal symptoms, drowsiness
Hyoscine hydrobromide	Motion sickness and vertigo.	Anticholinergics Sedating antiemetic with anti-muscarinic effects	200–600 μg IV/IM/SC Transdermal patch 1 mg/72 h 150–300 μg orally 30 min prior to travel	*Cautions*: Down's syndrome, children/elderly, gastro-oesophageal reflux, hypertension and conditions where a tachycardia would be detrimental *Contraindications*: Myasthenia gravis, pyloric stenosis, paralytic ileus *Side effects*: Constipation, bradycardia, dry mouth, flushing, drowsiness
Cyclizine	Useful in motion sickness, vertigo and nausea associated with opiates	Antihistamines	50 mg IV/IM/PO maximum 150 mg/24 h (Painful intramuscularly).	*Cautions*: Cardiac failure *Contraindications*: angle closure glaucoma. *Side-effects*: Drowsiness, blurred vision, hypertension, tachyarrhythmias following injection
Ondansetron	Ineffective in motion sickness. Useful in GI tract associated causes e.g. opiates, gastric irritation	5-HT$_3$ antagonist	4–8 mg IV/IM, maximum 32 mg/24 h	*Contraindications*: Long QT syndrome *Side-effects*: hypotension, headache, flushing

Table 23.2 Anti-arrhythmic drugs.

Drug	Indication	Mechanism	Dose	Side effects/ contraindications
Adenosine	Cardioversion of paroxysmal supraventricular tachycardias (including re-entry/ accessory pathways)	Blocks conduction at AV node (ECG monitoring and resuscitation equipment essential.)	6 mg bolus. 2 × 12 mg at 1–2 min if required	*Cautions:* Left main coronary artery stenosis; bundle branch block; stenotic heart valves; recent myocardial infarction; pericardial effusion; hyovolaemia; cerebrovascular disease. *Contraindications:* 2nd or 3rd degree AV-block, sick-sinus syndrome, long QT syndrome, cardiovascular compromise, obstructive lung disease. Pregnancy: Foetal toxicity. *Side-effects:* Chest discomfort, flushing and nausea. Arrhythmias (severe bradycardia and asystole), flushing, angina, dyspnoea, headache. Occasionally: metallic taste, hyperventilation, weakness, blurred vision. Rare: transient worsening of intracranial hypertension, bronchospasm, and convulsions.
Amiodarone	Haemodynamically stable atrial and ventricular tachyarrhythmias. Synergistic with DC cardioversion	Prolongs cardiac action potential and refractory period	Loading: 300 mg (or 5 mg/kg) IV over 10–60 min (dilute with 5% dextrose), 900 mg/24 h	*Cautions:* Ideally via central catheter. Multiple interactions with antibiotics and other anti-arrhythmics. *Contraindications:* Thyroid dysfunction, iodine sensitivity, circulatory collapse, severe hypotension, cardiac failure or cardiomyopathy, avoid bolus dose in respiratory failure. *Side-effects:* Thyroid dysfunction, nausea, vomiting, taste disturbances. Long term use: elevated transaminases, pulmonary toxicity. Rare: worsening of arrhythmia, bronchospasm, ataxia, benign intracranial hypertension, headache, vertigo, haemolytic/aplastic anaemia or thrombocytopenia
Atropine	Bradycardia or AV block causing haemodynamic instability.	Blocks vagal effects on SA and AV node: increasing automaticity	500 μg IV bolus, repeated to total of 3 mg	*Cautions:* Acute angle glaucoma, Downs syndrome, hypertension, gastro-oesophageal reflux. *Contraindications:* Myasthenia gravis, pyloric stenosis, paralytic ileus. *Side-effects:* Blurred vision, dry mouth, urinary retention, reduced oesophageal sphincter tone.
Atenolol (β1) Metoprolol (β1) Propanolol (β1/β2) Esmolol (short acting β1)	Narrow-complex regular tachycardias (e.g. atrial flutter/fibrillation) when ventricular function preserved.	β-adrenoceptor antagonism	5 mg IV/ 5 min, repeat if necessary. 2–5 mg IV at 5-min intervals Max 15 mg 100 μg/kg IV over 5 min Repeat: max 10 mg. 500 μg/kg over 1 min loading Infusion 50–200 μg/kg/min	*Cautions:* Verapamil therapy, known bronchospasm. *Contraindications:* 2nd/3rd degree heart block, hypotension, severe cardiac failure. Pregnancy: Neonatal hypoglycaemia and bradycardia. Infant observations required if used in labour. Labetalol relatively safe. *Side-effects:* Hypotension, bradycardia, bronchospasm, AV conduction delay
Lidocaine	Ventricular tachyarrhythmias if resistant and involving a re-entry pathway.	Increases threshold potential of the cardiac action potential, decreases duration and refractory period	1 mg/kg, then 1–4 mg/min	*Cautions:* Reduced dose in cardiac failure. *Contraindications:* Atrioventricular block, acute porphyria, severe myocardial depression. *Side-effects:* Dizziness, paraesthesia, confusion, tinnitus. High levels: seizures and cardiac arrest
Magnesium sulphate	Tachyarrhythmias (associated with ↓K+, ↓Mg+). Torsade de pointes. Digoxin toxicity	Facilitates neurochemical transmission. Intrinsically linked to potassium	2 g IV over 10 min Max 4 g	*Cautions:* Myasthenia gravis and muscular dystrophy *Side-effects:* CNS depression, hypo-reflexia, hypotension, muscle weakness. Potentiates neuromuscular blockade
Verapamil	Stable, regular, narrow complex tachycardias or rate control in atrial fibrillation.	Calcium channel blocker. Slows AV conduction, increases refractory period: terminating re-entrant arrhythmias. Controls ventricular rate	2.5–5 mg IV over 2 min 5–10 mg repeat every 15 min, max 20 mg	*Cautions:* Concurrent B-blockade – risk of complete AV block, hypotension and bradycardia. Risk of cardiovascular collapse with known severe LV dysfunction (reduced contractility). *Contraindications:* Wolf-Parkinson-White syndrome (accessory pathway predominates). Cardiac failure. Pregnancy: Reduces foetal blood flow. *Side-effects:* Flushing, nausea, vomiting, AV block, hypotension and cardiac failure. Rare: Stevens–Johnson syndrome

AV, atrioventricular.

Uterine relaxants

Tocolytic use in major antepartum haemorrhage should be discussed with a senior obstetrician case by case. Indicated in the very preterm: allows administration of corticosteroids and/or transfer to a facility with neonatal intensive care. Nifedipine should be avoided because of associated hypotension. Tocolysis is contraindicated in placental abruption.

In preterm labour the use of tocolysis has no clear evidence of benefit to prevent perinatal/neonatal morbidity or neonatal mortality and as such it is reasonable not to use them. Consider if it facilitates completion of therapy or transfer.

Nifedipine is used in preterm labour because of its smooth muscle relaxing effects (unlicensed indication). It does have several benefits: oral medication; simple dosing; comparable effectiveness to Atosiban; better neonatal outcome when compared to the β_2 agonists and fewer side effects.

- Cautions
  - atosiban: abnormal placental site increases risk of PPH.
  - β_2 agonists: pre-eclampsia, hypokalaemia, diabetes.
  - nifedipine: poor cardiac reserve/ heart failure, acute porphyria, diabetes. Risk of pulmonary oedema in multiple pregnancy
- Contraindications
  - atosiban: severe pre-eclampsia.
  - β_2 agonists: cardiac disease, severe pre-eclampsia, cord compression
  - nifedipine: cardiac disease (especially aortic stenosis).
- Side-effects
  - atosiban: nausea and vomiting, headache, chest pain and dyspnoea. Irritation at injection site
  - β_2 agonists: palpitations, headache, tremor, chest pain and dyspnoea. Rarely, pulmonary oedema
  - nifedipine: flushing, palpitations, nausea and vomiting, hypotension
- Dose
  - atosiban bolus 6.75 mg IV over 1 minute. Infusion 18 mg/h for 3 hours then 6 mg/h for up to 45 hours (maximum 330 mg).

After a loading dose titrate the following to uterine activity:

- nifedipine 20 mg orally, then 10–20 mg three or four times per day
- salbutamol 10 µg/min increased by 5 µg/min every 10 minutes. Maximum 45 µg/min for 1 hour then reduced by 50% every 6 hours; followed by 4 mg three times a day orally for 24 hours.

Antiemetics

Antiemetics act on the afferent supply to the vomiting centre (VC). The VC has multiple afferents with numerous receptors. A conscious patient lying flat in a helicopter, for example, is at high risk of feeling nauseous and will potentially vomit due to motion sickness. Hyoscine (anticholinergic at muscarinic receptors) and cyclizine (antihistamine – H_1) will be effective as both these receptors are present in the vestibular apparatus inputs. Conversely the 5-HT$_3$ antagonist ondansetron will be ineffective in motion sickness but will be very effective if opiates are used or gastric irritation is present, for example paralytic ileus, as these receptors are in abundance in the gastrointestinal tract. In the latter situation hyoscine would not be effective and potentially will exacerbate the symptoms! Adjunctive therapies such as hydration and gastric drainage with a nasogastric tube will be synergistic in reducing the symptoms. The commonly used drugs are summarised in Table 23.1.

Anti-arrhythmics

The anti-arrhythmic drug of choice will depend upon: cardiovascular stability; presumed origin on ECG (ventricular, supraventricular or re-entrant); 'tachy' or 'brady' arrhythmia; regular versus irregular; whether other drugs have failed to resolve the problem. The indications, mechanism of action, contraindications and dosage of the common anti-arrhythmics are summarised in Table 23.2.

In addition many post-surgical patients and those with sepsis are prone to new onset atrial fibrillation. In this scenario chemical cardioversion with amiodarone would be very appropriate as the probability of clot formation and subsequent emboli is very low, compared with the cardiovascular compromise caused by a rapid atrial rate. Conversely if they are known to have a paroxysmal tachyarrhythmia which has been exacerbated by their acute condition then verapamil or a beta-blocker could be considered to rate control rather than cardioversion.

Some scenarios dictate a specific antiarrhythmic. Magnesium for example is indicated in calcium toxicity, digoxin toxicity and torsade de pointes. Its membrane-stabilising capability is also very useful in the post cardiac arrest patient who is having multiple ectopics and rhythm disturbance during transfer en route to a facility that can provide definitive care.

Further reading

Smith AH, Laird C, Porter K, Bloch M. Haemostatic dressings in prehospital care. Emerg Med J [cited 2013 May 25]; Available from: http://emj.bmj.com/content/early/2012/11/16/emermed-2012-201581.

Roberts I, Shakur H, Afolabi A, Brohi K, Coats T, Dewan Y, et al. The importance of early treatment with tranexamic acid in bleeding trauma patients: an exploratory analysis of the CRASH-2 randomised controlled trial. Lancet 2011;377(9771):1096–101, 1101.e1–2.

Royal College of Obstetrics and Gynaecology. *Postpartum Haemorrhage, Prevention and Management (Green-top 52)* April 2011 [cited 2013 May 25]. Available from: http://www.rcog.org.uk/womens-health/clinical-guidance /prevention-and-management-postpartum-haemorrhage-green-top-52.

Royal College of Obstetrics and Gynaecology. *Preterm Labour, Tocolytic Drugs (Green-top 1B).* Feb 2011. [cited 2013 May 25]. Available from: http:// www.rcog.org.uk/womens-health/clinical-guidance/tocolytic-drugs -women-preterm-labour-green-top-1b.

Mortazavi M, Romeo A, Deep A. Hypertonic saline for treating raised intracranial pressure: literature review with meta-analysis. J Neurosurg 2012;116:210–21.

Resuscitation Council. *Advanced Life Support – 6th Edition.* Resuscitation Council, London 2011.

Section 5

The Transfer Team

CHAPTER 24

Managing and Leading a Transfer

D. Ellis[1,2,3] *and S. Mazur*[2,3,4,5]

[1]MedSTAR Emergency Medical Retrieval Service, South Australian Ambulance Service, Australia
[2]Emergency Medicine Department, Royal Adelaide Hospital, Australia
[3]School of Public Health and Tropical Medicine, James Cook University, Queensland, Australia
[4]South Australian Ambulance Service, Australia
[5]PreHospital and Retrieval Medicine, MedSTAR Emergency Medical Retrieval Service, Australia

---

OVERVIEW
- Clinical coordination is the key to managing a retrieval effectively
- High-quality, effective leadership is essential in pre-hospital and retrieval medicine
- Situation monitoring augments effective teamwork
- Clinical handover plays an important role in pre-hospital and retrieval medicine.

There are two distinct aspects to effectively managing a retrieval:

1 the role of clinical coordination
2 the role of the operational (retrieval) team.

By combining these two areas, a retrieval service is aiming to optimise both the use of retrieval resources and team performance. This ensures safe, high-quality patient care and that there is no step down in that care during the retrieval process.

Clinical coordination

The key to retrieval medicine lies in good-quality clinical coordination. Ideally the clinical coordination team should be led by a senior physician specialist who is clinically active in the retrieval (and preferably in addition the pre-hospital) arena. This physician should have a background in a critical care specialty and be supported by a team of ambulance and nursing colleagues who together will coordinate every aspect of the patient journey. The clinical coordination team should be contactable by a single common telephone number and must have the relevant technology to facilitate multi-party conference calls, use telemedicine and radio networks as well as secure appropriate transport platforms for use by the retrieval team. The role of the clinical coordination team is highlighted in Box 24.1. A clinical coordination team at work can be seen in Figure 24.1.

ABC of Transfer and Retrieval Medicine, First Edition.
Edited by Adam Low and Jonathan Hulme.
© 2015 John Wiley & Sons, Ltd. Published 2015 by John Wiley & Sons, Ltd.

Box 24.1 **The role of the clinical coordination team**

Receive the initial call requesting patient retrieval/transfer

Document patient's clinical problem, reason for retrieval, precise current clinical condition

Accurately decide on an appropriate retrieval timeframe (e.g. immediate versus 2 hours versus 24 hours)

If required, involve the specialist physician coordinator for high level telephone/telemedicine medical support and advice (e.g. a small general hospital at the weekend is likely to benefit from this advice whereas a tertiary ICU may not)

Ensuring the 'referring' facility attempts adequately to prepare the patient for transfer

Activation and briefing of the dedicated retrieval team in the most appropriate transport platform

Ongoing clinical and logistical support to the retrieval team. (Can be beneficial even for very experienced retrieval teams)

Timely liaison with the 'receiving' facility to ensure the appropriate teams are ready to receive and treat the patient

The operational (retrieval) team

There are many iterations of the retrieval team using a combination of physicians, nurses and paramedics. Many services have a physician led team paired with either a critical care nurse and/or paramedic.

Whilst it is sometimes feasible for one clinician to perform the retrieval on their own, many services accept that the two person team carries a distinct advantage, especially for critically unwell patients.

In addition to this two person generic medical team, there are other personnel who may feature in the operational team (Box 24.2). This is relevant as all team members will form part of the retrieval response and will need to be managed as part of the team.

Box 24.2 **operational team members**

Pilots – fixed wing, rotary wing
Drivers – ambulance/support vehicle
Technicians – e.g. extra-corporeal membrane oxygenator, extra-corporeal life support
Third team member – students, trainees, observers

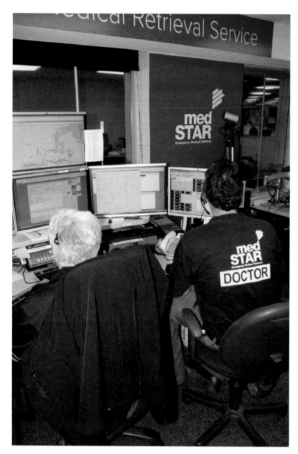

Figure 24.1 Clinical co-ordination team at work.

Leadership

As in all highly functioning teams, a retrieval team requires good leadership. A good team leader will articulate clear goals and recognise the need to draw on the strengths of the members of the team and will make key decisions accordingly. Retrieval teams operate in a high-risk, high-consequence environment. Teams in this kind of environment achieve good outcomes for their patients due to shared mental models, mutual trust, clear roles and responsibilities, all coupled with adaptability. Team members will be comfortable in being able to speak up and voice concerns if appropriate and a good team leader will hear and acknowledge those concerns.

For the retrieval team a key component of both leadership and teamwork, is situation monitoring (Box 24.3).

Box 24.3 **Components of situation monitoring**

STEP – Components of Situation Monitoring
Status of the patient
Team members
Environment
Progress towards goal

One of the key components of situational monitoring is team member welfare and safety. It is imperative that team members take responsibility for their own safety but also look out for other members of the team. A helpful tool in this regard is the "I'm SAFER Checklist" (Box 24.4) which can help with important decisions around both fitness to fly and fitness to work.

Box 24.4 **'I'm SAFER' checklist**

Illness
Medication
Stress
Alcohol and Drugs
Fatigue
Eating and elimination
Risk

Fatigue management can be a particularly difficult issue for retrieval teams. Retrieval taskings that occur at the end of a shift can be especially challenging as the tradition of continuing on for the supposed greater good of the patient has a strong hold in medical culture. Interestingly, the pilot of your aircraft will be bound by strict regulations that will stipulate when they can or cannot fly which will be irrelevant to the clinical condition of the patient. If there is a need for aircrew rotation en route, the medical team would be advised to consider their own fitness to continue with the transfer. In order for teams to maintain their fatigue safety, retrieval services should have a documented fatigue policy that is actively supported by the service.

Retrieval leadership can be considered through five key areas:

1 coordination
2 pre-departure
3 at the referring facility
4 en route
5 at the receiving facility.

Coordination
The key leadership function of appropriate task and resource allocation has been described above.

Pre-departure
In stand-alone retrieval services, the retrieval team is predetermined and solely designated for retrieval (and perhaps pre-hospital) tasks at any given time. This means the retrieval team will have been working together within the organisation and will be familiar with all aspects of the service. This will include equipment, medication, uniform/PPE, transport options, communications and tasking process. The team should have started the shift together and had the opportunity to check and prepare equipment and have a clear understanding of their roles for that shift. Some retrieval teams are drawn from other roles (e.g. the duty intensivist or anaesthetist) and such services should have processes in place to allow the retrieval

team to be easily extricated from ongoing hospital based clinical commitments. Likewise, in some retrieval situations, there will not be a clinical coordination team in which case the roles of clinical coordination team will fall to the retrieval team. The additional challenges this brings to an already complicated task should not be underestimated, and additional time should be factored in for this.

At the referring facility

On arrival at the referring facility, the retrieval team should aim to arrive at the patient's location together, *as a team*. The team leader should introduce the team to the clinical lead and state clearly the name of the patient they have come to retrieve and the destination facility. The retrieval team and the referring team should then make their way to the patient's bedside. The retrieval team should note the initial clinical condition of the patient and then take a handover utilising an appropriate clinical handover tool (Box 24.5). It is important for the team to listen attentively to the handover. It is increasingly apparent that handover is an area of high risk in medical practice and critical information can be lost, potentially leading to patient harm. It is important for the referring clinician to feel engaged and a part of the ongoing process. In addition to professional courtesy, this will have benefits for the retrieval team and for future relationships between referring clinicians and retrieval services. At this stage, the team leader should ensure that the patient (and/or relatives where appropriate) have been involved in the discussions and are aware of the plan. At all times, the retrieval team should verbalise their plans and ensure that everyone is clear about the objectives and has the same mental model. If the retrieval service has separate clinical coordination then they must be kept up to date with the plan and its timings. In the absence of clinical coordination, the retrieval team must make contact with the receiving hospital to ensure an appropriate reception is waiting.

Box 24.5 ISBAR handover tool

Introduction – your team, your patient and your role
Situation – patients presenting complaint
Background – past medical history, medications, allergies
Assessment – teams clinical findings and differential diagnosis
Response and **r**ecommendation – what the team has done and outstanding issues

---

En route

The process of transporting a critically unwell patient from the relative safety of a hospital to an ambulance and then perhaps into an aircraft en route to definitive care requires careful planning and close attention to detail. Patient movements on and off transport platforms is a team responsibility but is usually led by the designated aircraft or ambulance crew members. It is important that communication, role delineation and leadership is clear during these critical phases. At all times, the retrieval team leader needs to focus on good clinical care for the patient, as well as operational matters and logistics. This can be overwhelming and a good team leader will ensure key tasks are appropriately delegated whilst maintaining overall situational awareness. Good communication and regular updates are essential at this stage in the retrieval. This is also the stage at which unexpected events can derail even the best laid plans. Retrieval organisations should have in place standard operating procedures and training packages for dealing with unexpected occurrences en route. For some critical situations, it may be relevant to have 'action cards' to highlight the immediate course of action. It is during these periods of intensely stressful unexpected activity that the time and energy invested in team resource management training, within a formal clinical governance structure, will pay dividends. Most categories of "unexpected" emergencies can be anticipated (Box 24.6) and therefore the benefits of having a potential course of action prepared in advance should not be underestimated. Familiarity with the retrieval service, its equipment and its protocols will minimise the chances and impact of unexpected incidents.

Box 24.6 Unexpected situations during retrieval

Medical
Cardiac arrest
Falling ETCO$_2$
Sudden drop in blood pressure
Accidental extubation
Hypoxia

Logistics/aviation
Controlled ditching
Emergency warning light
Sudden pressure loss
Communications failure
Ventilator/monitor failure
Oxygen supply failure

At the receiving facility

On arrival at the receiving facility, the patient and the team should aim to arrive together at bed space or location allocated to the patient. The receiving clinician should be located and a handover given, focussing initially on any immediate needs. This handover should have been practised prior to arrival to ensure it is succinct and well presented. This also allows other members of the team an opportunity to contribute to handover content ensuring no valuable relevant information is missed. Whilst giving a synopsis of the patient's history is important, the retrieval team may need to make it clear that they have only been caring for the patient for the duration of the transfer and more in depth previous history can be obtained from the notes or from the referring doctor. A final set of observations should be documented upon patient handover. The retrieval team should then leave a copy of the retrieval record and extricate themselves from the location. This is important to allow the receiving team the opportunity to take charge of their patient but also to allow the retrieval team to prepare themselves for any potential follow on tasks. Once the team has repacked their equipment it is beneficial to return to the patient's room to see if there are any questions that may have become apparent to the receiving team prior to the retrieval teams final departure.

Further reading

MedSTAR Emergency Medical Retrieval Service, Adelaide, Australia.
EMRS Scotland, Glasgow, Scotland.
Ellis and Hooper. *Cases in Pre-hospital and Retrieval Medicine*. Churchill Livingstone.
TeamSTEPPS course.

CHAPTER 25

Teamwork and Communication

C. McQueen[1] and K. Thies[1,2,3]

[1]Midlands Air Ambulance; West Midlands Ambulance Service, Medical Emergency Response Incident Team (MERIT), UK
[2]Birmingham Children's Hospital, UK
[3]Mercia Accident Rescue Service (MARS) BASICS, UK

OVERVIEW

- Effective communication and team management are transferable, adaptable skills that should be applied to the challenging and unpredictable environments encountered in transfer and retrieval settings
- An understanding of the core components of team resource management is essential for practitioners working in transfer and retrieval teams
- The transfer and retrieval team often provide the fulcrum around which effective communication and information transfer pathways are organised
- An understanding of the ways in which such pathways can be established and supported is key to effective communication and teamwork in transfer and retrieval teams.

Introduction

The ability to work in multidisciplinary teams and communicate effectively are multifaceted skill sets that are integral to efficient and safe operations in transfer and retrieval medicine. Within transfer and retrieval services, team composition can change on a regular basis. Transfer and retrieval personnel are also required to integrate with members of other teams involved in patient care. Whilst the concepts described below are relevant to other fields of medicine, this chapter focuses specifically on clinicians working in transfer and retrieval services. Members of such teams should have an adaptable, informed approach to teamwork alongside individuals from varying healthcare backgrounds. The approach to the challenges that are faced by clinicians working in this field, is underpinned by an understanding of the importance of clear and effective team resource management (TRM), and the skills of both leadership and followership. Clinicians should therefore endeavour to develop and maintain transferrable and adaptable skills in communication and team management that can be applied to challenging and unpredictable environments. Through this approach, standards of patient care can be optimised, and common sources of error identified and minimised.

ABC of Transfer and Retrieval Medicine, First Edition.
Edited by Adam Low and Jonathan Hulme.
© 2015 John Wiley & Sons, Ltd. Published 2015 by John Wiley & Sons, Ltd.

Team resource management

TRM (sometimes referred to as crew resource management) describes the concept of a framework for an approach to working within teams that has at its heart an understanding of the factors that contribute to safe and effective interpersonal interaction. TRM has been derived from concepts first pioneered in the aviation industry, with emphasis given to factors that affect human performance, the functioning and safety of teams and wider organisations.

In order for TRM strategies to be maximally effective, complete involvement is required at an organisational level. Transfer and retrieval services should promote a culture of awareness and understanding of how factors encountered in operational settings can limit performance of individuals and teams, predisposing them to error. Strategies to optimise the efficiency of teamwork, identify and scrutinise chains of events that result in suboptimal performance and error should be embedded within the management and governance structures of the organisation. This identifies solutions that prevent recurrence.

Effective teamwork

An informed understanding of the factors that influence team dynamics and cohesion is required in order to coordinate effectively the transfer of critically injured/unwell patients in challenging environments. Factors that can contribute to resource management of teams are summarised in Figure 25.1.

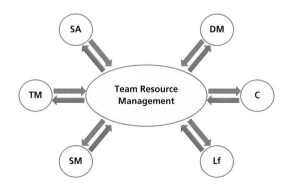

Figure 25.1 Schematic diagram illustrating the factors that contribute to team resource management. SA, situational awareness; DM, decision-making; C, communication; Lf, leadership and followership; SM, stress management; TM, task management.

Clinicians must understand how these factors can influence team dynamics and efficiency. Effective TRM is derived from the ability of individuals to identify and manage the various elements that contribute to the cohesion and dynamics of teams. Such attributes are commonly referred to as 'non-technical skills'. The coordination and execution of effective teamwork requires members to identify factors that contribute to potential for poor performance and error, and then implement solutions to address them.

Leadership/followership and authority gradients

He who has never learned to obey cannot be a good commander – Aristotle

Clear and effective leadership within teams is fundamentally important to the overall efficiency and safety of their operations. The qualities of a good team leader however involve the ability to follow direction or instruction from other team members when required. In the context of TRM the term 'authority gradient' is often used to describe the relationship between team leaders and members. The aim of effective team leadership is to flatten the authority gradient between individuals so that all members of the team feel empowered to contribute to its leadership and strategic direction.

Adopting a flattened authority gradient promotes a culture in which individual team members are encouraged to contribute to management decisions and highlight sources of error that are anticipated or have been encountered already. Leadership roles within teams should therefore be encouraged to be fluid in order that the entire team contributes to and understands a shared strategic direction for the teams' efforts. The lead clinician should encourage feedback and input from all team members involved in the transfer.

The team 'leader' role in these contexts then becomes that of a facilitator; an individual who coalesces the aims and expectations of team members into a common goal. The challenge with this approach is to ensure that clear and effective leadership is maintained at all times and all members understand the aims and objectives of the team; a process known as 'shared mental modelling'. A culture promoting and supporting such a leadership style should be encouraged and supported at an organisational level.

Communication

Clear and effective pathways of communication are vital for the co-ordination and delivery of high quality care throughout a transfer. Clinicians must therefore have a robust framework for integrated communication with a wide variety of individuals and agencies. Pathways of communication must be established and maintained (Summarised in Box 25.1):

> Box 25.1 **Summary of different pathways of communication**
>
> Inter-team communication: communication between the transfer team and the referring team that have been providing immediate/stabilising care for the patient, and the receiving hospital team
>
> Intra-team communication: communication between members of the transfer team
>
> Supra-team communication: communication with ambulance service control/operations base
>
> Communication with supporting agencies: communication with other agencies including police/fire/specialist rescue services (e.g. at scene or within the wider context of strategic oversight such as in a major incident)
>
> Communication with patients and relatives: at scene/in hospital/during transfer

A framework that optimises pathways of communication without leading to fragmented transfer of information is fundamental to the effective coordination and delivery of good quality care. An example of a model for clear and effective communication is called the 'communication web', illustrated in Figure 25.2.

Within this model one individual from the transfer/retrieval team acts as the fulcrum around which all pathways of communication are supported. All personnel need to participate in the exchange of information by communicating effectively, by both listening and speaking. The team leader facilitates this by providing

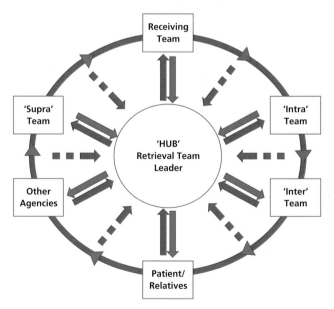

Figure 25.2 Schematic diagram of the 'communication web'.

informative and complete feedback as the case evolves, sharing information among the team members and communicating any changes in plans. In this capacity the team leader can ensure that the needs and expectations of all of the different components of the clinical case are understood and addressed. This approach is designed to reduce the potential for fragmented transmission of vital information, and minimises the potential for conflict or misunderstanding between individuals or organisations involved in the management of the patient. It also ensures completeness of handover between the different teams involved in the patient journey. Direct communication between individuals or agencies is possible, but should be fed back to the coordinator to ensure that the flow of information remains centralised.

Clinicians working in transfer and retrieval teams must ensure that they are adept at managing multiple pathways of communication simultaneously using a variety of tools and communication devices. A framework for the transfer of key information that is reproducible and easily understood by all of the teams involved in patient transfer is of great importance. An example is given in Box 25.2.

Box 25.2 The AT-MIST handover tool

Age (estimated if not confirmed)
T – time of injury
M – mechanism of injury
I – injuries identified
S – signs and symptoms
T – treatment provided

Identifying and addressing communication difficulties

Ineffective communication can result in the potential for delays in transfer and the provision of critical care interventions for patients. Confusion and misunderstanding between members of different teams, the patients themselves and their relatives can be sources of potential conflict during transfer missions. Clinicians must be able to identify circumstances in which communication and teamwork can be improved to avoid conflict and ensure that standard of clinical care provided to patients is not compromised. Strategies to improve communication and teamwork often focus on interventions in a number of key areas (Box 25.3).

Team debriefing

Debriefing is an effective way of improving future team performance and can be achieved by running an open discussion at the end of the transfer. It must be non-punitive and led by a member of the team using a structured approach. All team members need to have the opportunity to contribute at the same hierarchical

---

Box 25.3 Strategies to improve communication within a team

Role allocation: clear identification of roles within teams that are appropriate for the training and experience levels of individuals to avoid confusion and misunderstanding regarding management responsibilities

Communication pathways: the establishment of chains of communication (as shown in Figure 25.2) so that the pathways for transfer of information between individuals and teams are clear and effective

Management goals: the promotion of clear and achievable goals for patient management at each phase of the care pathway so that all team members have a common understanding

Timeline establishment: the identification and communication within the team of clear points for interventions to be performed.

Misunderstandings in any of the areas summarised above have the potential to lead to confusion and possible conflict. Team leaders should be mindful of this possibility and seek to address potential sources of conflict as they arise.

---

level and receive feedback in order to allow good actions to be acknowledged, errors corrected, areas of conflict resolved and lessons learned for future missions. Where possible, similar frameworks should be adopted for wider team debriefing including personnel from other teams and agencies involved.

The organisational level

Organisations should ensure that they operate in a culture that promotes safe and effective teamwork, encouraging clear and effective communication. In addition to offering training and development for staff in concepts such as TRM and communication skills, measures should be taken to ensure that operational performance and errors are monitored and investigated. A robust governance and case review structure should be established to highlight examples of best practice and identify development areas. At the heart of any such process should be the promotion of greater awareness and understanding of how factors encountered in transfer and retrieval operations can limit the performance of individuals and teams and predispose to error or adverse events. Error chains should be investigated thoroughly and reported as part of blame free, transparent process through which individual learning and organisational development opportunities are identified. This encourages high standards of operational efficiency and performance, thereby reducing sources of error.

Conclusion

Effective teamwork and communication are core skills in the armamentarium of clinicians working in transfer and retrieval environments.

Further reading

Budd HR, Almond LM, Porter K. A survey of trauma alert criteria and handover practice in England and Wales. Emerg Med J 2007;24(4): 302–4.

Carter AJ, Davis KA, Evans LV, Cone DC. Information loss in emergency medical services handover of trauma patients. Prehosp Emerg Care 2009;13(3):280–5.

European Trauma Course. European Resuscitation Council https://www.erc.edu/.

Lammers R, Byrwa M, Fales W. Root causes of errors in a simulated prehospital pediatric emergency. Acad Emerg Med 2012;19(1):37–47.

National NHS Syllabus Conflict Resolution Course Guidance Manual http://www.whnt.nhs.uk/document_uploads/Clinical_skills/CRTCourse GuidanceManual.pdf.

NHS institute for Innovation and Improvement. Communication Skills Training http://www.institute.nhs.uk/index

Yong G, Dent AW, Weiland TJ. Handover from paramedics: observations and emergency department clinician perceptions. Emerg Med Australas 2008;20(2):149–55.

CHAPTER 26

Non-technical Skills and Sources of Error

C. McQueen[1] and M. Horton[2]

[1]Midlands Air Ambulance; West Midlands Ambulance Service, Medical Emergency Response Incident Team (MERIT), UK
[2]Emergency Department, Heartlands Hospital, Birmingham, UK

OVERVIEW

- Clinicians working in transfer and retrieval teams must have a well-developed understanding of essential non-technical skills (NTS) that underpin the delivery of clinical care
- A variety of cognitive tools underpin effective resource management in dynamic challenging situations
- Frameworks should exist within organisations to support the development and application of NTS in operational practice.

Introduction

A range of factors can affect individual and team performance in transfer and retrieval environments, predisposing to error. Clinicians must have a mature and informed understanding of the ways these factors may impact upon clinical care, and possess the necessary skills to nullify or minimise their influence. The practical application of solutions by individuals requires an understanding of the cognitive tools that underpin effective resource management in dynamic, challenging situations. Organisational frameworks should exist that support the implementation of these skills in a functional model operationally.

Non-technical skills

Effective team resource management (TRM) can be adversely influenced by many factors. Time pressure, stress and fatigue have all been shown to predispose to failures in effective clinical management and lead to error. It is fundamental therefore that clinicians involved in transfer and retrieval operations have a highly developed, multifaceted skill set that can be utilised when challenging, unfamiliar or rapidly evolving situations are encountered. The term non-technical skills (NTS) is used to describe the framework of skills that can be utilised in these circumstances. NTS include the ability to recognise, interpret and manage the different elements that influence the performance of individuals and teams, summarised in Box 26.1.

ABC of Transfer and Retrieval Medicine, First Edition.
Edited by Adam Low and Jonathan Hulme.
© 2015 John Wiley & Sons, Ltd. Published 2015 by John Wiley & Sons, Ltd.

Box 26.1 The core themes of NTS

Situational awareness: the ability rapidly to assess and assimilate stimuli from the working environment into a mental model that is then utilised to identify and categorise problems, whilst formulating potential solutions

Decision-making: the ability to make clear, informed decisions and formulate appropriate management plans based on the nature of the identified problem

Communication: clear communication within a team ensures that problems and potential solutions are shared with other team members

Leadership/followership: facilitating the execution of management plans using available resources and personnel.

Task management: identification and allocation of appropriate tasks to team members to ensure that solutions are enacted efficiently and safely

Stress management: managing potential sources of stress and overload in oneself/others to ensure the team functions efficiently and safely.

When presented with external stressors the human brain can subconsciously utilise cognitive shortcuts (cognitive dispositions to respond (CDRs) or more colloquially 'intuition') in an attempt to streamline the processes of problem solving and decision making. When accessed subconsciously, CDRs are a potential source of cognitive error. Large numbers of CDRs have been identified, some of which are summarised in Table 26.1. Note the common theme of premature or inappropriate arrival at an endpoint or conclusion in critical thinking and problem solving, leading to inappropriate or misdiagnosis, or failures to identify potential pitfalls in management plans.

Expert management of challenging and rapidly evolving scenarios involves access of higher cognitive domains (summarised in Box 26.2) at each stage of the processes of recognising problems, formulating solutions and subsequently enacting plans. This allows for conscious problem processing, utilising appropriate CDRs where necessary to reach an applicable solution that has been carefully considered in terms of the context of the encountered environment. NTS are utilised at each stage of this process to influence and guide cognitive processes and minimise error.

Table 26.1 Examples of CDRs commonly encountered in clinical practice.

Cognitive disposition to respond	Description	Consequences
Ascertainment bias	A physician's thinking is pre-shaped by expectations of what they expect to find- relying on pre defined 'labels' for patients to assist decision making- e.g. the patient with a history of previous heart attack presenting with chest pain 'must' have angina	Prejudgement may lead to over or under assessment of patients
Availability and non-availability	'common things are common'- conditions are judged more likely if they are common and vice versa	Disproportionate estimates of the frequency of a particular diagnosis or condition
Confirmation bias	To only look for information that confirms the initial hypothesis and discount any that does not	Preservation of incorrect hypotheses. Correct diagnoses may be missed
Multiple alternatives bias	Decision making becomes more challenging when more possible choices are available: clinicians may revert to 'simple' decisions between only two options and discount the others	Irrational decisions and missed diagnoses due to decision overload
Outcome bias	The tendency to judge the decision made based on its likely outcome- i.e. to prefer decisions that will lead to desirable outcomes	In the ED this may mean choosing a decision that will achieve an objective (e.g. meeting a target) rather than focussing on the correct diagnosis
Premature closure	Accepting a diagnosis before consideration of all of the other alternatives	Arrests further thinking in problem solving
Search satisficing	Arresting the problem solving process once a diagnosis is made despite the possibility of additional diagnoses	Missed diagnoses

---

Box 26.2 Higher cognitive domains

Meta-recognition: the ability consciously to assimilate and interpret the physical stimuli from scenes/clinical scenarios into a recognised cognitive model, identifying key goals and expectations of subsequent management plans

Meta-cognition: 'thinking about thinking'; the ability consciously to evaluate and scrutinise the processes used to formulate a decision regarding the most suitable response to the identified problem

Meta-planning: the ability consciously to interpret the anticipated consequences of the planned response and adapt it where necessary (e.g. concept of a 'Plan-A'/'Plan-B'/'Plan-C')

A schematic diagram summarising the different stages of 'meta-decision making' and the NTS that can be utilised at each point is shown in Figure 26.1.

Human factors

'Human factors' is the term used to describe the operational and organisational frameworks by which the rather abstract concepts of NTS are translated into working practice. All levels of operational practice should be underpinned by robust frameworks that support the implementation of skills required for safe and effective problems solving and decision making in challenging and rapidly changing environments.

Individual and inter-personal level

Transfer and retrieval services should endeavour to instil into working practices the concept of a shallow authority gradient in which the opinions all team members are respected and given credence. Team members should be encouraged to speak out regarding issues related to decision making, with the team leader acting as a coordinator/facilitator. Central to this approach is the concept of shared mental modelling within teams; that is, the ability of team members to interpret and recognise problems and potential solutions collectively with a common understanding of the aims and objectives of the team, and potential to achieve them. Clear and effective pathways of communication are therefore required throughout the transfer. This approach needs to be balanced with the need for the team leader to retain overall strategic direction and oversight of management decisions that are shared with the rest of the team. This approach aims to ensure that potential sources of error are highlighted and acted upon swiftly and effectively.

Environmental and operational level

Patient transfer involves exposure of the patient and team to rapidly changing clinical/environmental conditions that contribute additional stress to all. Utilisation of checklists and standard operating procedures (SOPs) for complex interventions and procedures can provide clinicians with a well rehearsed framework and structure to standardise practice, thereby reducing the possibility of error. Regular training, including simulation and formalised drills for known or expected untoward incidents can prepare teams for their occurrence and ensure that they can be managed swiftly and effectively if they occur.

Organisational and cultural level

Transfer and retrieval schemes should have embedded within them a system for frank and effective multidisciplinary team debriefing after complex or challenging clinical incidents. Individuals should be encouraged to identify and reflect upon sources of error, and examples of good quality practice, in a culture that does not seek to apportion blame. Robust processes for error investigation that are transparent and impartial must be in place to ensure that untoward incidents or errors can be used to guide further developments in

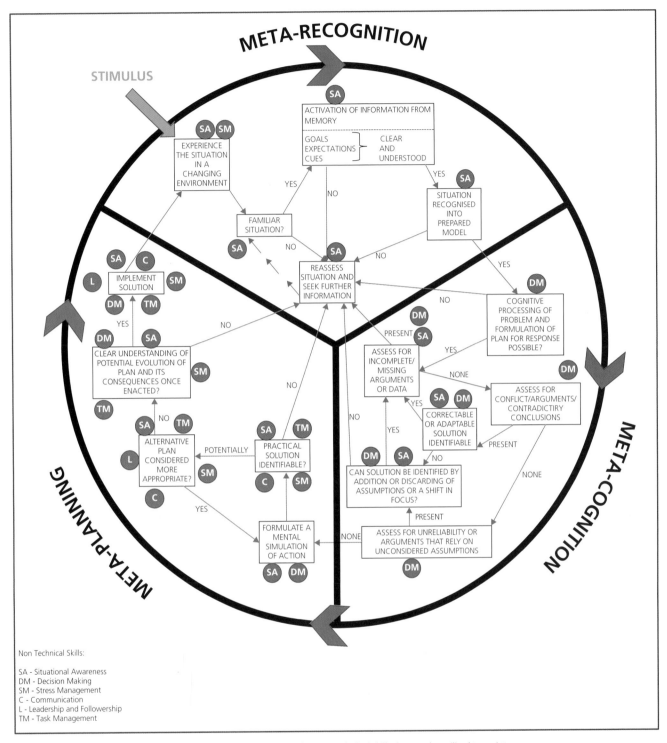

Figure 26.1 The cognitive processes involved in decision making and the non-technical skills that can be utilised to assist.

practice across the whole organisation. In this way future repetition of the same error chain can be avoided.

Practical application of the human factors approach into a working model for transfer and retrieval service operations will promote a culture in which potential sources of error can be swiftly identified and avoided by teams.

Training in non-technical skills and human factors

Human factors and NTS have been cornerstones of training and development in the aviation industry and military settings for many decades. Recently the United States military has developed 'Tactical

Decision Games' as a training tool to promote the development of cognitive awareness and NTS in decision making for officer recruits. These training tools have been applied in other sectors associated with high risk operations including Fire Rescue Services and the offshore drilling industries. The transferability of the model to medical settings shows significant promise as a method of encouraging the development of enhanced decision making and problem solving skills in teams involved in the management of patients in stressful, time pressured environments and requires further research.

Conclusion

Clinicians working in transfer and retrieval teams require a well-developed understanding of NTS and the ability to utilise them appropriately to underpin safe and effective operations. Both individuals and wider teams need to have conscious awareness of the skills required at each stage of planning and management processes involved in patient transfer, being adept at having adaptable and transferable frameworks of the application of those skills in practice. Clinical work must be underpinned by a robust operational model that promotes the concepts of human factors amongst individuals and the wider organisation.

Further reading

ANTS System http://abdn.ac.uk/iprc/ants.

Chalwin RP, Flabouris A. Utility and assessment of non-technical skills for rapid response systems and medical emergency teams. Intern Med J 2013;43(9):962–9.

Clinical Human Factors Group http://wwwchfg.org/.

Fletcher G, Flin R, McGeorge P, Glavin R, Maran N, Patey R. Anaesthetists' non-technical skills (ANTS): evaluation of a behavioural marker system. Br J Anaesth 2003;90(5):580–88.

Flowerdew L, Gaunt A, Spedding J, Bhargava A, Brown R, Vincent C, Woloshynowych M. A multicentre observational study to evaluate a new tool to assess emergency physicians' non-technical skills. Emerg Med J 2013;30(6):437–43.

Larsson J, Holmström IK. How excellent anaesthetists perform in the operating theatre: a qualitative study on non-technical skills. Br J Anaesth 2013;110(1):115–21.

Riem N, Boet S, Bould MD, Tavares W, Naik VN. Do technical skills correlate with non-technical skills in crisis resource management: a simulation study. Br J Anaesth 2012;109(5):723–8.

CHAPTER 27

Standard Operating Procedures, Checklists and Documentation

S. Sollid[1,2,3] and O. Uleberg[1,4]

[1]Norwegian Air Ambulance Academy, Norwegian Air Ambulance Foundation, Norway
[2]Air Ambulance Department, University Hospital, Norway
[3]University of Stavanger, Stavanger, Norway
[4]Department of Aeromedical and Clinical Emergency Services, St Olavs University Hospital, Norway

---

OVERVIEW

- Challenges of documentation and its importance in retrieval medicine
- Manual versus automated documentation, benefits and challenges
- The importance of standard operating procedures and to what extent they guide or rule medical care
- Benefits and challenges with checklists.

Documentation

Documentation is an essential part of good medical practice, but also a legal requirement in most systems. Good documentation ensures that vital information about the patient is transferred from one provider to another. In retrieval medicine this is imperative since handovers occur with every patient at least twice, with the potential for important information to be lost, predisposing to error. The transfer team needs to make sure that all relevant data from the delivering institution and documentation from the transport phase are reliably relayed to the receiving institution. All relevant patient records should follow the patient. If not available at the time of transfer, the delivering institution should provide them as soon as possible, securely, to the receiving institution (e.g. fax, telephone or electronic patient system). Informed consent may not always be attainable due to the patients' critical condition/inability to obtain this from next of kin. In these situations, the need for transfer and specialised care should be anticipated, documented and authorized.

Besides the name, gender and date of birth, the patient records should contain medical details about the patient. A patient identification band should be secured pre-transfer, and match all transferred medical records. Transfer records should contain a brief summary of the patients' clinical status prior to, during and after transfer; and relevant pre-morbidities, environmental factors, vital signs, clinical events and therapy given during transport. In secondary/tertiary transfers, records should

also include reason for transfer and names of the referring and receiving physician.

Traditional documentation is performed manually, either as a written, freeform description or as a series of data points in a predefined diagram (or a combination of both). The obvious weakness in manual documentation is that it relies on the ability of the person documenting to register and interpret data (e.g. vital signs or symptoms) correctly, and document relevant, important data (Box 27.1). Manual documentation also allows for selection bias: the documenter can omit data either willingly or unwillingly. From a medico-legal perspective omitted or missing data in records related to errors or patient harm can be incriminating for the provider (e.g. hypoxemia during endotracheal intubation as a result of poor pre-oxygenation).

Box 27.1 Weaknesses of manual documentation

Relies on ability of person documenting to register and interpret data correctly
Prone to selection bias: data omitted willingly or unwillingly
Difficult to maintain records up to date under high workload.

Another challenge is maintaining updated records, when transferring seriously ill or injured patients who require en route medical interventions. The priority should always be on maintaining quality patient care, but adequate documentation MUST be completed before leaving the receiving institution.

With improving technology, documentation can be automated, thereby eliminating selection bias. Most modern medical equipment is fitted with data-out ports where monitoring data can be transferred to storing devices or directly into software dedicated for the purpose of documentation. This kind of software and hardware solution has been available for a decade and is now finding its way from the operating room and intensive care unit to the pre-hospital environment. Modern portable diagnostic tools (e.g. ultrasound or point-of-care testing devices) also allow for data storage and transfer that can be used for documentation in retrieval medicine. Other technologies like radio frequency identification can improve medication tracking and documentation. Despite the advantages of these new technologies to improve documentation, they also pose practical challenges (Box 27.2). Foremost is selecting the

---

ABC of Transfer and Retrieval Medicine, First Edition.
Edited by Adam Low and Jonathan Hulme.
© 2015 John Wiley & Sons, Ltd. Published 2015 by John Wiley & Sons, Ltd.

appropriate data amount to store (e.g. continuous vs. interval data storage) and filtering out artefacts that can mimic pathology. The latter is a well-known issue with continuous data sampling of vital parameters where the benefit of objective data sampling is potentially lost in the follow up work of annotating artefacts to avoid misinterpretation.

Box 27.2 **Challenges of automated documentation and data sampling**

Finding the appropriate data sampling rate
How to filter and treat data artefacts that can mimic pathology
Defining the appropriate data points

Selecting the correct data is just as much a question of what data points should be stored and documented. Traditionally each retrieval or EMS service has predefined documentation standards, mostly a mix of mission and patient history data. Predominantly, the main goal is to document which medical interventions have been performed during transport and the patients' clinical response and behaviour. Some systems also document for quality purposes and in order to investigate if the service actually helps improve survival, or at least does not inflict unnecessary damage. Many services describe specific documentation needs, which also results in numerous different systems and templates, based on different definitions for each variable. In an isolated service this poses few problems, but data are not necessarily comparable across services or systems. Some initiatives have sought to change this and there are currently several templates available based on consensus processes where the goal is to generate templates for capturing comparable data across systems, for quality assurance and to allow for collection of research data across systems. Retrieval services should therefore strive to adapt their documentation systems to existing data templates. In this sense, the tools for documentation are less important; it is the data collected, recorded and documented that matters. Documentation attained prior and during the transport phase, in most systems serves as medico-legal documents and should be kept adequately filed and securely stored according to local judicial requirements.

Standard operating procedures

Standard operating procedures (SOPs) are mostly established as a reference to standardised/best practice, and should guide operations within a system to ensure that they are carried out in the same manner, independent of provider. They can cover many aspects of operations, including administrative, medical interventions and utilisation of specialist equipment SOPs. If SOPs are established, they should be easily available for the providers at the site where they apply, e.g. at the workstation or in the ambulance.

The tradition for using SOPs in healthcare is relatively new and there is still an unresolved debate in many systems as to how binding they are for each provider. For example, physicians are in most countries regarded as having independent responsibility for the care that they provide and are therefore not bound by SOPs *per se*, as long as they adhere to best or common practice guidelines. In these cases,

SOPs can be regarded as guides but not absolutes, and the physician can freely choose to deviate from the SOP according to his/her professional judgement. Some systems however demand that any deviation from the SOP should be documented, explained and justified. The last one is probably the best practice from a medico-legal perspective. In cases of medical error or patient harm, deviation from any SOP that is not documented and explained may be the basis for litigation. Although the legal binding of SOPs is often unclear, they should be regarded as binding unless otherwise stated. When establishing SOPs, the organisation must therefore have a clear attitude to how binding they are for the provider, and state this in every document.

The use of dedicated retrieval teams is often based on the need for ensuring high-quality care throughout the whole transfer process. Adherence to common SOPs both by the transport team, delivering and receiving institutions may induce higher efficiency and quality. In many transfers, medical interventions often need to be performed prior to departure. Interventions such as ensuring a patent airway, ventilator settings, intravenous lines, infusions, vasopressors and others may well be secured before the arrival of the transfer team, reducing turnaround time for the transfer team. Some systems use a form of central clinical coordination, which communicates on-line with the delivering and receiving institution as well as the transfer team en route.

Checklists

Checklists are often an extension or a result of SOPs. Checklists are much used in other high-risk safety conscious industries (e.g. aviation, oil or nuclear industry). They can be regarded as aide-memoires to ensure consistency and completeness of tasks. There are different types of checklists, from simple 'to-do' lists, to advanced sequenced work lists for carrying out complex tasks (Figure 27.1).

The promotion and understanding of the importance of checklists for multidisciplinary healthcare teams has increased with the demonstration of significantly reduced adverse outcomes in perioperative care that resulted in the publication of the World Health Organization (WHO) Surgical Safety Checklist.

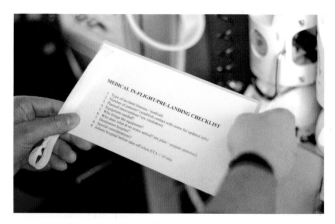

Figure 27.1 An example of a checklist used in HEMs missions.
(Source: Gunnar Vangberg, St. Olavs University Hospital, Trondheim, Norway. Reproduced with permission).

The main reason for using checklists is to ensure that critical sequences, items or tasks are not omitted. They are just as important in routine as in emergency settings. A typical example of a routine checklist in retrieval medicine is a pre-transport checklist that ensures that critical and vital items, tasks and procedures have been completed before transport is initiated (see Appendix 5). Checklist for pre-hospital intubation is an example of an emergency action checklist to ensure that the procedure is carried out safely and that no critical items are forgotten before or during the procedure. Whilst checklists are there to avoid complacency, they may *induce* complacency, so called 'checklist complacency' (Box 27.3). This occurs when checklists are hurried through, the interaction between call-out and call-back is not conscious or items on the checklist are not actually checked but assumed to be all right. Checklists should also be clear and not allow for interpretation or assumptions of what the items the list covers are: 'all equipment and personnel secured in the cabin?' is a better checklist item and call-out than "cabin clear?'

Box 27.3 **Signs of checklist complacency**

Checklist is hurried through (let's get on with it, we're in a hurry!)
Lack of conscious interaction between call-out and call-back (I know the drill, I'll call back what I always do)
Items are not actually checked, but assumed to be right (It was OK the last time and probably is now too).

Further reading

AAGBI. *Section 9: Documentation and handover*. In AAGBI Safety Guideline: Interhospital transfer. London: The Association of Anaesthetists of Great Britain and Ireland 2009:13–14

Hales, BM, Pronovost PJ. The checklist – a tool for error management and performance improvement. J Crit Care 2006;21(3):231–5.

Haynes , et al. on behalf of the Safe Surgery Saves Lives Study Group. A surgical safety checklist to reduce morbidity and mortality in a global population. N Engl J Med 2009;360(5):491–9.

Kruger AJ, Lockey D, Kurola J, et al. A consensus-based template for documenting and reporting in physician-staffed pre-hospital services. Scand J Trauma Resusc Emerg Med 2011;19:71.

Sollid SJ, Lockey D, Lossius HM, A consensus-based template for uniform reporting of data from pre-hospital advanced airway management. Scand J Trauma Resusc Emerg Med 2009;17(1):58.

CHAPTER 28

Audit, Medicolegal and Ethical Aspects of Transfer Medicine

G. Evetts[1], S. Cox[2,3], and R. Tipping[4,5]

[1]Intensive Care & Anaesthesia, Royal Air Force, Imperial College School of Anaesthesia, UK
[2]Critical Care and Aeromedical Transfer CEGA Air Ambulance, UK
[3]General Intensive Care Unit, University Hospital Southampton NHS Foundation Trust, UK
[4]University Hospitals Birmingham NHS Foundation Trust (Queen Elizabeth Hospital), UK
[5]West Midlands Ambulance Service NHS Foundation Trust Medical Emergency Response Incident Team (MERIT), UK

OVERVIEW

- Legal and regulation activity of patient transfer providers
- Cross-border and practitioner jurisdiction challenges
- Clinical governance and liability
- Regulation of transfer equipment
- Necessity of audit
- Ethical dilemmas of patient transfer.

Introduction

The transfer of patients by any mode of transport can present new challenges, risk and decisions that may not be present in a familiar hospital environment. These challenges are present on regional transfers and even more so on international transfers, particularly since these will usually be undertaken by an air platform. These may also involve a road transfer in a foreign country with its own rules and regulations. Reconfiguration of specialist healthcare services increasingly necessitates all forms of transfer, but the risks and benefits must still be weighed up by the transfer team.

Patient, staff, transport, permits to travel and equipment factors are all subject to scrutiny if any incident should occur. All organisations should have a clear mission statement, stipulating the goals of the service, led by a medical director who has overall responsibility for the patient and the transfer team. However, local, country and international regulations all impact upon transport of patients, irrespective of transport modality. Healthcare providers who are facilitating a transfer must be aware of how these regulations affect their choice of transport vehicle, as well as their legal responsibilities before, during and after the transfer.

Legal considerations and regulatory bodies

Fixed-wing air ambulance and helicopter emergency medical services regulation

All transportation services will be bound by specific regulatory authorities regardless of country of operation. These bridge the medical and the transportation element and have clear legal standing within the country of operation with their aims of patient safety regardless of modality. Some are summarised below.

National Advisory Committee for Aeronautics Score

It must be remembered that in the UK and Europe, until an air ambulance has a patient on board, it is an ordinary aircraft which is not given any enhanced priorities within aviation. Commercial airports operating within the UK and Europe utilise the National Advisory Committee for Aeronautics Score (NACA score; Box 28.1). This classifies the patient in terms of their illness and therefore designated platform air priority. In the USA, a far more relaxed approach is used, with any medical platform, whether staging or with the patient on board, is given a medical/coastguard call sign, always allowing priority.

Box 28.1 summary of the NACA score

NACA score

I   Minor disturbance, no medical intervention required
II   Slight to moderate disturbance. Outpatient medical investigation
III   Moderate to severe but not life threatening
IV   Serious incident where rapid development into a life threatening condition cannot be excluded
V   Acute danger
VI   Respiratory or cardiac arrest
VII   Death

Civil Aviation Authority and Care Quality Commission

The Civil Aviation Authority (CAA) regulates all aspects of air operation in the UK, abiding to the European Aviation Safety Agency (EASA), and so all helicopter emergency medical services (HEMS) and fixed-wing air ambulance (FWAA) providers using G-prefix registered aircraft must be certified by the CAA, and comply to their regulations. This also applies to use of G-registered commercial airlines as a patient platform. The Care Quality Commission (CQC) regulates health and social care providers in the UK, and thus providers must register with them and be subject

ABC of Transfer and Retrieval Medicine, First Edition.
Edited by Adam Low and Jonathan Hulme.
© 2015 John Wiley & Sons, Ltd. Published 2015 by John Wiley & Sons, Ltd.

to their guidance (Box 28.2). A memorandum of understanding between the CAA and the CQC exists in order to facilitate regulation of patient air transport, allowing sharing of information and collaboration, which together with a British Standard Institute (BSI) working party helps integrate both aviation and medical law in respect of patient air services.

Box 28.2 **A summary of regulatory bodies.**

The CAA regulates all aviation activity

The CQC regulates all patient care providers

The NACA defines air ambulances in terms of patient illness severity (UK only)

A memorandum of understanding and a British Standard Institute working party exists to aid collaboration between CAA and CQC

Care providers can register with worldwide voluntary organisations which function to provide standards for patient care

---

Voluntary organisations

Several organisations across the globe also function to regulate and provide standards for medical air operations including:

- European Aero-Medical Institute (EURAMI): regulates air operation and medical crews within Europe and worldwide
- Commission on Accreditation of Medical Transport Systems (CAMTS): additionally regulates road ambulances.

Cross-border patient transport

Particular planning and attention must be paid when performing international patient retrieval, and wider consideration must be undertaken to include multiple transport modalities and clearing customs and immigration. Medical crews must have appropriate visas issued to them to travel across borders and to allow access to the patient at the bed space of the receiving hospital. Without these they may not be able to leave the boundaries of the airport necessitating a 'tarmac handover' (Box 28.3). Transfer of responsibility is not complete until the staff on the receiving unit have received a full report of the patient's status, and appropriate documentation with information about the patient's next of kin, how to contact them and what they are aware of.

Box 28.3 **the risks associated with tarmac handovers**

Handover in potentially distracting situation

Receiving team unable to assess necessity/fitness to travel before patient leaves a place of safety

Multiple handovers of patient care may lead to distortion or omission of important information, and poor continuity of care for patients and relatives

Can be necessary for practitioner jurisdiction limitations

Sometimes vital for speed of urgent transfer

Medication during transportation

Within England, Scotland and Wales, companies and individuals need to apply for Home Office licenses if they wish to possess, import or export 'controlled drugs' across European and international boundaries by road or air.

Controlled drugs are named in the Misuse of Drugs legislation and grouped in schedules that were updated in 2014 and include common opiate-based pain relief. The Home Office will issue a personalised scheduled of medication allowed to be taken abroad. Other countries may have their own import regulations for controlled drugs and prescription medicines; therefore, before any European or International transfer, it is essential to check this with the appropriate embassy/High Commission/Consulate of the country/countries that you are travelling to/through. In addition to controlled drugs, consideration must also be undertaken if carrying medication on a non-dedicated air ambulance platform. Normally passengers may only take liquids that measure no more than 100 mL past security search points in a clear transparent bag that must not be greater than 1 litre in volume. Each individual airline and individual airport must be contacted if extra liquids are to be carried, and additional screening may be required at all airports transited. Further screening must be undertaken for hypodermic needles and syringes.

Clinical governance frameworks

Medical crew: liabilities, governance framework, and indemnity
Professional registration and professional development
As with any clinical practice, all medical crew must abide by their governance framework, which must be open to objective evaluation. This includes relevant qualifications with upkeep of registration with requisite councils (e.g. General Medical Council (GMC), Nursing Midwifery Council (NMC), and Health and Care Professionals Council (HCPC)). Specialties may also have their own colleges or associations which provide standards for patient transport (e.g. the Association of Anaesthetists Great Britain and Ireland (AAGBI), which publishes guidelines for transport of critically ill patients as does the Intensive Care Society (ICS)). These organisations also provide personal accident insurance for physicians when undertaking transfers. Services are responsible for ensuring that their healthcare providers have the relevant qualifications and experience, together with the necessary training specific to the company or platforms. Individuals should comply with revalidation and be able to show adequate continual professional development for their role, with regular appraisals. All practitioners should ensure that they have adequate professional indemnity with an appropriate organisation specific to their workload and mode of transport, and care providers should confirm this. The country of registration and qualification of practitioners is essential as this may not license the medical crew to work globally, and each professional body will provide guidance. The medical crew on a specific mission may not be licensed to work or practice at the hospital the patient is collected or delivered to, or indeed in the country at all. Airports are designated international space, thus in these countries tarmac transfers may be necessary.

Within the UK the practice exists that allied health professionals undertake transfers without the guidance of a registered medical professional. In this instance the practitioner should seek guidance through organisation-generated patient group directives; the medical director will always maintain overall responsibility.

Liability and risk: medical crew and medical director

Every transportation service must have an appointed medical director who will have the overarching authority and final responsibility for patients within its care. The medical directorate will monitor the governance, safety and risk stratification of all transfers (Box 28.4). With all transfers there is a measurable amount of risk, that must be considered in conjunction with the medical crew undertaking the transfer, and ultimately the medical director. If a commercial plane is utilised, fitness to fly certification is required. It is essential that the passenger's physician sends adequate details well in advance of the flight to the carrier. Most airlines have medical advisors who provide advice and 'clear' passengers as fit to fly and require information about the nature of the individual's condition and their severity/stability; medication being taken; and any pertinent information about mobility. The CAA Aviation Health Unit (AHU) provides guidance with this.

Box 28.4 Responsibilities of a medical director

A registered doctor within the country and specialty of practice
Leadership to clinical service and its design
Overarching responsible professional for clinical transfers and the treatment given by its employees
Clinical guidance to the multiprofessional teams
Creation of multi-professional protocols
To ensure quality assurance and clinical governance is adhered to
To lead on clinical teaching

If an incident occurs during retrieval or transfer either in the UK or on a UK registered aircraft, the investigation would fall under the jurisdiction of the CQC and the individual company's safety management and clinical governance systems. Conversely if death occurs during transportation there are no clear guidelines on how to manage this legally, and each case must be judged on its individual rights. Nevertheless, the transport crew must notify the local medical examiner of the county in which the patient died. This may involve, within air transport, air traffic directing the plane to a divisional airfield in the region the death has occurred, or to continue the resuscitation attempts until within the airspace of the destination and then to notify authorities. The patient is then taken to the nearest hospital. Advance directivities and do not attempt resuscitation orders are only legally valid in the country and county issued, which could have ramifications especially for non-physician global palliative transfers.

Equipment regulation

All equipment utilised with transportation should be appropriately certificated for use within the mode of transport it is within, and safely secured at all phases of transportation. Different standards of conformity exist globally when an air platform is used. Within Europe there is a two-part standard developed by CEN/TC 239 'rescue systems', which outlines the requirements necessary for air ambulances and medical equipment to be used aboard air ambulances.

EN 13718 (Part 1 -2008) specifies general requirements for medical devices carried in air ambulances, where the ambient conditions can differ from normal indoor conditions. This EN does not cover the requirements for approval and registration of the vehicle, or the training of the medical crew. These aspects are the responsibility of the authority/authorities in the country where the ambulance is registered.

EN 13718 (Part 2 – 2008) specifies the requirements for design, performance and equipping of air ambulances used for the transport and treatment of sick or injured persons. This European Standard is applicable to air ambulances capable of transporting at least one person on a stretcher. Requirements are specified for categories of air ambulances based on the different intended use. These are the HEMS, the helicopter intensive care medical service (HICAMS) and the fixed-wing air ambulance (FWAA).

The location of where the equipment is placed must be discussed with the driver or the pilot who will undertake load, weight and balance calculations to ensure safe performance and also that they are secured for all phases of transportation. All medical crews must be trained and certificated to use the equipment for patient care, and this equipment must be maintained by a certified engineer to the manufacturer's schedule, with clear dates when the equipment must not be used after. In addition any equipment that has a device error must be reported to the Medicines and Healthcare Regulatory Agency (MHRA), which is responsible for regulating all medicines and medical devices in the UK. Manufacturers and distributors are also licensed directly by MHRA. Medical devices are approved by private sector organisations called 'Notified Bodies'. Their approval is needed before a CE mark can be put on the device, although the manufacture of low risk devices is simply registered with the MHRA. The MHRA has overall responsibility and audits the performance of Notified Bodies.

Consideration must also be undertaken if carrying electrically powered medical equipment on a non-dedicated air ambulance platform. The airline and airport must be contacted to ensure they know you will be carrying the medical equipment and consideration taken that most airlines do not provide an aircraft electrical supply for passenger medical equipment. Therefore, there may be a requirement for it to be battery powered, which must meet the airline's requirements for carriage particularly in the case of lithium batteries.

Audit

As with any clinical department, to comply with governance (Box 28.5), regular audit of recognised standards is important to highlight areas for improvement that may have arisen, particularly with the extra challenges and considerations that patient transfer provides. Changes or protocols can be implemented in order to attempt to reach the targets set, and a completed cycle of re-audit can occur as confirmation that any change has created the desired outcome (Figure 28.1).

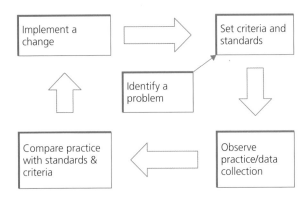

Figure 28.1 The audit cycle

Morbidity and mortality reviews

Any situation that occurs and impacts on a patient's well-being, either disease outcome or death, must have an open review of the care received, and the events that took place in order to identify any areas of concern that may require either further evaluation or 'lessons' that should be learnt for further cases of that nature. It should be in an entirely no-blame environment, and usually takes the form of a case presentation by the practitioners involved, followed by a discussion of the decisions on care made, and any resultant changes that should occur. These could be to implement an audit, perform an equipment check/service, add further items to a medical kit or such like.

Box 28.5 **Essentials: clinical governance of practice**

Revalidation & continual professional development of practitioners
Regular audit of clinical practice against desired standards
Maintenance and regulation of equipment as per legal standards
Regular morbidity and mortality review of patient care in a no-blame environment.

Ethical considerations

All care and patient intervention should be subject to consideration of a risk–benefit ratio, and whether it will result in the desired outcome in terms of care targets, patient and at times relative wishes.

Any transfer of a patient is the same from the ongoing care provided during transport to the decision to transfer the patient. There are times when transporting a patient is necessary for clinical reasons to a place able to provide necessary care of a specialist nature or where they are entitled; there are also non-clinical reasons, which may be a bed resource issue, or simply to a place such as a home country or area of abode near to a family support network. At times decisions to transfer patients can be clear cut, particularly with a stable, well patient. However, with a critical, unstable patient both the decision and the timing of a transfer must be justified as in the patient's best interests. This can sometimes not be straightforward, and may facilitate discussion between doctors, nurses, paramedics, family members and the patient if possible, in order to agree on a course that allows patient wishes, safety and medical need to be prioritised and satisfied (Box 28.6).

Box 28.6 **Essentials: ethics**

Any transfer must be in the patient's best interests
Where able, patient consent should be gained
Relatives/next of kin are often involved in decision-making
Critical patient transfer for non-clinical reasons poses dilemmas with no easy answer.

Further reading

Memorandum of understanding between the civil Aviation Authority and the Care Quality Commission.
http://www.caa.co.uk/docs/17/20110810MemorandumOfUnderstanding BetweenCAAAndCareQualityCommission.pdf
Framework for a High Performing Air Ambulance Service 2013
http://www.associationofairambulances.co.uk/resources/events/AOAA -Framework%202013-OCT13-%20Final%20Document.pdf
EURAMI Standards
http://www.eurami.org/eurami-standards-4-0/
CAMTS accreditation standards
http://www.camts.org/Approved_Stds_9th_Edition_for_website_2-13.pdf
Home Office Drug licensing
https://www.gov.uk/controlled-drugs-licences-fees-and-returns
British Standards Institution CH/239 Rescue Systems
http://standardsdevelopment.bsigroup.com/Home/Committee/50081158

CHAPTER 29

Training for Transfers

J. Warwick[1,2] *and D. Quayle*[2]

[1] Oxford University Hospitals NHS Trust, UK
[2] Air Medical Ltd, London Oxford Airport, UK

OVERVIEW

- Training for retrieval and transfer medicine should reflect the changing landscape of specialised healthcare and its growing demands

- Most Critical Care Networks in the UK hold their own generic training courses; the requirements of air ambulance organisations and specialist medical groups will build on this foundation

- Adult, postgraduate learners prefer a collaborative learning style where they are treated as colleagues and acknowledged for the skills and attributes they bring

- Continuing professional development is key to the successful expansion and progress of an organisation and its transfer teams.

Introduction

We are on the cusp of exciting times with respect to transfer and retrieval training. The increasing requirement for specialist healthcare, and the increasing centralisation of specialist services for all medical disciplines, has resulted in significant growth in patient transfer events. This chapter is based on our experience in the UK, although readers from different countries should recognise the themes and be able to relate this content to the particular regulatory environment in their own country.

The creation of Critical Care Networks (CCNs) throughout the UK has seen the development of transfer and retrieval courses by numerous hospital Trusts that has started to address this need for training. More recently, four factors will fuel the requirement for a continued expansion in this aspect of medical education for doctors:

1 the pre-hospital emergency medicine (PHEM) sub-specialty curriculum development, and the need to undertake both primary and secondary transfers as part of that process

2 the intensive care medicine (ICM) certificate of completion of training (CCT) contains a new sub-specialty module in transfer medicine

3 the provision within existing curricula (e.g. anaesthesia) for trainees to gain experience of transfer medicine

4 the creation of a Diploma in Retrieval and Transfer Medicine by the Royal College of Surgeons, Edinburgh.

This chapter will visit some important components of training for transfer and retrievals and the principles of adult learning.

Composition of the medical team

The composition and skill set of the transferring medical team should be competent to deal with any predicted complication of the patient's injury or disease process. The precise composition of this team will depend on the nature of the transfer operation and the types of patient encountered. There is a wide range of medical personnel involved in retrieval practice (Box 29.1 and Figure 29.1). In general, the dispatch of the most senior team available at the time will ensure redundancy of capabilities to manage unpredicted complications. Transfer services must therefore establish their own guidelines for minimum experience levels.

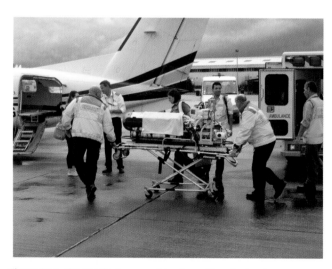

Figure 29.1 The transfer team consists of a multi-professional group.

ABC of Transfer and Retrieval Medicine, First Edition.
Edited by Adam Low and Jonathan Hulme.
© 2015 John Wiley & Sons, Ltd. Published 2015 by John Wiley & Sons, Ltd.

The role of regulatory bodies for retrieval personnel

The General Medical Council (GMC) was established in 1858 following the Medical Act and registers all doctors to practice medicine in the UK. Entitlement to practice now depends on successful 5-yearly revalidation based on evidence reviewed during annual peer appraisal. The GMC publication 'Good medical practice 2013' provides the framework that underpins the core values expected. All four domains of 'Good medical practice' are of fundamental importance to retrieval personnel:

- knowledge, skills and performance
- safety and quality
- communication, partnership and teamwork
- maintaining trust.

Clinicians have a duty to ensure that they are not engaged in work outside their areas of expertise.

In turn, the GMC is overseen by the Professional Standards Authority for Health and Social Care, established under the Social Care Act 2012, and is an independent body accountable to parliament. The Authority oversees a total of nine regulatory bodies, including the Nursing and Midwifery Council and the Health and Care Professions Council (Box 29.2).

The medical Royal Colleges in the UK provide the standard teaching framework for doctors in training. Medical transfers form a component of the syllabus for this training in disciplines such as anaesthesia, intensive care medicine and emergency medicine. In addition, specialist organisations (e.g. ICS and the AAGBI) have published important guidelines relating to transfer and retrieval practice (see Appendix 6).

The Care Quality Commission (CQC) was established in 2009 and is the independent regulator of all health and social care services in England, both NHS and private. In addition to hospitals, GP surgeries and care homes, ambulance services also came under

their responsibility from 1 April 2011. This includes air ambulance services, and it provides an important regulatory framework for their operation. The remit of the CQC is to ensure the service delivers safe, effective, compassionate and high-quality care. It does this by setting standards of quality and safety, and examines the service from the patients' perspective.

Two organisations provide voluntary accreditation of medical transport services: CAMTS was established in the USA in 1991. It audits and accredits rotary, fixed-wing and also ground ambulance services. EURAMI was established in Frankfurt for air ambulance (both rotary and fixed wing) programmes in 1992, with significant revision of its standards and accreditation process in 2013. Both are acknowledged worldwide as badges of quality.

Initial training

Most stakeholders have developed their own transfer and retrieval courses to meet local needs. A typical induction course that addresses the generic issues and teaches a systematic approach will be a 1–2 day programme, with subsequent sessions that focus on more specialised areas (Box 29.3). It is generally assumed that core medical and nursing knowledge is taught elsewhere.

The main aims are to provide candidates with the necessary knowledge and skills to manage the transfer of critically ill patients, and to avoid the common pitfalls. Considerable time, effort and expertise has been invested by clinicians to design courses to raise the standard of care for their patients requiring transfer, whether intra- or inter-hospital.

Box 29.3 **Transfer and retrieval training requirements**

Generic induction

The indications for patient transfer

Communication

Patient stabilisation and optimisation for transfer

The stressors and physiological effects of transfer

Patient preparation and packaging, familiarity with trolley/bridge systems

Monitoring and equipment

- Contents of transfer medical kit and drug bags
- Syringe pumps and volumetric fluid systems
- Transport ventilator and gas requirements

Familiarity with the transfer vehicle and loading systems

Management of complications en route

Record keeping, quality assurance and audit

Ethics of patient transfer

Aeromedical transfer

Indications for air transfer

Aeromedical physiology and its implications

Helicopter and aircraft safety

Safe patient loading and unloading

The aircraft cabin environment

Emergency procedures (including ditching and evacuation drills)

Crew resource management

Specialist patient requirements

Courses to address the requirements of specific patient groups, e.g.

Neonatal transfers

Paediatric patients

Obstetric patients

ECMO transfers

Bariatric patients

Infectious disease (e.g. H1N1 pneumonia).

Courses may consist of a series of lectures, interactive workshops, discussion groups and hi-fidelity simulation training. Although conventional medical and nurse training is often undertaken within professional groups, there is significant benefit in transfer training if learning can be accomplished together as a multiprofessional team. Training alongside medical clinicians can be motivational for nurses and paramedics; clinicians also learn from their peers in other professional groups. Team working is extremely important during transfer and joint training will help to build this dynamic.

Effective communication and learning in such multiprofessional groups will require a teaching style that:

- establishes early group rapport
- understands the job role of the receiver
- creates an open, non-threatening discussion forum
- responds rapidly and positively to points raised.

Adult, postgraduate learning theory suggests that individuals learn best in an environment that is problem-based and collaborative (Table 29.1). Scenario-based simulations are extremely useful exercises for transfer team training.

In air ambulance operations, joint training of medical crew with aircrew for subjects such as team resource management (TRM)

Table 29.1 Characteristics of adult learners.

Characteristic	Description
Autonomous and self-directed	Prefers to be actively involved in their own learning, and in directing learning goals
Brings life experiences and knowledge	Adult learners will have past experiences, knowledge and opinions
Goal orientated	Motivated to learn when they can see the need to acquire specific knowledge to address a real-life problem or situation
Relevancy orientated	Adults learn best when they can relate the task to their own goals and objectives
Practical	Will allow adult learners to apply learned theory to real life experiences and settings

and non-technical skills (NTS) can be very productive. Both the medical and aviation industries are highly pressured and regulated disciplines; the human factors involved in accidents and incidents can display many common themes. During mandatory annual ground and refresher training for air ambulance flight crew, there may be good opportunity for shared learning if TRM can be scheduled together with medical crew.

The development of hi-fidelity medical simulation has enabled realistic scenario teaching by training providers. Acute patient deterioration and medical emergencies can be simulated in patients 'en-route', and the team can rehearse how they would manage the case in real time and with their actual equipment available. In addition, team dynamics, communication, logistics and standard operating procedures can all be experienced, evaluated and developed. The post-scenario debrief for the whole group is often the most important aspect of the exercise, and requires careful and sensitive guidance from the teacher. Many simulator centres run 'train the trainer' courses that aim to equip clinicians with the necessary skills to manage debrief sessions effectively (Figure 29.2).

The challenge of continuing professional development

How do busy clinicians find the time and opportunity to keep up to date? The challenge is to incorporate a continued learning culture

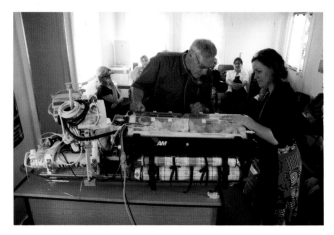

Figure 29.2 Simulation training for neonatal transfers.

into the organisation so that continuing professional development (CPD) becomes routine activity. A hallmark of professionalism is high performance through self-regulation and self-improvement that flows from a commitment to CPD.

Although each individual has responsibility for identifying, planning and undertaking CPD, the transfer/retrieval organisation also has responsibility to coordinate and resource training activity for all staff. Unfortunately, the current economic climate may place significant restrictions on this activity. The use of e-learning can improve accessibility for staff and reduce cost.

CPD is not just about attending lectures, courses and workshops. Activity that makes the most difference to practice is a culture of open dialogue, support, peer review, coaching and reflection by all team members; the leadership must encourage an ethos of continued learning. Some suggested strategies are presented in Box 29.4.

Box 29.4 Strategies for CPD

Role of the organisation
Foster a culture of continued learning
Create an annual program of CPD activity
Nominate key restrictive training and ensure compliance
Promote activities such as mentoring, shadowing and peer support

Role of the individual
Maintain a personal logbook/diary of all transfers
Reflect on each case following post-mission team debriefs
Identify areas of strength or weakness
Feedback suggestions for organised CPD events
Summarise objectives in a personal development plan
Maintain a personal database of all CPD activity

Modern learning places great emphasis on personal reflection after CPD. It should occur as soon as possible following the activity to ensure as much recollection and meaning as possible. An example of a template to facilitate the documentation of this reflection is summarised in Box 29.5.

Fitness to practice

In addition to maintaining a high standard of up-to-date knowledge and skills, personnel must be very mindful of their physical and mental health in order to be safe. Retrieval and transfer

---

Box 29.5 Reflective template for CPD activity

Title and description of activity/event
Date
Type of activity (e.g. general information, review of practice, feedback)

What have you learned?
Description of key points
Link to 'Good Medical Practice' domains (see earlier)

How has this influenced your practice?
Changes to knowledge, skills, behaviour?
Changes to personal practice?
Changes to team/organisational working practice?

Looking forward, what are your next steps?
Further development needs
Set objectives
How will objectives be met?

---

often occur during unsocial hours and the work can be arduous and exhausting. The isolated environment may place a greater need to be aware of one's physical limitations than a traditional hospital-based role (see Box 29.6). Long-haul international repatriation involving prolonged shift patterns and irregular sleep, food and drink may further impair personal fitness.

Box 29.6 Conditions that may influence fitness

Motion sickness
Acute viral illness
Traveller's diarrhoea
Stress and fatigue
Pregnancy
Chronic conditions, e.g. diabetes, epilepsy

Further reading

General Medical Council. Good Medical Practice 2013. Available at: www.gmc-uk.org/static/documents/content/GMP_2013.pdf_51447599.pdf.

General Medical Council. Continuing Professional Development: guidance for all doctors, June 2012. Available at: www.gmc-uk.org/CPD_guidance_June_12.pdf_48970799.pdf.

Knowles M, Holton EF III,, Swanson RA. *The Adult Learner: The definitive classic in adult education and human resource development* (6th ed). Burlington, MA: Elsevier, 2005.

Section 6

Neonatal and Paediatric Transfers

CHAPTER 30

Anatomical and Physiological Considerations

S. Revanna

Kids Intensive Care & Decision Support, Birmingham Children's Hospital, West Midlands, UK

> **OVERVIEW**
>
> - Neonates and children differ from adults anatomically and physiologically
> - Awareness of these changes allow for safe management during transfer
> - Practitioners must know normal physiological variables to appreciate abnormality.

Introduction

Children are not small adults: they vary enormously both anatomically and physiologically from birth to 16 years of age. It can be daunting for a healthcare professional to manage this diverse group of patients safely and competently. It is the aim of this chapter to describe the anatomical/physiological differences with emphasis on differences in airway, breathing and circulation. For ease of better understanding, neonates are considered separately in this chapter.

Airway

The anatomy of a young child's airway differs in many respects from that of an adult, impacting on airway manoeuvres and intubation.

The infant's tongue is large in proportion to the mouth, thus more easily obstructing the airway. The relatively larger head with prominent occiput and a short neck makes airway management more challenging. The head should be maintained in the neutral position for intubation (Figure 30.1).

The small oral cavity with large tongue and large, posterior placed epiglottis may make the Cormack and Lehane view at intubation difficult. There may also be loose deciduous teeth. The high anterior larynx in infants means it may be easier to intubate this age group using a straight blade. The larynx is funnel shaped and the airway is at its narrowest at the cricoid cartilage. The epithelium is loosely bound to the connective tissue underneath, making it prone

to oedema. Care should be taken to allow for some leak if using an uncuffed endotracheal tube.

The trachea is short and soft which makes tube displacement easy. Always confirm tube position with X-ray and ensure the tube is securely strapped pre-transfer.

Breathing

The lungs are relatively immature at birth with fewer and smaller alveoli. After birth, alveoli rapidly multiply from 20 million saccules to 300 million by 8 years of age. Thereafter alveolar expansion is mainly by increase in size. Because of the smaller alveolar surface area there is reduced gas exchange and children can tire more easily. Smaller alveolar radius predisposes to collapse, thus in a mechanically ventilated child it is very important to provide external PEEP.

In children both upper and lower airways are small and can get easily obstructed with secretions. The airway enlarges in diameter and length with age but the growth of distal airways lag behind proximal, during the first 5 years of life. As resistance to flow is inversely proportional to the fourth power of the radius (Poiseuille's law – see Chapter 19) seemingly mild obstructions can cause significant difficulty in ventilation.

Compliant chest wall with immature intercostal and diaphragm muscles (fewer fatigue-resistant type 1 fibres) makes them more prone to exhaustion and respiratory failure. They are unable to increase tidal volume and so minute volume is altered predominantly by respiratory rate (Table 30.1 and Box 30.1).

Note – do not wait for the child to be exhausted or near collapse to intubate, intervene earlier.

Table 30.1 Normal values by age (APLS 4th edition).

Age (years)	Resp rate (breath/min)	Systolic BP (mmHg)		Pulse (beats/minute)
		50th centile	5th centile	
<1	30–40	80–90	65–75	110–160
1–2	25–35	85–95	70–75	100–150
2–5	25–30	85–100	70–80	95–140
5–12	20–25	90–110	80–90	80–120
>12	15–20	100–120	90–105	60–100

Source: Advanced Paediatric Life Support: The Practical Approach, 5th Edition (2011) John Wiley & Sons, Oxford.

ABC of Transfer and Retrieval Medicine, First Edition.
Edited by Adam Low and Jonathan Hulme.
© 2015 John Wiley & Sons, Ltd. Published 2015 by John Wiley & Sons, Ltd.

Box 30.1 **Endotracheal tube size in relation to age.**

Internal diameter of ETT – *uncuffed* = (age ÷ 4) + 4
Internal diameter of ETT – *cuffed* = (age ÷ 4) + 3.5
Oral - Length of ETT (in cm) at lips = (age ÷ 2) + 12
Nasal - Length of ETT (in cm) at nares = (age ÷ 2) + 15

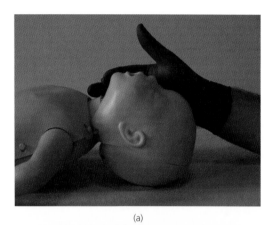

(a)

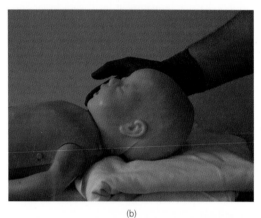

(b)

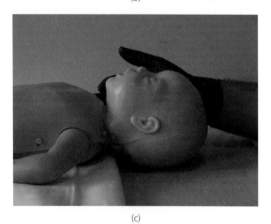

(c)

Figure 30.1 Correct positioning of the neonate/infant's head for airway management. (a) The head is too flexed (due to the large head) and airway occluded. (b) The head is over extended, the airway will be difficult to manage (c) Optimal positioning in the neutral position. A towel or sheet under the shoulders as shown may help with positioning. (Source: With thanks to Paul Slater, West Midlands CARE Team).

Circulation

At birth the ventricles are small, there is decreased sympathetic innervation, decreased β- adrenoceptor concentration and fewer contractile elements in the cardiac myocytes. Cardiac output is mainly dependent on increasing heart rate. Ionised calcium plays a central role in the maintenance of myocardial contractility. Deficiency in intracellular calcium contributes significantly to myocardial dysfunction and therapeutic manipulations of these parameters can directly influence the force of contraction. Myocardial contractility increases over the first few months of life, as do the numbers of sympathetic nerve fibres within the myocardium and the total concentration of endogenous noradrenaline (norepinephrine).

In low cardiac output states, commonly used inotropes are dopamine, adrenaline and noradrenaline. It is important to note that sustained use of catecholamines can lead to down regulation of β-receptors and therefore decrease in the efficacy of catecholamines (Table 30.2).

Vascular access

Children have small blood vessels buried under thick pads of subcutaneous tissue; vascular access can be challenging. Any attempts at siting a peripheral cannula should be restricted to three and intraosseous access should be obtained early. **All drugs including inotropes can be given intraosseously.**

Neurology

It can be challenging to assess neurology in a young child. In a child with altered level of consciousness, age-appropriate Glasgow Coma Scales should be used. Infants and children have limited glycogen stores and higher metabolic demands, thus are prone to develop hypoglycaemia quickly. Glucose level should be checked early and maintenance fluid should contain dextrose.

Sedation and muscle relaxants

Sedation for ventilated children is usually achieved with morphine infusion, and midazolam is added for children over 6 months of age. Propofol is not routinely used in critically ill children due to the risk of developing propofol infusion syndrome. Use of a muscle relaxant infusion for transfer is recommended to aid ventilation and prevent accidental dislodgement of the endotracheal tube by coughing/movement.

Psychological considerations

Children vary enormously with their emotional response. Infants less than 6 months of age are not usually upset by separation from

Table 30.2 Variation of normal blood volume with age.

Age	Blood volume
Newborn	85–90 mL/kg
6 weeks to 2 years	85 mL/kg
2 years to puberty	80 mL/kg

PAEDIATRIC GLASGOW COMA SCALE (PGCS)			
	> 1 Year	**< 1 Year**	**Score**
EYE OPENING	Spontaneously	Spontaneously	4
	To verbal command	To shout	3
	To pain	To pain	2
	No response	No response	1
MOTOR RESPONSE	Obeys	Spontaneous	6
	Localizes pain	Localizes pain	5
	Flexion-withdrawal	Flexion-withdrawal	4
	Flexion-abnormal (decorticate rigidity)	Flexion-abnormal (decorticate rigidity)	3
	Extension (decerebrate rigidity)	Extension (decerebrate rigidity)	2
	No response	No response	1
	> 5 Years	**2-5 Years**	**0-23 months**	
VERBAL RESPONSE	Oriented	Appropriate words/phrases	Smiles/coos appropriately	5
	Disoriented/confused	Inappropriate words	Cries and is consolable	4
	Inappropriate words	Persistent cries and screams	Persistent inappropriate crying and/or screaming	3
	Incomprehensible sounds	Grunts	Grunts, agitated, and restless	2
	No response	No response	No response	1
TOTAL PAEDIATRIC GLASGOW COMA SCORE (3-15):			

Figure 30.2 Age-appropriate Glasgow Coma Scores.

their parents and will more readily accept a stranger. Children up to 4 years of age are upset by the separation from their parents, unfamiliar people and surroundings. School age children are more upset by the surgical procedure, its mutilating effects and the possibility of pain. Adolescents fear narcosis and pain, the loss of control and the possibility of not being able to cope with the illness. Age appropriate communication is essential.

Other important differences

Weight
The average birth weight of a neonate is 3.5 kg, by the end of 1 year an infant triples the birth weight, and there is a pubertal growth spurt during adolescence.

In emergency situations where it is not possible to weigh the child, weight can be calculated using the formulae in Table 30.3.

Fontanellae
The fontanellae, commonly known as the soft spot, is an anatomical feature of an infant's skull. It comprises of a membranous gap between the incompletely formed cranial bones. It is present to facilitate rapid brain growth in infancy.

The anterior fontanel is located between the growing frontal and the parietal bones. It is the largest, diamond shaped and most used in clinical assessment. It closes between 18 months to 2 years of age, the posterior fontanel located near the occiput closes at 2–3 months of age and the smaller sphenoid and mastoid fontanellae between 6–12 months of age.

Clinical significance of fontanellae:

- bulging anterior fontanel: think of raised ICP
- depressed anterior fontanel: think of dehydration (Table 30.4)
- delayed closure/large fontanellae: hypothyroidism, rickets, hydrocephalus, IUGR
- early closure of fontanellae: craniosynostosis.

Temperature regulation
Owing to a high body surface area to weight ratio, children lose heat quickly. They also have an immature hypothalamic system and less able to compensate for extremes of temperature. Temperature

Table 30.3 Calculations to estimate weight according to age.

Weight	Formula
0–12 months	Weight (in kg) = (0.5 × age in months) + 4
1–5 years	Weight (in kg) = (2 × age in years) + 8
6–12 years	Weight (in kg) = (3 × age in years) + 7

Table 30.4 Segar and Holliday calculation of maintenance fluid requirements in 24 hours.

<10 kg	100 mL/kg
10–20 kg	50 mL/kg
>20 kg	20 mL/kg

should be closely monitored and any non-physiological variations promptly managed.

Renal system

Renal blood flow and glomerular filtration are low in the first 2 years of life due to high renal vascular resistance. Tubular function is immature until 8 months so infants are unable to excrete a large sodium load. Urea, creatinine and serum electrolytes should be closely monitored in a critically ill child and maintenance fluid calculated.

Urine output should be monitored and targeted at 1–2 mL/kg/h.

Hepatic function

Liver function is initially immature with decreased function of hepatic enzymes. Barbiturates and opioids for example have a longer duration of action due to the slower metabolism.

Immune function

At birth the immune function is poor and young infants are prone for infection. In the first 6 months maternal antibodies acquired across the placenta provide some protection. As the immune system matures these antibodies are replaced. Babies who are breastfed have better protection against respiratory and gastrointestinal infections.

Additional special considerations in neonates

Foetal circulation

In the foetal period the lungs are not expanded and gas exchange occurs through the placenta. Oxygenated blood from the placenta flows through the umbilical vein into the IVC via the ductus venosus; 30% of this oxygen-rich blood passes through the foramen ovale into LV through LA and supplies the coronaries and the brain. The venous blood from the SVC drains into the aorta through right ventricle, pulmonary artery and ductus arteriosus.

Changes in the circulation at birth

At birth, with the first breath, the lungs expand, pulmonary vascular resistance (PVR) falls and blood flows through the pulmonary arteries. With increase in pulmonary venous return there is an increase in left atrial pressure and the foramen ovale closes. The rise in oxygen tension closes the ductus arteriosus and over the ensuing weeks there is a drop in PVR.

In vaginal deliveries, as the baby passes through the birth canal, squeezing of the chest results in better drainage of the lung fluid via lymphatics. This aids in the initial expansion of the lungs. With the lung expansion and drop in PVR, there is reduced ventilation perfusion mismatch.

Breathing

Neonates preferentially breathe through their nose; the narrow nasal passage may be easily obstructed by secretions or damaged by nasogastric tubes.

Minimal handling

Particularly in preterm infants excessive handling can make them stressed, leading to desaturations, apnoea, bradycardia and vasoconstriction.

Temperature regulation

Babies have minimal subcutaneous fat stores, are unable to shiver to generate heat and tend to lose heat rapidly because of the large surface area to body weight ratio. Hypothermia is a serious, yet easily preventable complication.

Simple measures like minimising exposure during procedures, removing any wet blanket and where appropriate use of polythene wrapping, socks, hats and gloves to keep them covered helps in preventing this. Central temperature should be monitored at all times. Consider infant heating mattresses/ incubator for transfer.

Fluid and electrolytes

Neonates have immature kidneys; their capacity to concentrate urine or excrete sodium and water loads is limited. This makes them easily susceptible to fluid overload and dehydration. Gestational age and weight appropriate maintenance fluid should be given.

Pain and analgesia

Neonates suffer pain: analgesia and sedation should be used before intubation, and for painful procedures like arterial line insertion. Morphine is an effective analgesic with sedative properties and widely used in neonatal intensive care and transport.

Immunity

Neonates, particularly preterms, have deficiency in both cellular and humoral immunity. A high index of suspicion for infection should be maintained, and where necessary, appropriate antibiotics used. Preterm neonates are particularly susceptible to necrotising enterocolitis.

Haematology

At birth the predominant haemoglobin is HbF, it binds avidly to oxygen but releases it slowly, hence at birth babies are relatively polycythaemic (Hb 18–20 gm/dL). There is also deficiency of vitamin K-dependent clotting factor (remember to check that a newborn has received vitamin K at birth, which prevents haemorrhagic disease of the newborn).

Further reading

Advanced Paediatric Life Support: The Practical Approach (APLS) 5th Edition
Roberton's Textbook of Neonatology. Elsevier Science Health Science Division, 4th edition.
Roger's Textbook of Paediatric Intensive Care. Lippincott Williams & Wilkins, 4th edition.
Paediatric Cardiac Intensive Care. Chang, Hanley, Wernovsky.
Paediatric Intensive Care (Oxford Specialist Handbooks in Paediatrics). Barry, Morris, Ali.

CHAPTER 31

Neonatal Medical Transfers

Lesley Jackson

West of Scotland Neonatal Transport Service, Yorkhill Hospital, UK

OVERVIEW

- Neonates require transfer to specialist centres for various clinical indications, ranging from complications of prematurity to specialist management of congenital anomalies. Such transfers can be required on an emergency or elective basis
- Knowledge of neonatal physiology and the circulatory changes during the transition from the *in utero* to *ex utero* environment are fundamental to understanding the principles of clinical management
- Neonatal transport requires the combination of practical procedural abilities and good diplomacy skills which are necessary to promote consistent communication between families and clinicians across different centres.

Introduction

Centralised neonatal services and Managed Clinical Networks (MCNs) throughout the UK have promoted regional neonatal transport service development. When clinical care beyond local expertise is required, transfer to another unit with appropriate clinical skills and equipment for ongoing care becomes necessary. Neonatal transport seeks to emulate the neonatal intensive care unit environment, aiming to provide seamless clinical care from the referring hospital to the destination unit.

Infants requiring tertiary-level care can require transfer on an emergency or elective basis for medical, surgical or postpartum complications beyond the remit of the referring unit. The most frequent clinical reasons for *emergency* neonatal transport are outlined below.

Prematurity

Premature infants delivered from borderline viability (23–24 weeks) to 28 weeks gestation for tertiary-level intensive care management. Stabilisation prior to and during transfer can be challenging and complex. Issues requiring consideration include the following.

Respiratory support

Intubation, ventilation and exogenous surfactant administration to improve pulmonary compliance is often required in respiratory distress syndrome (RDS), a common condition complicating prematurity characterised by a 'ground glass' CXR appearance (Figure 31.1).

Clinical indications prompting decision to intubate are further summarized in Box 31.1. ETT position must be confirmed radiologically. Ventilation modes are summarised in Box 31.2.

Oxygen carrying capacity

A haemoglobin concentration >12 g/dL should be maintained to maximise oxygen delivery. Red cell transfusion may be required.

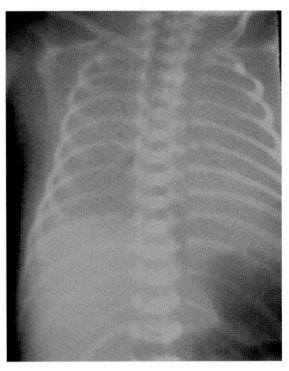

Figure 31.1 Chest X-ray appearance of RDS (ground glass appearance with air bronchograms).

ABC of Transfer and Retrieval Medicine, First Edition.
Edited by Adam Low and Jonathan Hulme.
© 2015 John Wiley & Sons, Ltd. Published 2015 by John Wiley & Sons, Ltd.

Vascular access

Central line insertion (venous and arterial umbilical catheters) for haemodynamic management, drug administration and ventilatory monitoring requires technical skills. Confirm line placement radiographically pre-transfer and document line position.

Cardiovascular support

Maintaining mean systemic blood pressure $\geq$ gestational age (in weeks) in the first day of life is accepted good practice. Inotropes are frequently required to achieve this. Cardiovascular parameters, tissue perfusion, urine output and serum lactate require monitoring.

Neurological assessment

Cranial USS to assess for intraventicular haemorrhage (IVH) influences the decision to transfer and prognosis. *Ex utero* transfer is known to increase the risk of IVH in extremely immature neonates.

Necrotising enterocolitis

Premature infants may require emergency transfer for assessment of necrotising enterocolitis. Abdominal distension, with potential bowel perforation, impairs gas exchange and haemodynamic stability. Discussing drain insertion with neonatal surgeons and adjusting ventilator settings can optimise ventilation. Sepsis is common and broad-spectrum antibiotic cover is advised. Analgesia is essential and IV morphine is required pre-transfer.

Term infants with respiratory failure

Term infants with respiratory failure can require consideration of extracorporeal life support (ECLS). Transport teams require an awareness of the location of ECLS centres and their facilities/equipment.

Meconium aspiration syndrome

Meconium aspiration syndrome (MAS) typically affects postmature infants and is associated with ventilation/perfusion mismatch and a pneumothorax risk through excessive pulmonary expansion. Such infants require sedation and muscle relaxation for transfer. Treatment with exogenous surfactant (200 mg/kg) and aiming for a mean systemic pressure >50 mmHg, which may require inotropes, may reduce the development of persistent pulmonary hypertension of the newborn (PPHN). Hydrocortisone (2 mg/kg bd) can be administered for hypotension but takes several hours to become effective.

PPHN when present is often severe. Echocardiography, to quantify pulmonary and systemic pressures, is diagnostic and provides knowledge of ductal flow. Inhaled nitric oxide (iNO) commenced at 20 ppm and titrated can reduce the need for ECLS in term infants with MAS, but methaemoglobin monitoring is required, accepting a concentration of <2%. Methylene blue can be administered if methaemoglobinaemia develops.

Sepsis

Sepsis, most frequently caused by Group B *Streptococcus*, is often complicated by hypotension and coagulopathy. Antibiotics should be administered to all infants with respiratory distress prior to transfer based upon local sensitivities.

Hypoxic ischaemic encephalopathy

When hypoxic ischaemic encephalopathy (HIE) is confirmed using standard criteria, inducing systemic hypothermia for 72 hours (target rectal temperature 33.5°C) improves outcomes in term/

near-term infants. Bradycardia (80–90 beats/minute) is expected at target temperatures. Monitoring alarms require limits adjusted during transport. Sedation is mandatory during cooling. Seizures may require phenobarbital or phenytoin and cerebral function monitoring provides additional prognostic information during transport. Coexistent hepatic and renal injury are common and cardiovascular support is often required.

Congenital anomalies

Centrally cyanosed newborns may have congenital cardiac anomalies. Echocardiography can provide a provisional diagnosis to inform discussions with Paediatric Cardiology. Increasingly, neonatal units have access to telemedicine links that can be utilised by transfer teams and paediatric cardiologists to assist in management decisions.

Transposition of the great vessels
Circulation is dependent on the patent ductus arteriosus (PDA) and foramen ovale (PFO). Ductal patency should be maintained with a prostaglandin infusion (Dinoprostone, 5 ng/kg/min). Where possible, avoid intubation. Emergency septostomy may be indicated when echocardiography suggests an intact atrial septum. In such cases communication is essential between the transport team and the paediatric cardiology service as septostomy may be necessary prior to transfer.

Hypoplastic left heart syndrome
These clinically complex cases involve balancing systemic and pulmonary circulation flow, avoiding pulmonary hyperperfusion and consequent systemic hypoperfusion. Central access is required for infusions and monitoring. Maintain ductal patency via a prostaglandin infusion (Dinoprostone, 5 ng/kg/min) and avoid intubation as this further unbalances the pulmonary and systemic circulations, (accepting target $PaCO_2$ 7–8 kPa and target oxygen saturations 75–80%). Systemic vasodilators (Milrinone, sodium nitroprusside) may be used when peripheral perfusion deteriorates, indicated by a pink baby with oxygen saturations >90%, a rising serum lactate and worsening base deficit. Monitoring haemodynamics with near infrared spectrophotometry (NIRS) may benefit this group of patients during transport.

Surgical

Congenital diaphragmatic hernia
Congenital diaphragmatic hernia (CDH) babies are often profoundly hypoxic and ECLS may be required. If not already established by the referring centre, immediate intubation, sedation, muscle relaxation and decompression of the gut via nasogastric tube are indicated prior to transfer. CDH lungs are at risk of pneumothorax and a 'gentilation' ventilation strategy (tidal volumes 3–4 mL/kg vs. 6–8 mL/kg in other infants) is recommended. Mean systemic blood pressures >50 mmHg should be the aim in term infants. PPHN, defined as pre/post-ductal oxygen saturation difference of >5% (frequently >20%) commonly complicates CDH. Inhaled nitric oxide is of benefit.

Anterior abdominal wall defects such as gastroschisis (Figure 31.2)
Defects should be carefully inspected. Signs of ischaemia (black, poorly perfused bowel) should prompt urgent neonatal surgical advice and enlarging defects to restore bowel perfusion may be recommended before transfer. Urgent transfer, aiming for neonatal surgical review by age 4 hours is desirable. Infant position during stabilisation and transport is important: nursing the neonate right-side down relieves pressure on the mesentery. A nasogastric tube should be passed and 'cling film' applied to the lesion to maintain temperature and reduce fluid loss. Avoid saline soaks. Maintain circulatory volume during stabilisation and transfer by replacing estimated volume fluid losses from the defect, monitoring trends in capillary perfusion, toe/core temperature gap and serum lactate. Losses of 20–60 mL/kg are common in the first 6 hours of life.

Neural tube defects
Assess lower limb neurological, anal and bladder function. Cover the lesion (Mepitel dressings), prescribing antibiotics as per local protocol if CSF is leaking. Early transfer to a neonatal surgical centre is indicated with the infant nursed prone for transfer with appropriate monitoring.

Term infants with bilious vomiting
Malrotation or volvulus should be assumed until proven negative by contrast studies. The gut should be decompressed with a nasogastric tube, systemic perfusion assessed and indicators of tissue perfusion (e.g. lactate) monitored. Management is time-critical and antibiotics should be administered to cover for sepsis.

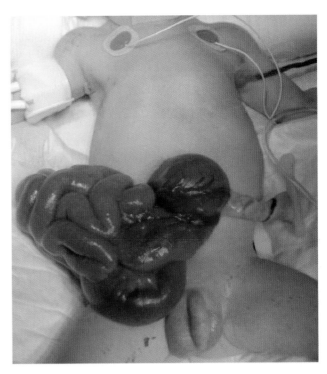

Figure 31.2 Infant with gastroschisis.

Oesophageal atresia and/or tracheo-oesophageal fistula

A Replogle tube (Sherwood Medical, Tullamore, Ireland) should be placed in the blind-ending oesophagus. These double-lumen tubes have a lumen for aspirating oesophageal contents and another irrigation channel to loosen secretions. Infants with tracheo-oesophageal fistula (TOF) are usually stable and should be positioned slightly head-up during transfer to minimise aspiration of excessive secretions. Ventilation should be avoided unless comorbidity exists: ventilation when a distal fistula is present can lead to abdominal distension, diaphragmatic 'splinting' and worsening respiratory distress. An abdominal drain may be required if respiratory embarrassment develops, in this situation discussion should take place with the neonatal surgical team prior to insertion. Associated congenital anomalies, such as anal atresia, radial anomalies and hemivertebrae are common and merit careful clinical examination.

In utero transfers

Wherever clinical circumstances permit *in utero* transfer (IUT) is preferable to an *ex utero* transfer (EUT) following birth. A considered and coordinated approach is vital in the organisation of IUTs and EUTs to ensure efficient and appropriate neonatal intensive care cots use. These transfers are discussed further in Chapter 38.

Repatriation or 'back to base' transfers

Neonates are moved back to their base hospital for ongoing care on an elective basis when specialist care is complete. Elective transfers require careful communication and planning to ensure the family and base hospital teams are prepared.

Elective transfers

Neonates are regularly electively moved between hospitals for pre-arranged surgery and investigations such as MRI and EEG. Such transfers are normally booked well in advance.

Neonatal transport-specific issues to consider

Thermal control

Extremely premature infants may weigh <600 g at birth, with immature skin prone to large insensible losses of up to 40 mL/kg. These excessive losses persist over the first week of life in extremely premature infants.

Thermal control during transport can be difficult due to environmental conditions. Servo-controlled incubators, chemical mattresses (e.g. Transwarmers, Advanced Health Technology, Herts, UK) and humidification can be utilised to maintain thermal control. Table 31.1 summarises suggested incubator temperature settings for neonates by gestation and weight.

Therapeutic hypothermia during transfers

Trials have demonstrated neurodevelopmental and survival benefits from 72 hours of controlled hypothermia in term infants with

Table 31.1 Suggested initial incubator settings for neonates.

Weight	Initial temperature setting (°C)
>2500 g	33
1500–2500 g	35
1000–1500 g	36
<1000 g	39

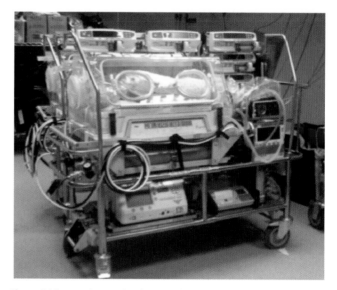

Figure 31.3 Intensive care incubator with servo-control cooling equipment.

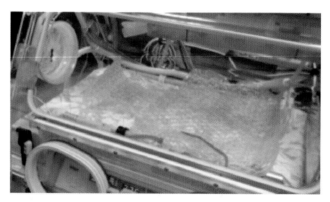

Figure 31.4 Cooling mattress for systemic hypothermia during transport.

hypoxic-ischaemic encephalopathy (HIE). Controlled systemic hypothermia is recommended by NICE and the BAPM but requires prompt initiation (within 6 hours of delivery or preferably earlier) for best efficacy and is therefore best commenced by referring institutions before transport team arrival. 'Passive' cooling may be beneficial in units not offering this technology. Transport teams now have servo-controlled cooling equipment to deliver hypothermia during transfer (Figures 31.3 and 31.4).

Further reading

Barry P, Leslie A. *Paediatric and Neonatal Critical Care Transport*. London BMJ Publishing Group, 2003.

Bowman E, Doyle LW, Murton LJ, Roy RN, Kitchen WH. Increased mortality of preterm infants transferred between tertiary perinatal centres. BMJ 1988;297:1098–100.

British Association of Perinatal Medicine. Standards for hospitals providing neonatal intensive care and high dependency care and categories of babies requiring neonatal care. 3rd ed. London: British Association of Perinatal Medicine, 2011. (www.bapm-London.org).

Fenton A, Leslie A, Skeoch C. Optimising neonatal transfer. Arch Dis Child Fetal Neonatal Ed 2004;89:F215–19.

Parmanum J, Field D, Rennie J, et al. National census of availability of neonatal intensive care. BMJ 2000;321:727–9.

Position Statement on therapeutic cooling for neonatal encephalopathy. British Association of Perinatal Medicine, 2010.

CHAPTER 32

Paediatric Medical Retrievals

S. Ray and E. Polke

Children's Acute Transport Service, Great Ormond Street Hospital for Children NHS Trust, London, UK

OVERVIEW

- The transfer environment exposes the infant/child and team to an additional risk of incidents
- Application of specific clinical guidelines to the stabilisation and transport environment is beneficial
- Ideally there should be local policy for the transfer of such patients
- The risk–benefit ratio of local versus specialist transfer team must be considered
- Adequate preparation prior to transport will prevent/reduce critical incidents and ensure safe transfer of critically ill children.

Introduction

The majority of paediatric intensive care transfers in the UK are undertaken by specialist intensive care transport teams. There are however occasions when non-specialist teams will be required to expedite the transport of an acutely unwell child (e.g. neurosurgical emergency/surgical abdomen), where time is of the essence.

Preparing for transport

The principles of safe transfer of children are not different from those described for adults.

Specific consideration must be made to calculating age/weight-specific drug doses and equipment sizes that may be needed in transit.

Mechanically ventilated children

Children needing ventilatory support need careful preparation for transport.

If the child is already intubated it is important to ensure that you are prepared for reintubation (Box 32.1). Ensure that you have the capacity to hand ventilate the child using either a self-inflating bag or, if trained in its use, an Ayres T-piece, with a correct size face

---

ABC of Transfer and Retrieval Medicine, First Edition.
Edited by Adam Low and Jonathan Hulme.
© 2015 John Wiley & Sons, Ltd. Published 2015 by John Wiley & Sons, Ltd.

Box 32.1 **The following items should be carried ready to hand when transferring a ventilated child**

Correct size endotracheal tube (including a smaller and larger size)
Introducer/guide/bougie
Lubricating gel
Guedel airway
Magills forceps
Laryngoscope handle and appropriate blade(s)
Suction catheters
Securing device/tapes, scissors

---

mask attached to a full cylinder of oxygen. Always test your cylinder prior to transfer ensuring it is turned on and remember to turn it off when not in use.

Troubleshooting

If there is a sudden change in ventilation status during transfer, a systematic approach must be used to diagnose the problem. The mnemonic DOPES is a useful aide memoir.

D displaced ETT
O obstructed ETT – try physiotherapy and suction down the ETT
P pneumothorax
E equipment problems: check gas supply and ventilator including tubing
S stomach: non-invasive and bag-mask ventilation will inflate the stomach and compromise diaphragmatic excursion, increasing the risk of aspiration of stomach contents in an unprotected airway. The child must have a nasogastric tube, aspirated and on free drainage.

Common paediatric problems needing transport

Respiratory distress

Respiratory problems are the commonest reasons for children needing an emergency transfer to an intensive care unit. The disease process may involve the upper airway (croup), large airways (asthma), small airways (bronchiolitis) or alveoli (pneumonia).

Key points

- In severe upper airway obstruction the most senior anaesthetist, paediatrician and ENT surgeon should be available to secure the airway. It is safest to use a gas induction, even though this may require a transfer to the operating theatre
- Higher ventilator pressures may be necessary if a smaller than expected tube size is needed for upper airway obstruction. Viral croup may have a component of small airways disease, so wheeze may also be concurrent – try bronchodilators
- In asthma, venous return can be compromised with lung hyperinflation and vasodilation during anaesthetic induction. Adequate circulatory resuscitation is therefore essential
- In asthma and occasionally in bronchiolitis, mechanical ventilation can become difficult with air trapping. Ventilation should be adjusted to deliver a low I:E ratio (**low rate** to allow a long expiratory time). The rate should be adjusted allow the capnograph to plateau (Figure 32.1)
- A pneumothorax can cause a sudden cardiovascular and respiratory deterioration. Teams should have equipment for emergency thoracocentesis readily available at all times as this can be life saving
- Cuffed endotracheal tubes should be considered if difficult ventilation is anticipated.

Circulatory shock

Circulatory shock is common in critically ill children. Sepsis is the commonest aetiology of circulatory shock. Myocarditis or cardiomyopathy are rare, but the management is slightly different. Acute crises in sickle cell disease may present with dissociative shock, which will need specialist management (therefore seek appropriate telephone advice if unsure).

Key points

- The management of sepsis needs to be prompt and aggressive. The American College of Critical Care Medicine (ACCM) paediatric life support guideline puts a timeline on the fluid resuscitation of children that should be followed with continued reassessment. The aim is to reverse shock: failure to do so increases the likelihood of death
- Inotropes should be started early (after 40 mL/kg of fluid), especially if there are signs of myocardial dysfunction (hepatomegaly or developing pulmonary oedema)
- Intubation and ventilation should be undertaken early for haemodynamic management (even though the child may still be alert). Delaying intubation will lead to a more hazardous induction later
- Resuscitation doses of adrenaline should be prepared in advance, and fluid should be drawn up.

Ventilation with PEEP is necessary to prevent ongoing pulmonary oedema.

- If shock is resistant to fluid and inotropes a 1–2 mg/kg of hydrocortisone should be considered (but there is not adequate evidence to support this routinely currently.)
- Antimicrobials are needed for definitive therapy if sepsis is suspected. A broad spectrum cephalosporin will provide adequate empirical cover for most children. Aciclovir and a macrolide should be considered in addition if encephalitis is suspected. In neonates acyclovir and amoxicillin should be considered as they are more susceptible to herpes simplex and listeria infection
- Myocarditis/cardiomyopathy can be very difficult to distinguish from children with sepsis. Continued fluid resuscitation will not reverse shock and is likely to be detrimental. *Hepatomegaly and pulmonary oedema in response to a small volume of fluid is a good indicator of a failing heart.* Cardiomegaly on chest X-ray, when present, may suggest primary cardiac pathology, but has a poor negative predictive value
- Arrhythmias are not uncommon in the failing heart. A defibrillator must be available for transfer and preferably pads should be applied on the chest in preparation
- Children with acute sickle crises may need aggressive treatment as the crisis may rapidly evolve. A blood transfusion may be necessary to slow the sickling, and may need to be given en route.

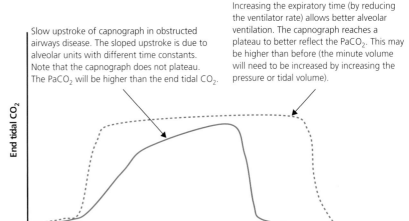

Figure 32.1 Capnograph pattern in a child with obstructed airways disease (asthma, bronchiolitis). The dotted line shows difference once the expiratory time has been increased, along with an increase in minute ventilation using the pre-set peak pressure or tidal volume.

Slow upstroke of capnograph in obstructed airways disease. The sloped upstroke is due to alveolar units with different time constants. Note that the capnograph does not plateau. The $PaCO_2$ will be higher than the end tidal CO_2.

Increasing the expiratory time (by reducing the ventilator rate) allows better alveolar ventilation. The capnograph reaches a plateau to better reflect the $PaCO_2$. This may be higher than before (the minute volume will need to be increased by increasing the pressure or tidal volume).

A risk benefit assessment may need to be made according to the clinical situation regarding waiting for cross matched blood or using emergency universal donor blood. Oxygenation and hydration needs to be maintained.

Abnormal neurology

Abnormal neurology can present as a part of any critical illness. Status epilepticus is a common presentation in children. The need for intensive care arises in order to protect the airway, when airway protective reflexes are lost, and to control intracranial pressure (ICP), by controlling physiological parameters closely.

Patients with abnormal neurology also need intra-hospital transfer for brain imaging. CT scans are quick, but CT scanners provide an unfamiliar environment with restricted access to the patient. MRI should not be used as a scanning modality in an emergency, as ventilated patients need specialist monitoring, equipment and personnel to facilitate the scan, and access to the patient can be very restricted.

The aim is to 'neuroprotect' these children. As in adults, this involves:

- maintaining adequate perfusion and oxygenation to the brain
- the adequate drainage of blood and cerebrospinal fluid from the brain
- reducing the cerebral metabolic rate.

This is achieved in the same way as in adults. The specific cerebral perfusion pressure targets for children are set out in Box 32.2.

Box 32.2 **The cerebral perfusion pressure (CPP = mean arterial blood pressure – intracranial pressure) targets**

55 mm Hg in infants
60 mm Hg in pre-school age children
70 mm Hg in older children
If the ICP cannot be measured, but is likely to be raised, estimate it as 20 mmHg.

Key points

- Pupils should be examined frequently for any changes
- The conscious level may fluctuate: if the GCS is ever less than 8, the patient should be intubated and neuroprotected
- The benefits of paralysing the child (ICP control, preventing accidental extubation) outweigh the risk of being unable to monitor neurology during transfer
- Children with traumatic brain injury should be managed along the same principles as adults, within the local trauma network. If there is any suspicion of the ICP rising (relative bradycardia and hypertension and/or pupillary changes), then aim to reduce it with:

  ◦ boluses of opioids or sedatives
  ◦ 2.7% sodium chloride (2–5 mL/kg) or mannitol (0.5 g/kg)
  ◦ hyperventilation will decrease the ICP albeit by reducing cerebral blood flow – this can be used temporarily if brainstem herniation is imminent.

- If urgent neurosurgical intervention is needed, it is usually quicker for a team from the local hospital to transfer the child to the neurosurgical centre, rather than waiting for a specialist retrieval team. While the decision is being made, the local team should prepare for transfer. The team should take 2.7% sodium chloride or mannitol for use en route in case of impending brainstem herniation
- Non-accidental injury (NAI) must be considered as a possible cause for the brain injury, especially in younger children
- For suspected inborn errors of metabolism, check the glucose, ammonia and lactate levels to help with a possible diagnosis. Correct hypoglycaemia with a bolus of 10% glucose followed by a dextrose infusion (however avoid hypotonic solutions – children with metabolic encephalopathy are at risk of cerebral oedema). Hyperammonaemia (ammonia >150 mmol/L) needs urgent treatment – liaise early with your local metabolic team.

Fluid and electrolyte imbalances

Diabetic ketoacidosis is the commonest metabolic derangement in children necessitating transfer to a HDU or ICU setting.

Key points

- The risk of cerebral oedema in paediatric diabetic ketoacidosis is high. The level of acidosis may be very severe but the aim is to correct parameters slowly. Most children will hyperventilate to compensate for their metabolic acidosis. Mechanical ventilation should be avoided if possible as this compensatory mechanism is taken away
- Dehydration should be corrected slowly over 48 or 72 hours. Fluid boluses should be kept to a minimum (less than 30 mL/kg total)
- Insulin should be started as an infusion (0.05–0.1 units/kg/hour) after rehydration has been started. Boluses should not be given
- 0.9% sodium chloride should be used, with added potassium (as the serum potassium will drop once the insulin starts)
- Glucose should be added to the fluid once the blood glucose is below 14 mmol/L or if the blood glucose is dropping rapidly (5 mmol/L over 1 hour)
- The measured plasma sodium should be corrected for the glucose level using the following formula: Corrected [Na]= measured [Na] + (0.4 × measured glucose in mmol/L) –5.5
- If the corrected sodium is rising (more than 5 mmol/L over 4 hours) then the rate of rehydration needs to be increased. If the corrected sodium falls too quickly (5 mmol/L over 4 hours) then the rate of rehydration should be decreased

- Avoid bicarbonate administration – this may increase the risk of cerebral oedema
- If the child complains of a headache or becomes confused, cerebral oedema is developing; 2.7% sodium chloride should be given after discussion with the local intensive care retrieval team.

Further reading

British Society of Paediatric Endocrinology and Diabetes Guideline: Diabetic Ketoacidosis, available at: www.bsped.org.uk/clinical/docs /DKAGuideline.pdf. Last updated 2009.

Dellinger RP, Levy MM, Rhodes A, et al, Surviving Sepsis Campaign: international guidelines for management of severe sepsis and septic shock, 2012. Intensive Care Med 2012;39(2):165–228.

Lampariello S, Clement M, Aralihond AP, et al. Stabilisation of critically ill children at the district general hospital prior to intensive care retrieval: a snapshot of current practice. Arch Dis Child 2010;95(9)681–5.

CHAPTER 33

Paediatric Trauma Retrievals

Mary Montgomery

KIDS (Kids Intensive Care and Decision Support), Birmingham Children's Hospital, UK

> **OVERVIEW**
>
> - Paediatric trauma, while relatively rare is the leading cause of death in children >1 year in the developed world
> - A structured approach to the management of paediatric trauma is essential for primary and secondary transfers
> - Anatomical differences result in a different injury pattern to adults based on the mechanism of injury
> - Follow local policies if concerned about non-accidental injury.

Introduction

This chapter will cover the key points relating to paediatric (birth to 16 years) trauma. Both primary and secondary transport considerations will be addressed where they are specific to paediatric patients. Knowledge of widely available paediatric and trauma resuscitation courses is assumed.

This chapter will highlight important differences and challenges relating to paediatric trauma. Basic principles of management of the transport of paediatric trauma are those of the transport of adult patients – the older the child, the more adult their management plan will be.

Paediatric major trauma is the commonest cause for mortality in children over a year of age in the Western world. The majority of children die before reaching hospital, and most emergency departments will rarely find themselves caring for children suffering from major trauma. Pre-hospital and Enhanced Care Teams (ECTs) are then crucial in the care pathway, with their expertise in robust systematic primary and secondary survey, resuscitation and stabilisation likely to be called upon for primary and secondary transfers.

Pre-hospital deaths in children have similar causes to those in adults (P. Hyde personal communication, UK) when data collection is robust. In the UK younger children present more frequently with burns, while those over 5 years suffer blunt trauma (RTC and falls) more commonly (Tarnlet, UK).

On-scene management and primary transfer is consequently a significant opportunity for impacting on outcome. Significant paediatric trauma is a relatively rare occurrence even in large paediatric and trauma centres and adherence to principles and a structured approach is crucial. Clear allocation of roles and responsibilities (TRM) is crucial given the rarity with which children present with major trauma. Transfer teams may provide telephone or bedside assistance in stabilisation for (secondary) transfer, with attention to comprehensive primary and secondary surveys being fundamental.

For pre-hospital teams, resuscitation and transfer often differ not only internationally, but nationally and regionally. Evidence exists that networked pathways of care with clear processes and triage for centralised management impacts on outcome. In the UK this has led to the institution of the National Trauma Networks. Triage tools provide direction for need for escalation, treatment and destination. Backing this up with access to telephone expertise via Regional Trauma desks/Specialist retrieval services provides additional avenues for trauma and paediatric advice as required. Early communication with receiving the facility via structured handover allows preparation of drugs, equipment and staff. If formal networked care delivery is not established make use of the principles of regular training, common tools and access to specialist telephone advice early.

Clinicians should be aware of the anatomical/physiological changes with advancing age (Chapter 29), but quick reference age/size guides are invaluable – the range of normal (from birth to 16 years) is huge and potentially unmemorable. Widely available apps on smartphones, are invaluable on scene.

Paediatric injury patterns

Head injury is the major cause of death in hospital following major trauma, and is associated with significant morbidity. Relatively larger head size contributes to higher incidence of injury. This, coupled with the immaturity of the cervical musculature and elasticity of ligaments, mean that cervical spine injuries without radiological abnormality (SCIWORA) are more common in younger patients. Physically dependent children are at risk of non-accidental injury (NAI). Toddlers suffer injuries related to curiosity and physical development outstripping cognitive maturity (scalds and falls). The younger the child, the more compliant the chest wall, and more exposed the abdominal viscera – be vigilant and consider

ABC of Transfer and Retrieval Medicine, First Edition.
Edited by Adam Low and Jonathan Hulme.
© 2015 John Wiley & Sons, Ltd. Published 2015 by John Wiley & Sons, Ltd.

concealed chest and abdominal injuries based on mechanism of injury. Remember compensatory mechanisms in children may result in delay in physiological evidence of ventilator or circulatory insufficiency, with sudden transition from 'seemingly ok' to peri-arrest.

Older children suffer from injuries which reflect the natural risk-taking behaviours present during adolescence (and beyond). Self-harm becomes more common during teenage years. Physiological and psychological maturity potentially lag behind physical maturity.

Pay attention to parents and caregivers – they can be a valuable resource if supported to manage their own distress.

Equipment considerations

The equipment list for paediatric trauma transfers is as for adults, but size appropriate according to age.

Knowledge of anatomical differences will underline the need for straight-bladed laryngoscopes in babies and infants in order to visualise the anterior larynx. Cuffed endotracheal tubes are NOT contraindicated in pre-pubertal children. Use secure fixation – strong tape with good adhesive qualities resistant to softening by secretions – such as the 'red tape strapping' method (Figure 33.1). In failed intubation needle cricothyroidotomy is preferable to a surgical airway in children under 10 due to risk or subsequent subglottic stenosis.

C-spine collars in small children are notoriously difficult to fit effectively – other methods may be more effective for c-spine immobilisation, with combinations of towels, bags of fluid, and taping potentially more secure.

Spine boards used for extrication do not allow for the large occiput and lumbar lordosis of smaller children – consider the use of a vacuum mattress.

Adequate access to circulation can be challenging in younger children particularly, and early use should be made of intraosseous modes of access.

Initial triage/assessment (5–10 seconds)

A rapid overview is taken to gauge how critical the child is. Is the child crying/moving – signs of consciousness. Is the airway patent and ventilation effective? Is there obvious catastrophic haemorrhage or significant circulatory compromise? Immediately respond to life threatening findings. Box 33.1 summarises danger signs in paediatric cases. Read the scene and establish mechanism of injury – thereby predicting potential injury patterns (Table 33.1).

Box 33.1 **Danger signs**

Bradycardia
Bradypnoea
Hypotension
Lethargy
Tolerance to procedures
Grey skin colouration (poor perfusion)
Cyanosis

Table 33.1 Injury risk stratification according to anatomical differences and important considerations during transfer.

Common issues	Consequences
Relatively large head	Trauma to head more common, greater forces on neck
Fontanelles fuse by 2 years of age	Intracerebral haemorrhage may be significant proportion of blood volume in traumatic brain injury
Upper airway anatomy	Obstruction + risk of foreign body. Difficult laryngoscopic view. Multiple attempts at laryngoscopy may compromise airway patency – resultant oedema. Large adenoids = risk of bleeding with NP airway insertion
Compliant chest wall	Hidden injuries. Energy wasted. Increased work of breathing. Chest commonly impacted in car vs child. Clinical evidence of injury = significant force through the thorax
Abdominal organs exposed	Soft abdominal wall musculature, and organs less well protected by chest wall – higher risk of splenic and liver injuries
Relatively high circulating blood volume Small total blood volume	Small losses have significant cardiovascular effect. Importance of accurate estimation of blood loss on scene and early haemorrhage control
Long bones	Significant force required to break a long bone. Greenstick fractures more common. Involvement of growth plate will impact subsequent growth
Emotional impact of resuscitating sick child	Disturbance of personal and team practice through fear and upset
High metabolic rate Small glycogen stores	Rapid use of reserves Hypoglycaemia

Primary survey (allow <2 minutes)

Pay attention to deviation from normal physiological values throughout.

Catastrophic haemorrhage

Address major haemorrhage rapidly utilising a stepwise approach of direct compression, haemostatic dressings and tourniquets.

Airway with C-spine control

Immobilise C-spine manually initially. Use bags of fluid, blocks and tape, and common sense to effect spinal immobilisation, particularly if the child is combative (risk vs. benefit). Visually inspect mouth and suction for vomit/teeth/other debris. If required insert oropharyngeal airway with downward pressure on tongue (insert correct way round (not upside down and rotate as in adult) to prevent causing soft palate trauma and bleeding.

If the airway needs to be secured and reflexes are present, drug assisted intubation (RSI) may be required if training, assessment and advice suggests safe/effective to do on scene.

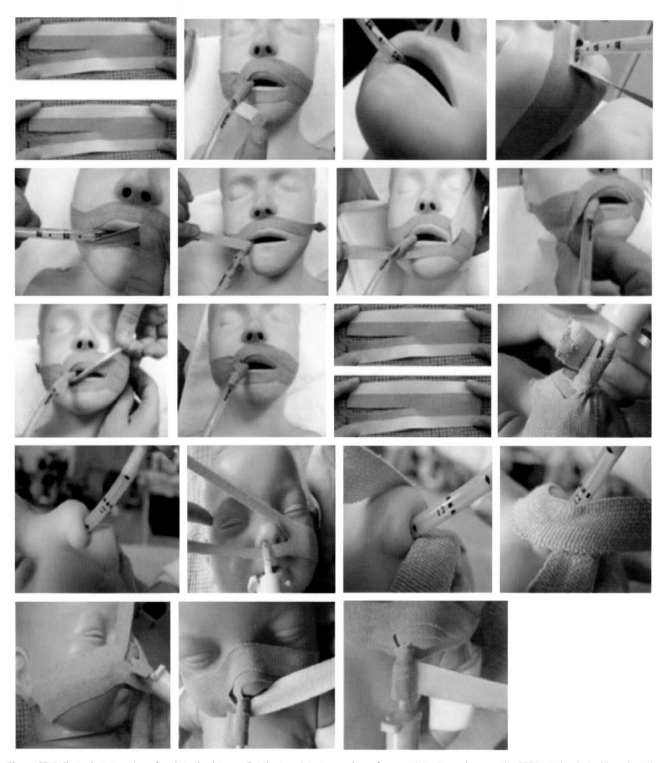

Figure 33.1 Elastoplast strapping of endotracheal tapes. Cut the tape into trouser legs of appropriate size and ensure the ETT is at the desired length at the corner of the mouth. Avoid areas of broken skin and ensure the tape is not placed over the lips. At least 2 cm of ETT is left free above the tape. Use two pieces of tape as illustrated in the sequence of photographs. (Source: Fiona Reynolds and Chris Timmins, Birmingham Children's Paediatric Intensive Care Unit. Reproduced with permission).

Breathing

Apply high-concentration oxygen as per local protocols. Look for evidence of increased work of breathing, external injury, abnormal chest wall movement (pneumothorax/haemothorax/rib fractures). Young children tolerate chest injury poorly – compliant chest wall results in high energy expenditure with increased work of breathing (and relatively low energy stores). Have a high index of suspicion of concealed chest injury. Palpate for discomfort/crepitus. Auscultate for lack of sounds/additional sounds/asymmetry. Consider augmenting ventilation early (bag/mask/high flow O_2) – children can tolerate/conceal impending decompensation. **Bradypnoea is pre-terminal**.

Circulation

The child who looks well, is interactive, warm and well perfused has adequate circulation. Having addressed obvious haemorrhage, feel for (brachial) pulse rate and volume. Consider concealed losses – intra-abdominal, intra-thoracic, long bone/pelvic fractures and immobilise. Tachycardia is sensitive (non-specific) for inadequate circulatory volume. Bradycardia is pre-terminal. Blood pressure is preserved until loss of ≥ 40 mL/kg, so hypotension is a danger sign. Obtain access using same techniques as adult – low threshold for use of intraosseous technique (caution with respect to growth plates). Use aliquots of 5 mL/kg of volume for fluid resuscitation (on the basis that this might prevent rebleeding of delicate haemostasis of bleeding points) – aim for normalisation of heart rate, blood pressure and signs of adequacy of end organ perfusion (perfusion, pulse pressure, GCS). Following administration of 40 mL/kg of resuscitation fluid (isotonic crystalloid) with ongoing haemodynamic instability or evidence of blood loss, consider administration of blood and blood products. Note that evidence-based protocols for timing and proportionate delivery of blood and blood products for massive transfusion in children is absent, and most centres use adult-based guidelines. Advanced warning should be given to receiving hospital from the primary transfer team if blood products are anticipated to be needed. Aim for physiological normality for circulatory status – early operative management is indicated for ongoing loss/instability.

Disability

Trauma and immediate care are frightening – communicate clearly with the child and reassure (parents as well). Use AVPU to assess consciousness in children who are unable cognitively to respond for GCS. Consider the use parents or familiar adults to help with assessment of consciousness in younger children. Note pupillary size/reactivity and abnormalities of limb movement or asymmetry (ask for wiggling of fingers/toes). Confusion/agitation may be signs of inadequate circulation as well as head injury. Check blood glucose if not A on AVPU.

Exposure

Heat loss is rapid (large surface area vs size) with negative impact on outcome. Pay attention during examination to reduce hypothermia risk by limiting exposure, removing wet clothing, and using suitable packaging.

At this point it should be evident if injuries are time critical. Over-triage is an accepted part of paediatric trauma. Use telephone advice to risk assess and assist with decision making regarding extending on scene time, addition of expertise to the scene, or transport of child to expertise.

Secondary survey

This is a systematic, head to toe examination of the child for less critical/concealed injuries. This may be performed on scene if assessed as non-time critical at completion of primary survey; en route (if safe to do so), or in the emergency department if time critical transfer is being performed. Figure 33.2 summarises a typical

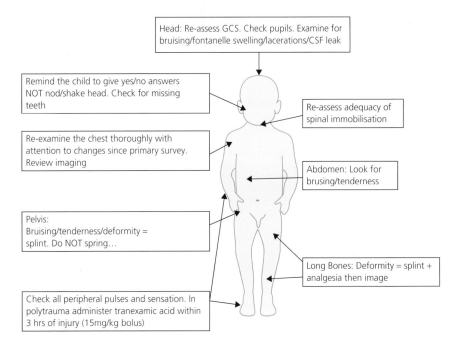

Head: Re-assess GCS. Check pupils. Examine for bruising/fontanelle swelling/lacerations/CSF leak

Remind the child to give yes/no answers NOT nod/shake head. Check for missing teeth

Re-assess adequacy of spinal immobilisation

Re-examine the chest thoroughly with attention to changes since primary survey. Review imaging

Abdomen: Look for bruising/tenderness

Pelvis: Bruising/tenderness/deformity = splint. Do NOT spring…

Long Bones: Deformity = splint + analgesia then image

Check all peripheral pulses and sensation. In polytrauma administer tranexamic acid within 3 hrs of injury (15mg/kg bolus)

Figure 33.2 Secondary survey.

secondary survey. Note presence of pain and treat adequately with a multimodal approach (including intravenous administration of morphine as per local guidelines).

Packaging for primary transport

Pay particular attention to exposure and safe immobilisation. Use a pelvic splint if indicated (NB SAM splint may be ineffective, but other splints will fit, e.g. Prometheus™). Remember to cut away all clothing before applying splints to avoid underlying pressure sores. A systematic review is advisable after every patient move (i.e. scene to vacuum mattress to ambulance, etc.). Thorough assessment as outlined above is necessary while minimising on scene time. Ensure lines and tubes are accessible and suitably secured. Do not try to clear the C-spine on scene unless very confident that there is no injury. Fear and anxiety, along with cognitive immaturity, make clearing the C-spine difficult.

Parents will often want to accompany the injured child – this must not interfere with safe delivery of care to the child, but can be useful in reassuring anxious children. Ensure meticulous documentation of injury pattern and treatments given.

Secondary transfer

For time-critical transfers

Use established pathways for referral to expedite transfer and obtain advice on resuscitation and stabilisation pre-transfer. Note: if the patient cannot be adequately stabilised prior to transfer, consider local emergency intervention – keep the patient's best interests at the forefront of decision making.

A structured approach to the patient and management of transfers in children is recommended, as in adults, supported by the use of a standardised pre-departure checklist.

Speed of transport – progress through traffic rather than high speed should be the aim. Acceleration/deceleration and hard cornering impact negatively on physiological stability of the patient and escort, and increase the risks of accidents. Avoid convoys of emergency vehicles travelling using exemptions (e.g. police escort of ambulance) – this is extremely dangerous (other road users do not expect the second emergency vehicle – it is this one which is usually involved in incidents). Longer journeys may be more appropriately performed by air – caution if multiple transfers between modes of transport are required (no helipads on site) as this may negate the benefit of the speed of the helicopter.

Non-time critical transfers

More care and attention can be paid to pre-transport stabilisation. This minimises the risks of decompensation en route. In addition to the above, the secondary survey should be completed prior to transfer.

Burns

See Chapter 36 for more comprehensive discussion of acute management. The rule of nines is inadequate for children. Palmar surface equates to approximately 1% TBSA. Lund and Browder charts with age adjustments provide greater accuracy.

Specifically consider the following:

A. Early intubation – small airways so risk to patency with even mild swelling. Don't forget risk of trauma and potential need for c-spine control.

B. The work of breathing with respect to compliant chest wall, reduced respiratory reserve, and immature musculature means exhaustion can be rapid.

C. Circulatory access may be challenging as before. Fluid calculations – estimate weight (e.g. APLS/Broselow) and use a formula to assess fluid requirements. Adequate urine output for younger children is higher than for adults (aim 2 mL/kg/h).

D. Pain relief needs careful attention – use intravenous morphine/diamorphine/ketamine as per local guidelines. Ketamine or diamorphine can be given intranasally.

E. Temperature control is challenging – meticulous attention to limiting exposure and active warming. Consider NAI and need for child protection procedures to be implemented.

Non-accidental injury

Whilst deliberately inflicted major trauma is uncommon, children suffering from NAI will present to pre-hospital and transfer teams – be vigilant.

Children under the age of 2 years with head injury should raise a high index of suspicion of NAI, alongside other warning red flags (Box 33.2). If suspicious, share concerns with other members of the team and inform the paediatricians at the receiving unit. Ensure child protection procedures are instituted by the local paediatric team or other responsible clinicians. Document everything meticulously – including all visible marks and injuries, any sites of access/attempts at access, and conversations with parents or carers. Note that for the purposes of any potential court action, there is likely to be a need for proof or a chain of evidence – your notes/statements may well form a part of this.

Ensure that child protection processes are engaged. If parents or carers have potential to interfere or compromise care of the child, and attempts to prioritise care of the child are compromised, ask for help (police) in managing them. Parents may wish to accompany their child – where NAI is suspected this can be difficult for the clinical escort. Stick to local process – in some areas parents accompanying the child even in these circumstances may be accepted.

Box 33.2 Red flags for NAI

Repeat attendances to healthcare
Previous history of abuse
Known to social services
Younger age/prematurity
Young maternal age
Inconsistent history
unexplained injury pattern (bearing in mind age and physical development
History of domestic violence
Parental drug/alcohol abuse

Acknowledgements

The author would like to acknowledge and thank Birmingham Children's Hospital Paediatric Intensive Care Unit, Fiona Reynolds and Chris Timmins for their advice and support in preparing this chapter.

Further reading

Kanakaris NK, Giannoudis PV. Trauma networks: present and future challenges. Bmc Med 2011;9.

Litman RS, Maxwell LG. Cuffed versus Uncuffed endotracheal tubes in pediatric anesthesia the debate should finally end. Anesthesiology 2013;118(3): 500–1.

Luten RC, Zaritsky A, Wears R, Broselow J. The use of the Broselow tape in pediatric resuscitation. Acad Emerg Med 2007;14(5):500–1.

O'Connor RE. Trauma triage: Concepts in prehospital trauma care. Prehospital Emerg Care 2006;10(3):307–10.

CHAPTER 34

Additional Considerations

H. McNeilly[1] and J. Hegarty[2]

[1]West Midlands Deanery, UK
[2]Newborn Services, National Women's Health, Auckland City Hospital, New Zealand

---

OVERVIEW

- Paediatric and neonatal transfers provide unique challenges
- Additional specialist equipment and interventions may be required
- Thermoregulation poses a greater problem than in adults, particularly in transport situations
- Transport also presents a significant emotional challenge to the child.

Introduction

Paediatric or neonatal transfers and retrievals present unique challenges when compared to adult cases and often requires specialist equipment. These challenges range from maintaining normothermia, to the need to inform and support parents or carers, as well as transportation to the receiving institution. These so called 'additional considerations' are discussed in this chapter.

Environmental considerations

Thermal care

Infants and young children have much higher surface area:volume ratios than adults and therefore lose heat more rapidly. This is particularly relevant in a transport scenario where there may be significant seasonal and diurnal variation in ambient temperature.

Neonates are particularly vulnerable to heat loss and should be transported in incubators, usually at a temperature of 32°C. Premature neonates benefit from a humidified environment to minimise transcutaneous fluid losses.

Simply covering a child with an appropriate insulating layer can reduce heat loss by around 29% and this may be sufficient. Radiant heaters reduce heat loss by up to 77% in children. However, skin surface temperature must be monitored during use of radiant heaters to avoid overheating and burns (Figure 34.1).

Forced-air warming systems may also be used. Skin surface temperature should be monitored regularly. These systems are very effective, but bulk and weight limits their use in a transport setting.

ABC of Transfer and Retrieval Medicine, First Edition.
Edited by Adam Low and Jonathan Hulme.
© 2015 John Wiley & Sons, Ltd. Published 2015 by John Wiley & Sons, Ltd.

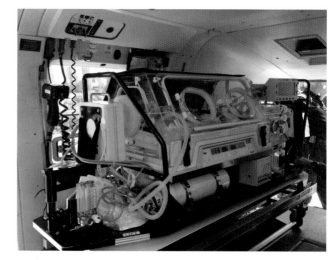

Figure 34.1 Incubators are an integral part of temperature management in neonatal transfers.

Specialized paediatric scenarios

Therapeutic hypothermia

Therapeutic hypothermia reduces mortality and improves neurodevelopmental outcome in neonates with hypoxic ischaemic encephalopathy. Therapeutic hypothermia requires intensive care support and therefore transport to a network Neonatal Intensive Care Unit (NICU) is often required. Therapeutic hypothermia should be initiated within 6 hours of the hypoxic insult. Infants may therefore commence cooling prior to transfer, either actively if the equipment is available, or passively by environmental exposure.

Active cooling involves the use of an enveloping wrap which circulates cold water under the control of a microprocessing system regulated by a rectal temperature probe. The infant is cooled to a rectal temperature of 33.5°C for 72 hours. Active cooling improves temperature stability and reduces stabilisation and transport time. Adverse sequelae are considered in Box 34.1.

Box 34.1 **Possible adverse effects of therapeutic hypothermia**

Sinus bradycardia (<80 bpm)
Thrombocytopenia
Cold-related damage to skin and subcutaneous tissues

Points to consider:

- Continual rectal temperature monitoring is vital. The rectal probe can be dislodged, particularly on moving the patient, and infants can be cooled excessively, causing increased adverse effects. Check placement regularly throughout the journey
- Rapid rewarming is associated with an increased risk of seizures and should be avoided
- Resting heart rate is considerably lower than normal in a cooled neonate, often in the range 90–110 bpm
- Cooling is uncomfortable and probably painful. Analgesia should be administered.

Nitric oxide

Inhaled nitric oxide (iNO) is administered via the endotracheal tube to neonates with PPHN (Box 34.2). iNO acts locally on the smooth muscle of the pulmonary vasculature increasing levels of cGMP, causing relaxation and vascular dilatation. This improves oxygenation by decreasing total pulmonary vascular resistance and by preferentially increasing blood flow to well-aerated areas of lung, decreasing ventilation-perfusion mismatch. The rapid breakdown of iNO prevents any systemic vasodilatory effect.

Box 34.2 **Nitric Oxide administration: some practical considerations**

Recommended starting dose is 20 ppm inhaled concentration
There is little evidence of increased benefit with higher concentrations
NO canisters are light green with a dark green neck and usually contain 1000 ppm. They are attached to the transport incubator via a console which provides constant-flow delivery of NO and gives readouts of NO, NO_2 and O_2 concentration. Most systems can deliver 0 – 100 ppm iNO, set via the console
Tanks must be well secured during transport. Ensure sufficient supply for the whole journey, as withdrawal of iNO can cause profound hypoxaemia
iNO may be administered during airborne transport. The canisters should be secured to the incubator itself.

Indication

- Term infant with clinical and/or echocardiographic evidence of PPHN, with oxygenation index >25.

Monitoring

- Continuous pre- and post-ductal oxygen saturation monitoring is required with separate saturation probes and a dual monitor/additional pulse oximetry monitor
- Aim to keep systemic blood pressure at the upper range of normal for gestational age to decrease right-left shunting across the PDA.

Side effects

- NO reacts with oxygen to form NO_2 with potential toxic effects. Concentration of NO_2 is monitored electrochemically within the delivery circuit. Minimise dead space in the ventilatory circuit to limit the proportion of NO oxidised prior to reaching the alveoli.

Additional considerations

- Occasional rebound hypoxia has occurred on commencing iNO. Ensure stability prior to transfer. Exclude potential complicating factors, e.g. pneumothorax in MAS
- PPHN may necessitate ECMO, which should be considered at oxygenation index (OI) > 35 and is necessary at OI >40; therefore consider appropriate destination with access to ECMO
- OI: $FiO_2 \times$ mean alveolar pressure/PaO_2

Vascular access

Vascular access is harder to achieve in a transport situation and is easily lost in neonates and children. Make sure you are happy with IV access (and how it is secured) before departure, siting new lines if necessary.

Neonates commonly have umbilical lines in situ. Make sure lines are clearly labelled as arterial or venous. Ensure you are happy with how the lines are secured as there are a number of methods in common use. A dislodged umbilical line can bleed significantly in a short period of time. Consider taking copies of imaging which confirm line placement for the receiving team.

Psychological aspects

Transportation of an unwell neonate or child can be an intimidating situation. However, with good preparation it can be a rewarding experience.

- Use the experience and expertise of other members of your team and pool your resources
- Ensure you are physically prepared before your shift – fatigue and stress affect arousal levels and performance
- Plan and prepare ahead for potential problems. In children fluids and most medications are calculated on weight, so prepare a chart of emergency drug dosages on current weight before departure
- Remember that this is an anxious and emotionally fraught time for both the child and the parents. Discuss the transfer step by step, including why it is necessary, and explain potential delays. Be as positive and reassuring as the situation permits. Answer questions as fully as possible
- Depending on the stability of the child (and mother if neonatal transfer), and the room available it may be possible to have one parent join the transport team in the ambulance. If not, parents often follow the ambulance in a car – make sure to remind them that they should not attempt to follow in a blue-light situation. If a parent is not going to be travelling with the child, a few quiet moments together before setting off are always appreciated.

Further reading

Anttonen H, Puhakka K, Niskanen J, Ryhänen P. Cutaneous heat loss in children during anaesthesia. Br J Anaesth 1995;74(3):306–10.
British Association of Perinatal Medicine. Position Statement on Therapeutic Cooling for Neonatal Encephalopathy, July 2010

Bloch KD, Ichinose F, Roberts JD, Jr., Zapol WM. Inhaled NO as a therapeutic agent. Cardiovasc Res 2007;75(2):339–348.

Chaudhary R, Farrer K, Broster S, McRitchie L, Austin T. Active versus passive cooling during neonatal transport. Pediatrics Peds 2013-1686; published ahead of print October 21, 2013, doi:10.1542/peds.2013–686

Finer NN, Etches PC, Kamstra B, Tierney AJ, Peliowski A, Ryan CA. Inhaled nitric oxide in infants referred for extracorporeal membrane oxygenation: Dose response. J Pediatr 994;124:302–8.

Jacobs S, Hunt R, Tarnow-Mordi W, Inder T, Davis P. Cooling for newborns with hypoxic ischaemic encephalopathy. Cochrane Database Syst Rev 2007;(4):CD003311. Review.

Steinhorn RH. Neonatal pulmonary hypertension. Pediatr Crit Care Med 2010;11(2 Suppl):S79–S84.

Section 7

Specialist Transfers

CHAPTER 35

Head & Spinal Injuries

R. Protheroe and F. Lecky[1,2]

[1]Salford Royal NHS Foundation Trust, UK
[2]University of Sheffield and Salford Royal NHS Foundation Trust, Greater Manchester, UK

OVERVIEW

- Transfer of head injured, brain injured and spinal injured patients will continue to occur from all acute receiving hospitals
- All brain injured transfers are time critical and should be transferred as a priority
- All other injuries should have been stabilised prior to transfer in agreement with the local neuroscience or spinal centre
- Good perfusion and oxygenation are the primary aims of management during the transfer
- Ensure that accompanying staff are trained and equipped to deal with potential deterioration of the patient.

Introduction

Isolated brain-injured patients, spinal injured patients and poly-trauma victims with brain and spinal injuries present to all acute receiving hospitals. Consequently, there is always a need to transfer these patients to the local regional neurosciences or spinal unit once the initial resuscitation, stabilization, investigation and diagnosis has taken place. The development of regional MTCs means that the majority of trauma cases should be transferred directly to a centre with neurosurgical and spinal support, but patients with vascular disease such as sub-arachnoid haemorrhage or stroke will still require transfer directly from ED, ICU or wards.

The need for transfer

The evidence supports treatment in specialist centres which leads to better outcomes, necessitating both primary and secondary transfer into the local regional centres. These neuroscience patients require time critical transfers, since there is a wealth of evidence demonstrating the worsening outcomes associated with delays in presenting the patient for early surgical treatment. There is also plenty of evidence supporting the need for rapid resuscitation and stabilization of the patient both prior to and during transfer, in order to

support cerebral or spinal perfusion and to rapidly correct or prevent hypotension and hypoxia.

There are now established criteria for referral to neuroscience centres for all categories of patients, that is trauma, stroke, sub-arachnoid haemorrhage and spinal injury (see Boxes 35.1, 35.2 and Table 35.1 illustrating the GCS). With the advent of the regional

---

Box 35.1 Criteria for referral of head injured patients

NICE criteria: local guidelines should be drawn up but transfer would benefit all patients with serious head injuries (GCS≤8), irrespective of the need for surgery
Intracranial haematomata (extradural, subdural and intracerebral)
Subarachnoid blood
Altered conscious level
Seizures
Focal neurological signs

Box 35.2 Information required by the specialist teams

Name and age of patient
Time of injury
Mechanism of injury
Initial GCS, post resuscitation GCS and current GCS
Pupillary size, discrepancy and response to light
Current status and stage of resuscitation, including vital signs, other injuries and medical interventions as well as significant deterioration
Past medical history
Drug history

Table 35.1 Glasgow Coma Score.

Score	Eyes	Verbal	Motor
1	None	None	None
2	Open to pain	Incomprehensible sounds	Abnormal extension to pain (decerebrate)
3	Open to voice	Inappropriate words	Abnormal flexion to pain (decorticate)
4	Open spontaneously	Confused speech	Normal Flexion to pain
5		Normal speech	Localises to pain
6			Obeys commands

ABC of Transfer and Retrieval Medicine, First Edition.
Edited by Adam Low and Jonathan Hulme.
© 2015 John Wiley & Sons, Ltd. Published 2015 by John Wiley & Sons, Ltd.

trauma networks and agreed criteria for bypass, some patients may be primarily transferred directly to a MTC; however, some patients may stop at trauma units for control of airway and/or major haemorrhage if this has not been possible pre-hospitally.

Preparation

The crucial element of transferring either a brain injured or spinal injured patient is both optimising current brain/spinal perfusion and oxygenation, whilst trying to pre-empt any expected deterioration or problems.

On receiving a patient into the resuscitation room of an emergency department, immediate resuscitation will have commenced along the recommended C-ABC approach with ongoing treatment of life threatening problems. When able, the history will be determined and appropriate essential investigations undertaken to establish a diagnosis.

As part of the resuscitation, intravenous access should have been established and isotonic intra-venous fluids commenced. A GCS <9 or falling more than 2 points demonstrates the need for sedation, muscle relaxation, facilitated intubation and ventilation controlled to normocapnia. Securing the oro-endotracheal tube should be carefully done so as not to exacerbate any jugular venous congestion (i.e. taped). Throughout this, adequate protection of the cervical spine should be maintained in view of the possibility of an injury.

A stable GCS >12 would permit an awake transfer, but precautions and preparations should be made to sedate, intubate and ventilate if problems such as falling GCS, seizures or respiratory failure occur during the transfer. It is inherent on the transferring team to ensure they are fully equipped with appropriate monitors, equipment and drugs to deal with all eventualities.

At this stage arterial access for monitoring and blood sampling is extremely useful, but central venous access is not necessary if large bore peripheral venous access has been established. Blood pressure should be restored to normal levels with fluid and peripherally active vasopressors such as ephedrine, metaraminol or diluted adrenaline (epinephrine) (e.g. 1:100,000). Orogastric decompression of the stomach and urinary catheterisation would be helpful if possible within the time constraints but should not delay transfer.

Basic monitoring should include standard ECG, pulse oximetry, invasive blood pressure (non-invasive if arterial line not established), capnography and regular pupillary checks in the absence of intracranial pressure monitoring.

In the event of the patient being a trauma victim, adequate spinal precautions should be established or if present checked for appropriate positioning and tightness. Hard extrication collars, particularly if poorly fitted or of the incorrect size are a common cause of raised intracranial pressure in these brain injured patients and should be carefully checked so as not to be causing any venous obstruction, as well as the ETT ties or tape. Provided the patient is protected with appropriately secure blocks and straps/tape, the extrication collar could be loosened to prevent further problems.

If possible the patient should be nursed head-up at an angle of 30 degrees to aid venous drainage. Not all transfer trolleys are able to be so positioned but consideration should be given to this if the trolley can be tilted while maintaining axial stability for the rest of the spine. Ideally the patient should be log-rolled off the hard, extrication spinal board, provided axial spine stability can be maintained. Scoop stretchers or vacuum mattress should be used in preference to extrication boards for transfer and are particularly useful for moving patients with unstable spinal injuries.

Drugs should be prepared to maintain or induce anaesthesia during transfer, including emergency drugs to maintain adequate blood pressure and cerebral perfusion pressure, as well as controlling seizures and other potential metabolic problems such as glycaemic derangement (see Box 35.3).

Spinally injured patients are particularly prone to a relative hypovolaemic hypotension due to the loss of autonomic (sympathetic) vascular control and bradycardias. Atropine, glycopyrrolate and vasopressors may all be required.

> **Box 35.3 Common intratransfer problems**
>
> Coughing – check ETT, analgesia, sedation and muscle relaxation
>
> Hypertension – check pupils, $ETCO_2$ and ventilation, sedation and muscle relaxation, consider mannitol/furosemide if worried that ICP may be increasing
>
> Hypotension – check for haemorrhage, increase IV fluids and consider peripherally active vasopressors, e.g. metaraminol
>
> Seizures – stop with appropriate hypnotics, e.g. bolus propofol, midazolam or thiopentone, check glycaemic status and correct as necessary.

All investigations and notes should be collated, or photocopied to be transferred over with the patient. These days most of the radiology images can be remotely accessed via the PACS system, but if not arrangements should be made for the images to be image-linked across or copied onto CD to go with the patient.

There should be established arrangements for local transfer teams to deliver the patients to the receiving hospital. Unfortunately, due to the time critical nature of these injuries, retrieval teams have not proved to be useful in most areas yet. The personnel accompanying the patient should be of sufficient seniority and experience to adequately undertake the management of these complex and frequently unstable patients. This usually means a registrar equivalent or greater grade of medical staff with both airway and resuscitative skills, that is anaesthesia, emergency medicine or critical care. They will require dedicated assistance drawn from nursing, operating department or paramedical staff. Ideally all of the accompanying personnel should have previously undertaken formal transfer training, although rotas, skill mix and ongoing needs in the transferring hospital can make this more challenging. All staff accompanying the patient will need to consider appropriate clothing (i.e. layers), money and telephones in order to cover various unpredictable eventualities.

Further reading

Intensive Care Society. *Guidelines for the transport of the critically ill adult*. Intensive Care Society 2002. http://www.ics.ac.uk/downloads/icstransport2002mem.pdf.

Neuroanaesthesia Society of Great Britain and Ireland and the Association of Anaesthetists of Great Britain and Ireland. *Recommendations for the safe transfer of patients with brain injury*. London: NASGBI and AAGBI, 2006.

NICE Guidelines. Head Injury: triage, assessment, investigation and early management of head injury in infants, children and adults. HMSO 2003. http://www.nice.org.uk

CHAPTER 36

Burns

T. Muehlberger[1], M. Büeschges[2,3], and C. Ottoman[2,3]

[1]Department of Plastic & Reconstructive Surgery, DRK-Kliniken, Germany
[2]Universitätsklinikum Schleswig Holstein Campus Lübeck, Germany
[3]Abteilung für Plastische Chirurgie, Intensiveinheit für Schwerbrandverletzte, Germany

OVERVIEW

• Awareness of criteria for referral to specialist burns centres
• Associated complication, particularly inhalational injuries
• Considerations for the resuscitation of acute burns injuries
• Transportation considerations.

Classification of burns by agent, size and depth

Burns are caused by exposure to flames, hot surfaces or contact with gases, electric shock and arcing, radiation and scalding with hot liquids. The extent of the burn will depend on temperature and exposure time. Cells are no longer able to compensate at temperatures above 45°C, with subsequent cell destruction and tissue necrosis following prolonged exposure. Initial cellular protein degeneration leads to protein denaturation, which develops into defined coagulation necrosis. Protein destruction and changes in protein structure result, and these protein fragments may have toxic, antigenic or immunomodulatory effects. This leads to local hypoperfusion, ischaemia and destruction of cell function. Even after the thermal exposure causing the burn has been removed, cell function will still be impaired until tissue temperatures are <40°C. The layperson's reaction of immediately cooling down the tissue around the burn may indeed lower the temperature around the burn more rapidly, but care should be taken in preventing patient hypothermia. Cooling also has an analgesic effect. Table 36.1 summarises categorisation of burns.

Guidelines for referral to a burn centre

• Adult patients: second-degree burns on more than 15% of the body surface
• Adult patients: third-degree burns on more than 10% of the body surface
• Children: second-degree burns on more than 10% of the body surface

Table 36.1 Thermal lesions are described in degrees of burn.

First degree (I)	The lesion is confined to the epidermis; the skin is red, painful, and swollen with oedema, but the burn will heal without scarring. One example is sunburn
Second degree (IIa):	Alongside superficial skin injury, the burn shows blistering hyperaemia in the wound bed, albeit with recapillarisation intact; the burn will heal without scarring as skin appendages and stem cells contained lead to full integrity restoration. This type of wound is very painful
Second degree (IIb):	Deep skin lesions show only some blistering on the skin since the fluid in the blister evaporates due to the intensity or time of exposure involved; this leads to delay or cessation in wound bed recapillarisation. The skin appendages and stem cells are affected, and scars will develop while healing. The area affected is moderately painful
Third degree:	Complete degradation of all skin layers – the skin is painless, dry, white and leathery

• Children: third-degree burns on more than 5% of the body surface
• Patients with inhalation injury
• Localisation to the face, hands, feet or genital area, including thermal damage caused by electric current
• Burns from blast trauma.

Pulmonary inhalation injury

Around 80% of those killed in fires die from toxic fume inhalation. Thirty per cent of patients treated in burn centres present with inhalation injury. Glottal oedema with thermal damage to the lower respiratory tract and carbon monoxide or cyanide poisoning are especially hazardous. Box 36.1 illustrates indicators for potential inhalational injury.

Unconsciousness and pulmonary inhalation injury indicate severe hypoxia and/or poisoning from carbon monoxide, cyanide or phosgene. Fumes and thermal cell destruction stimulate alveolar macrophages with chemotactic factor release causing a massive inflammatory response in the lungs. The inflammatory mediators released destroy the pulmonary mucosa and increase capillary perfusion, leading to capillary leak with formation of interstitial

ABC of Transfer and Retrieval Medicine, First Edition.
Edited by Adam Low and Jonathan Hulme.
© 2015 John Wiley & Sons, Ltd. Published 2015 by John Wiley & Sons, Ltd.

pulmonary oedema and pulmonary gas exchange obstruction. The negative impact of the mediators on pneumocytes gives rise to surfactant deficiency and alveolar collapse with atelectasis. Intubation conditions may initially appear favourable, but swollen soft tissues in the neck and face proceed to cause airway obstruction, rendering endotracheal intubation difficult or impossible; thus the need for endotracheal intubation and ventilation including positive end-expiratory pressure in any patient with suspected inhalation injury.

Carbon monoxide poisoning

Carbon monoxide (CO) poisoning is one of the most common immediate burn-related causes of death by CO–Hb formation. CO also blocks enzymes in the respiratory chain, leading to cell death. Patients complain of headaches, while the skin shows a rosy complexion. Convulsions and loss of consciousness increase with CO concentration. Without intervention, the outcome is usually fatal if CO binds more than 60% of the haemoglobin molecules. Pulse oximetry shows 100% oxygen saturation, even in patients with serious CO poisoning, due to the absorption spectra, and is therefore ineffective at determining CO poisoning. Controlled ventilation with 100% oxygen is the only form of primary treatment.

Cyanide poisoning

Plastic, nylon, polyurethane, paper, wood, silk and wool combustion generates cyanide fumes, so virtually every fire today involves cyanide gas liberation. Cyanide blocks the respiratory chain by inhibiting the cytochrome c oxidase enzyme, leading to cell death. Substantially elevated blood lactate levels are strongly indicative of cyanide poisoning; the patient should be ventilated with pure oxygen on suspicion of cyanide poisoning. On theoretical grounds, hydroxocobalamin is an attractive antidote for cyanide poisoning as cobalt compounds have the ability to bind and detoxify cyanide. Limited data on human poisonings with cyanide salts suggest that hydroxocobalamin is an effective antidote; data from smoke inhalation are less clear-cut.

Other irritants

Hydrogen chloride is generated during polyvinyl chloride (PVC) combustion, and various plastics also release nitrous gases while burning. All of these gases lead to severe respiratory irritation and potential lung injury; again, the treatment of choice is ventilation in 100% oxygen.

Interventions that can be undertaken prior to, and during, retrieval in the patient with major burns

Sterile wound dressings are sufficient at the scene of the accident; they should be dry to prevent hypothermia, such as with metallised films. Ointments should be avoided as they would otherwise complicate wound assessment at the burn centre. Ongoing wound care with blister removal should be left to the burn centre; however, deep burns will lead to dermal collagen shrinkage around the wound. Oedema in circumferential burns enhanced by high-voltage current may cause ischaemia in the extremities (compartment syndrome) or hinder thoracic respiratory excursion, so escharotomy may be necessary before transfer to a burn centre if the burn centre cannot be reached within the first six hours (Figures 36.1–36.3).

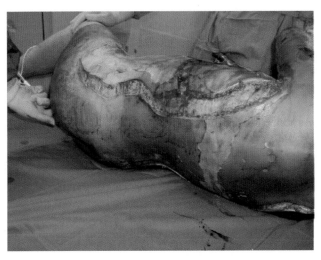

Figure 36.1 Burns escharotomy to the thorax and abdomen.

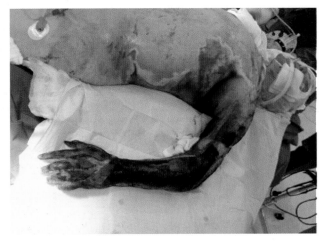

Figure 36.2 Escharotomy to the upper limb for compartment syndrome.

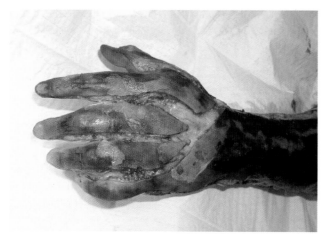

Figure 36.3 Escharotomy to the hand in third degree burns.

Fluid resuscitation

Cell decomposition caused by thermal injury causes highly potent vasoactive mediators to be released, which impact overall body circulation. Haemodynamic stabilisation should be high-volume since catecholamines restrict capillary circulation, leading to further cell damage in the zone of stasis. Attaining supranormal circulatory values improves survival and decreases morbidity in the severely traumatized patient. Cell breakdown product release leads to an increase in vascular permeability, with plasma proteins leaking into the interstitium. These proteins promote burn oedema formation in the interstitium due to fluid influx from increased colloid osmotic pressure, a process referred to as capillary leak. Crystalloids are given preference over hyperoncotic fluids in infusion therapy due to capillary leak: lactated Ringer's solution is ideal for fluid resuscitation. The simple instructions in the Nebraska Burn Manual should be followed where transfer to a burn centre will take less than an hour:

- Adults: 500–1,000 mL/h lactated Ringer's
- Children >5 years: 250–500 mL/h lactated Ringer's
- Children <5 years: 125–250 mL/h lactated Ringer's.

The cardinal rule is to make sure that the patient is admitted to a burn centre as soon as possible. Plan differential infusion therapy according to the Parkland formula (Box 36.2) in case of delayed transport. Use central venous catheters with a lumen as large as possible. Always make sure that the patient has a urine output more than 50 mL/h.

Box 36.2 **Parkland formula for fluid resuscitation**

4 mL × kg BW × %age of burned body surface per 24 h

- of that, 50% in the first 8 h, 50% in the following 16 h
- 50% increase in pulmonary inhalation injury
- Criterion: urine output >0.5 mL/kg BW/h

Analgesics, sedation, anaesthesia, haemodynamic stabilisation, nutrition

Dependent of the size and depth of the burn, intravenous analgesics and mild sedatives should be administered at the scene of the accident and in the hospital administering primary care. Ketamine S is well suited as an analgesic and sedative in burn-injured patients, co-administered with a hypnotic (e.g. midazolam) to avoid dissociative anaesthesia. Opioids are equally practical, their respiratory depressant effect is rare due to the increased respiration caused by pain/agitation. Avoid succinylcholine associated with intubation if you need to administer a muscle relaxant, as it may give rise to hazardous hyperkalaemia. Glucocorticoid administration is not recommended as it will not decrease the severity of pulmonary inhalation injury, and increased bronchopulmonary infections have been reported in patients during the further course of inpatient treatment. Untargeted sodium bicarbonate administration does not present any benefit to the patient for the primary care. Never administer diuretics during the shock phase, as laboured urine production can simulate a sufficient diuretic rate.

Initiate a high-calorie, fat-free diet by gavage to counteract intestinal villous atrophy and bacterial translocation within the first 24 hours of enteral nutrition. Add intravenous nutrition substitution to ensure sufficient calorie intake after capillary leak has subsided in patient transports lasting longer than twenty-four hours. Calculate the calorie requirement as follows:

$$25 \text{ kcal per kg BW} + 40 \text{ kcal/\% age burn surface}$$

Problems experienced during retrieval of the patient with major burns

Monitoring

Use the ECG's three or four-channel signal recording for continuous cardiac monitoring during transport. Conventional adhesive gel pads maybe difficult to apply in severe burns and may need to be sutured in place. Percutaneous oxygen measurement is indicated to detect hazardous changes in this phase. Controlled ventilation allows exhaled CO_2 measurement along with pulse oximetric oxygen saturation; apart from that, the high-volume therapy necessary often leads to concomitant pulmonary oedema requiring PEEP ventilation to ensure adequate oxygenation. Cuffed endotracheal tubes (uncut) should therefore be used; suture the tube to the gums or nasal septum as a temporary measure to support fixation during transportation. Wiring the tube to the teeth is a common technique, but more practical for the ICU. Temperature measurement especially during long transports provides information of an often underestimated value.

Choice of transport vessel

Patient transport by helicopter has been available in many industrialised countries for more than 30 years. There are countless air rescue stations in developed countries forming a cross-country network, thus only permitting limited applicability of data from US studies, in which greater distances play a decisive role. It is difficult to identify groups of patients who obtain a clear benefit from air transport. These probably include newborns, children with dyspnoea and polytraumatised patients. The results from studies of burn patients have either negated a positive effect of the use of a helicopter with regard to morbidity and mortality. There has not yet been a study to show any clear advantage in terms of time gained or improved prognosis. The objective of using a helicopter is shortening the interval of time before reaching the burn unit. An advantage in time by helicopter can only be achieved for a distance of more than 10 miles between the scene of the accident and the hospital, compared with an ambulance. The ground distance, taking the course of inner-city streets into account, is 1.3 times the distance as the crow flies. The time from the alarm until reaching the scene of an accident is shorter with a motor vehicle than by helicopter. Burn patients transported by helicopter are more often intubated, resulting in a higher probability of these burn patients developing hypothermia.

Further reading

Adams HA, Vogt PM. Die notfall- und intensivemedizinische Grundversorgung des Schwerbrandverletzten. Anästh Intensivmed 2010;51: 90–11.

De Wing MD, Curry T, Stepheneson E, et al. Cost-effective use of helicopters for the transportation of patients with burn injuries. J Burn Care Rehabil 2000;21:535–40.

James MF. Place of the colloids in fluid resuscitation of the traumatized patient. Curr Opin Anaesthesiol 2012;25(2):248–52.

Muehlberger T, Ottomann C, Toman N, et al. Emergency pre-hospital care of burn patients. The Surgeon 2010;(8):101–4.

Orgill DP, Piccolo N. Escharotomy and decompressive therapies in burns. J Burn Care Res 2009;30(5):759–68.

CHAPTER 37

Polytrauma and Military Retrievals

D. Keene[1] and O. Bartells[2]

[1]Specialist trainee Anaesthesia and Pre-Hospital Emergency Medicine, Department of Military Anaesthesia and Critical Care, UK
[2]Royal Army Medical Corps, Ministry of Defence Hospital Unit Northallerton, UK

OVERVIEW

After reading this chapter you should have a basic understanding of

• the definition of polytrauma
• key physiological considerations during polytrauma retrieval
• when military transfers occur and the unique challenges posed
• how military transfers are conducted and the key differences to civilian retrieval.

Polytrauma

Polytrauma is a significant cause of mortality worldwide leading to 5 million deaths annually. It is defined internationally as an Injury Severity Score (ISS) of >15 (range 1–75) (Box 37.1). Polytrauma occurs in both civilian and military settings, however significant differences exist.

Box 37.1 Injury Severity Score

Each injury is assigned an abbreviated injury score (AIS) from 1 to 6 (1 = Minor, 6 = Unsurvivable)
Each AIS is allocated to one of six body regions
(Head, Face, Chest, Abdomen, Extremities (including Pelvis), External Structures)
Only the highest score per area is used
The three most injured regions have their AIS squared and added together to give the ISS
An AIS of 6 in one area by convention equals an ISS of 75

Retrieval

Both primary and secondary movement of polytrauma casualties can be complex. By definition the casualties will have significant injuries to one or more areas of the body, leading to significant physiological derangement.

ABC of Transfer and Retrieval Medicine, First Edition.
Edited by Adam Low and Jonathan Hulme.
© 2015 John Wiley & Sons, Ltd. Published 2015 by John Wiley & Sons, Ltd.

Primary retrieval of the polytrauma casualty

The primary aim when preparing to move the casualty is to maximise physiological stability for transfer. All overt injuries should be identified and the possibility of concealed injuries considered, based on the clinical picture and mechanism of injury.

Polytrauma casualties may require multiple interventions prior to transfer, but remember:

• each intervention requires time
• the ideal management of one injury may impact negatively on that of another.

To minimise scene time injuries should be dealt with simultaneously utilising a team approach.

Physiological considerations

During the primary transfer of polytrauma casualties the physiological targets aimed for are dependant on organ systems injured. In the casualty with hypovolaemic shock the initial management is to allow 'permissive hypotension' (Box 37.2) (shown to reduce mortality). Permissive hypotension should not be continued indefinitely as prolonged hypotension will result in irreversible acidosis. Whilst there is no international consensus, a maximum of 1–2 hours is suggested.

Box 37.2 Permissive hypotension

Resuscitation to a palpable radial pulse or systolic >90 mmHg
Aim to reduce further clot disruption/reduce haemodilution
Causes ongoing tissue hypoperfusion
Contraindicated in head injury

In the head injured casualty hypotension is associated with significantly worse neurological outcome. In this group a mean arterial pressure (MAP) of >80 mmHg should be maintained to ensure adequate cerebral perfusion. However, in the pre-hospital environment confirming head injury as the cause of altered consciousness is difficult. Shock, hypoxia, hypoglycaemia, alcohol or drugs can also result in altered mental status. When the possibility of head injury and shock co-exist, the clinician must decide how best to manage blood pressure (Table 37.1).

Table 37.1 Challenges in managing head injured patients with polytrauma.

Head injury target	Conflict in polytrauma
MAP >80 mmHg	Hypovolemic shock requiring permissive hypotension
EtCO$_2$ 4.0 kPa or PaCO$_2$ 4.5 kPa	Protective lung ventilation in chest injury, management involves low tidal volumes and peak airway pressures (tidal volume 6–8 mL/kg, peak plateau pressure <30 cmH$_2$O). This may require permissive hypercapnia
No obstruction to venous drainage	Cervical collar for suspected cervical injury can reduce venous blood flow through internal jugular veins
Head up 30°	Spinal/pelvic injury contraindicates flexion at the waist
	If hypovolaemic this will worsen cerebral perfusion

Secondary transfer

As with primary transfer the aim when preparing the casualty is to maximise physiological stability. Casualties should be assessed in a stepwise manner to ensure all systems are reviewed prior to departure, utilising a transfer checklist (see Appendix 4).

All bleeding should be controlled and casualties should be cardio-vascularly stable and haemoglobin/clotting normalised prior to transfer. A baseline blood gas should be taken ensuring any significant abnormalities are corrected (Table 37.2).

Intercostal drains should be sited prior to transfer in ventilated casualties with pneumothorax or spontaneously ventilating patients with pneumothorax/haemothorax and respiratory compromise. All necessary imaging and medical notes should be available to transfer with the casualty.

Considerations during transfer

Head injured patients should be managed to minimise rises in intracranial pressure (Table 37.1). In the sedated and ventilated casualty the cervical collar should be loosened or removed but the head should remain immobilised in the neutral position (blocks/straps).

Careful rolling of casualties is necessary during long transfers to avoid pressure sores. In casualties who have had temporary surgical measures, such as abdominal packing or a pelvic binder for pelvic fracture, this may dislodge any primary clot leading to catas-

Table 37.2 Examples of abnormalities screened for on blood gas analysis in polytrauma.

Blood gas target	Reasons for abnormalities
Potassium <6 mmol/L	Soft tissue damage (rhabdomyalysis) and massive transfusion increase serum potassium
Calcium >1 mmol/L	Falls with blood product administration if products contain citrate.
pH/BE/lactate acceptable	Metabolic acidosis if under resuscitated
PaCO$_2$ 4.5–5 kPa	Confirm correlation with EtCO$_2$ value for accurate targeting in head injury management

trophic bleeding. While avoidance of pressure points would be ideal, cardiovascular stability takes precedence.

Polytrauma casualties are susceptible to chest injuries and if suspected protective lung ventilation strategies should be used:

- blunt chest trauma – pulmonary contusions
- blast Injury – blast lung
- transfusion – transfusion-related acute lung injury (TRALI).

The effect on respiratory function will depend on the time and severity of initial injury.

UK Defence Medical Services retrieval systems

UK Defence Medical Services (UK-DMS) has seen high levels of severe trauma over the last decade. In 2006–2007 ISS scores over 36 occurred in 51.3% of casualties compared to only 8.4% in the NHS. The mechanism of injury is significantly different, with penetrating/blast injury accounting for 83.7% in UK field hospitals in Iraq and Afghanistan. In contrast, motor vehicle crashes accounted for only 5.1% of injury compared to 56.3% in the NHS.

The differences in injury pattern and type along with ongoing combat operations at the point of wounding, has lead to key differences in casualty retrieval and treatment (Box 37.3).

> Box 37.3 **Principles of the Geneva Convention regarding medical evacuations**
>
> Protects medical vehicles, facilities and personnel from attack
> Must be marked with protective emblem – Red Cross, Red Crescent, Red Diamond
> Personnel and vehicles can have light armament for *personnel protection only*

Medical planning and lay down

In order to understand UK DMS casualty retrieval it is important to understand the overall aims of the deployed medical system and the stages that require casualty transfer. Medical facilities are divided into four roles/echelons of care, defined by NATO (Table 37.3). Casualties are transferred down the evacuation chain from Role 1 to 4. It is implicit in NATO doctrine that each Role not only extends the medical capability, but also retains that of the facility before it. This system developed from conflicts with a secure area (rear area) behind the front line, allowing freedom of movement of medical vehicles (Box 37.3) to enable MEDEVAC (Box 37.4). Casualty movement is by road or air dependent on distance and speed of evacuation required.

Medical time lines

Facilities are positioned to ensure treatment of casualties within specified time frames set by the NATO 1-2-4 rule (Box 37.5). During recent conflicts the UK-DMS has developed an approach of 'damage control resuscitation' (DCR) for treating major trauma.

Box 37.4 **Military evacuation definitions**

CASEVAC – primary casualty evacuation in a non-assigned vehicle (an aircraft of opportunity) which may not include in-transit care
MEDEVAC – Forward Aeromedical evacuation – transfer from the point of wounding to the initial medical treatment facility which may be anything from a R1 Regimental Aid Post to a R3 Field Hospital.
TACEVAC – Medical evacuation between treatment facilities within an operational area.
STRATEVAC – Medical evacuation primarily from an operational area to a home or allied nation.

Box 37.5 **NATO 1-2-4 rule**

1 – Primary surgery within 1 hour
2 – if unavailable DCR within 2 hours
4 – Primary surgery within 4 hours of DCR

DCR is defined by UK-DMS as 'a systematic approach to major trauma combining the <C>ABC (catastrophic bleeding, airway, breathing, circulation) paradigm with a series of clinical techniques from point of wounding to definitive treatment in order to minimise blood loss, maximise tissue oxygenation and optimise outcome.'

The elements of DCR are:

- permissive hypotension – minimise clot disruption and haemodilution

- haemostatic resuscitation – early delivery of blood products to reverse coagulopathy
- damage control surgery – stop haemorrhage/minimise contamination.

This shift has led to a change in clinical timelines that guide UK military medical planning. Assets are laid down in order to achieve timelines set by the 10-1-2 rule (Box 37.6).

Box 37.6 **UK-DMS 10-1-2 rule**

10 – bleeding and airway control within 10 minutes
1 – advanced airway, analgesia and IV access within 1 hour
2 – surgery within 2 hours

Primary retrieval

To achieve treatment timelines and project clinical assets forward, the Medical Emergency Response Team (MERT) was developed. On current operations, areas outside of established bases are deemed non-secure, prohibiting ground evacuation. Therefore MERT is a rotary-based asset, but this may vary on future operations.

Primary retrieval activation

There are several terms used to describe casualty evacuation (see Box 37.4). NATO doctrine directs that medical evacuation is controlled by a Casualty Evacuation Co-ordination Centre (PECC), part of the military command chain. Requests for casualty evacuation are initiated by a ground call sign (military unit) using a

Table 37.3 Nato-defined military medical echelons of care.

Role	Treatment aim	Equipment	Personnel
Role 1	Initial field resuscitation Primary health care	Non-invasive monitoring Non-refrigerated drugs	Combat medical technicians Regimental Medical Officer
Role 2 Light Manoeuvre (R2LM)	Damage control surgery and haemostatic resuscitation	Operating table Invasive monitoring Small blood product supply Short-term intensive care capability Plain X-ray/USS	Nursing staff Operating department practitioner Consultant surgeon and anaesthetists
Role 2 Enhanced (R2E)	Damage control surgery and primary surgery (deployed when Role 3 facility not required)	Operating tables Computed tomography Medical/surgical specialties Intensive care facilities Full laboratory and blood product support Basic rehabilitation services	Nursing staff Operating Department Practitioner Consultant Surgeons Physicians and Anaesthetists
Role 3	Primary Surgery to ensure stability prior to evacuation	Operating tables Computed Tomography Medical/Surgical Specialties Intensive Care Facilities Full laboratory and blood product support	Nursing staff Operating department practitioner Consultant surgeon and anaesthetists Physiotherapists Pain team
Role 4	Full spectrum of definitive medical care that cannot be deployed to theatre or is too time consuming to be *conducted there*	All medical/surgical subspecialties Full imaging capability Full rehabilitation services	Nursing staff Operating department practitioner Multiple consultants Physiotherapists Pain team

Table 37.4 The ATMIST report.

Line 1 Location (grid)

Line 2 Call sign and frequency

Line 3 Number of patients/priority:
Urgent (R2/R3 within 30 minutes)	Priority (R2/R3 within 24 hours)
Priority (R2/R3 within 4 hours)	

Line 4 Special equipment required:
None	Extrication equipment
Hoist	Ventilation

Line 5 Number of patients
Litter	Ambulatory

Line 6 Security at pick up site
No enemy	Enemy in area
Possible enemy	Hot pick-up zone

Line 7 Pick up zone marking method
Panels	None
Pyro	Other
Smoke	

Line 8 No. of patients by nationality
Coalition military	Non-coalition civilian
Civilian with coalition forces	Opposing forces/PW/detainees
Non-coalition security forces	Children

Line 9 Terrain/obstacles

Source: www.gov.uk/government/publications/jsp-999-clinical-guidelines-for-operations.

NATO '9-liner', augmented by an AT MIST report (see Table 37.4). Depending on the injury type/severity, an appropriate evacuation platform is tasked by PECC, including routine transport aircraft or specific medical airframes.

Comparison with civilian air ambulance services

Size

The current preferred aircraft is the CH-47 Chinook: seven stretchers can be placed on the floor and up to 23 casualties have been moved in a single lift. The aircraft itself can lift over 55 passengers, for a normal mission floor space, not weight, is the limiting factor. The MERT equipment is transferable between any Chinook in the fleet and does not rely on bespoke fittings (see Figure 37.1). In the event of an unserviceable aircraft a new one can be loaded in less than 15 minutes. Training is undertaken in other RAF aircraft as Chinooks will not always be available.

The US Army uses pairs of UH-60A Blackhawk aircraft which can carry two or three stretchers each, are unarmed and marked with a Red Cross (Box 37.3). The US Air Force uses pairs of specialist HH-60 Blackhawk aircraft which are armed and have night operations capability. These are not marked with a Red Cross and are designed for 'personnel recovery' tasks, but often perform conventional MEDIVAC missions.

Crew

MERT medical personnel are an emergency department nurse and two paramedics. MERT(E) includes the enhanced skillset of

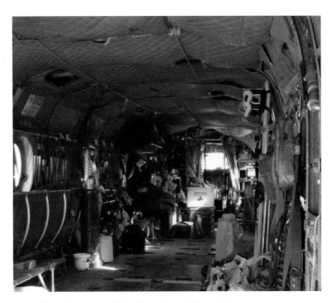

Figure 37.1 The inside of CH-47 configured for MERT use.

a pre-hospital consultant physician. Accompanying them are RAF Regiment soldiers, providing force protection. The medical crew will often work together on a daily basis, enhancing team cohesion.

Escorts

The MERT is accompanied by two AH-64 Apache Attack helicopters providing:

- improved air to ground communications
- fire support to the ground call-sign
- security for the helicopter landing site (HLS).

HLS

The ground call-sign, rather than the pilot, identifies the HLS and direction of approach. There is often significant dust leading to loss of visual contact between the aircrew and the ground call sign (further compounded by night evacuations). Security cannot be guaranteed so time on the ground is minimised. The rotors are kept running making the rear of the CH-47 the only safe approach. This produces significant noise making verbal handover almost impossible. A written AT MIST is passed with the casualty, often written on the casualty themselves as paper is liable to displacement in the down draft of the rotors.

In-flight treatment

The two most significant differences are:

- all medical treatment is carried out in the aircraft
- there are often multiple casualties making triage necessary.

The availability of space allows 360° access. However, vibration and the necessity to use blue light at night can hinder treatment. Resuscitation follows a <C>ABC approach with team members simultaneously treating the casualty, as with hospital-based resuscitation. When initially loaded the casualty will not have any monitoring attached, as equipment needs to be retained by the ground call sign. If required, RSI is carried out in-flight, manual in-line stabilisation is used only if specifically indicated. Packed red blood cells and fresh frozen plasma are carried on board and administered warmed from the outset in hypovolaemic casualties, initiating 'haemostatic resuscitation'.

Hospital handover

Similar to civilian HEMS services, handover utilises a structured format (e.g. AT MIST). Only lifesaving treatment of the casualty should occur during this time. Non-NATO casualties need to be searched to ensure no live ammunition or explosives are brought into the hospital. Handover may therefore occur prior to these casualties' arrival.

Secondary retrieval services

Secondary retrieval consists of TACEVAC and STRATEVAC (see Box 37.4). All casualty transfers are initiated by a Patient Movement Request (PMR) completed by the sending treatment facility. This contains a comprehensive summary of the patient's condition and treatment to date. It allows allocation of the appropriate transfer resources. For the UK this can be a Critical Care Air Support Team (CCAST) for high-dependency and ventilated casualties, or nurses and flight medics from the aeromedical evacuation squadron for the more stable/routine transfers. There are two CCAST immediately available (one based in the operational theatre), with a third on 6 hours' notice to move in the UK.

It is the responsibility of the Air Evacuation Liaison Officer (AELO) to provide an interface with Air Command in the UK to identify a suitable airframe and coordinate transfer within a clinically suitable timeframe. The preferred aircraft are C-17 Globemaster or Tri-star for STRATEVAC.

Team composition

The basic team consists of a consultant intensivist (and a trainee), two flight nurses (one of whom is team leader), a flight nursing assistant and a medical devices technician. Multiple casualties will see this team augmented depending on their individual condition. All clinical staff work in critical care areas in the UK, and before being cleared to fly undertake multiple training courses, including two weeks focusing exclusively on equipment.

Equipment

Typical equipment for a single casualty transfer weighs in excess of 500 kg. Any equipment used has to be cleared for flight on military aircraft prior to use and operate independently of aircraft power and oxygen supplies (for up to 12 hours), maximising flexibility and safety. I-Stat can provide routine blood results as well as blood gas analysis during transfer.

CCAST will transfer casualties with quantities of blood and FFP to continue haemostatic resuscitation during transfer after DCS. As with civilian transfers, lines and chest drains are placed prior to transfer.

Regional anaesthesia

For non-ventilated casualties with significant peripheral injuries, continuous infusion of local anaesthetic nerve blocks via elastomeric pumps have been successfully used over the last 5 years. They are also provided with a morphine patient-controlled analgesia (PCA) device in case of breakthrough pain.

Specialist capability

As well as the secondary transfer of battlefield casualties the Royal Air Force continues to provide a retrieval capability to the UK Armed Forces covering the rest of the world. They also provide the UK air-transportable isolation service to the Department of Health and can manage CBRN (Chemical, Biological, Radiation, Nuclear) casualties.

Clinical governance

The monitoring of performance is essential to ensure casualties are receiving the best available care, by clinical audit, incident reporting and trend analysis (including time lines for evacuation). At present this occurs in bi-weekly clinical governance meetings in theatre, and in the UK, where all patient report forms are analysed.

Disclaimer

The opinions expressed are those of the authors and not necessarily MoD.

Further reading

Bricknell M, Johnson A. Forward medical evacuation. JRAMC 157;4: S444–8.

Bricknell M, Kelly L. Tactical aeromedical evacuation. JRAMC 157;4: S449–452

Garner J, Watts S, Parry C, Bird J, Cooper G, Kirkman E. Joint Services Publication 999 Clinical Guidelines for Operations. Prolonged Permissive Hypotensive Resuscitation Is Associated With Poor Outcome in Primary Blast Injury With Controlled Hemorrhage. Ann Surg 2010;251: 1131–9.

Hodgetts TJ, Davies S, Russell R, McLeod J. Benchmarking the UK military deployed trauma system. J R Army Med Corps 2007;153:237–8.

Joint Doctrine Publication 4-03 Joint Medical Doctrine (May 19, 2011)

Kehoe A, Jones A, Marcus S, et al. Current controversies in military pre-hospital critical care. JRAMC 157;3: S305–9

Ryan's Ballistic Trauma: A practical Guide. 3rd Edition. Springer Publications 2011.

Turner S, Ruth M, Tipping R. Critical care air support teams and deployed intensive care. JRAMC 155;2:171–4.

CHAPTER 38

Obstetric Transfers

H. Simpson

James Cook University Hospital, South Tees Foundation Trust, UK

OVERVIEW

- The key principle for most obstetric transfers from the home environment is scoop and run
- If delivery is imminent prepare for it and ask for assistance from a midwife
- Be aware of the need for time critical transfer
- Always remember there are two patients and both need consideration and assessment for transfer.

Introduction

Transfer may be required from any place of delivery. Risk factors leading to transfer of mother *and/or* baby develop antenatally, during labour or postnatally. Evaluation of these, leads to a decision of whether to undertake immediate transport or conduct a delivery in the non-hospital environment. Table 38.1 summarises the key roles of staff involved in obstetric transfers.

Table 38.1 Key roles of staff involved in the transfer of obstetric patients.

	Paramedic/doctor	Midwife	Obstetrician/accepting unit via phone
Clinical condition	Assess	Assess	
Initial treatment	ALS Obstetric support	Assist ALS Obstetric expertise	Advice on treatment
Transfer	Transportation Liaise with accepting unit Advise accepting unit of expected time of arrival and clinical situation	Advice on appropriate accepting unit Liaise with accepting unit Advice on timing and need for transfer	Advise on appropriate accepting unit Advice on timing and need for transfer

Reasons for transfer

Transfer from home or other non-hospital environment without midwifery support

Unless delivery imminent, scoop and run, otherwise urgently request midwifery attendance depending on local policy (Box 38.1).

Box 38.1 **Possible reasons for transfer from home without midwifery support**

Labour ± delivery (term or preterm)
Haemorrhage: antenatal or postnatal (including miscarriage)
Abdominal pain other than labour
Eclampsia
Prolapsed cord
Non-obstetric reason, e.g. asthma, chest pain, trauma

Transfer from a home or midwifery standalone unit with midwifery support

In this case the decision for transfer has already been made by the attending midwife. The midwife will accompany the woman on the transfer and is responsible for any obstetric intervention (Box 38.2).

Box 38.2 **Possible reasons for transfer from a home delivery with midwifery support**

Concerns about labour progress
Fetal compromise
Concerns over maternal well being, e.g. raised BP, haemorrhage, risk of sepsis
Neonatal wellbeing.

Transfer from a consultant-led unit (Box 38.3)

A midwife (±medical staff) will accompany depending on clinical situation.

Box 38.3 **Reasons for transfer from a consultant-led unit**

Need for a neonatal cot due to prematurity or congenital abnormality
Maternal specialist care, e.g. ICU, liver unit, neurology HDU, CCU.

ABC of Transfer and Retrieval Medicine, First Edition.
Edited by Adam Low and Jonathan Hulme.
© 2015 John Wiley & Sons, Ltd. Published 2015 by John Wiley & Sons, Ltd.

Principles of obstetric emergencies

Overall assessment from the 'end of the bed' ('Quick Scan') and perform primary survey as detailed in the resuscitation and stabilisation chapter, using **<C>ABCDE plus F for fundus** (Box 38.4). If the baby has been delivered undertake a separate primary survey. There are **two patients** and rarely this may necessitate calling a second crew.

Box 38.4 **Quick scan and primary survey key points**

<C> Catastrophic haemorrhage: blood on the floor, bed linen, soaked clothes, bath towels. Volume loss usually significantly underestimated.

A. Provide high flow oxygen
    If needed, gold standard airway management is **intubation** which may be more difficult than usual due to:
    ○ presence of full dentition
    ○ short obese (oedematous) neck
    ○ engorged breasts
    ○ oedema of the upper airway (in pre-eclamspia)
    ○ risk of regurgitation during intubation

B. Tachypnoea is an early sign of maternal compromise. Ventilation can be more difficult due to splinting of the diaphragm by the gravid uterus

C. 15–30 degree left lateral tilt required after 20 weeks' gestation if supine, to relieve pressure from gravid uterus on inferior vena cava. NB: Physiological changes of pregnancy may mask early signs of shock associated with acute blood loss. Following trauma (e.g. road traffic crash) a woman may appear well but the foetus could be severely compromised. Immediately transfer pregnant patients to an obstetric unit/ED following crashes ≥ 50 kph (30 mph).

D. As for non-pregnant women

E. Has the baby been born, is the house clean and warm, are other children around, where is the woman located?

F. **F**undal height above umbilicus means pregnancy likely to be >24 weeks. If below the umbilicus, foetus unlikely to be viable.

Some transfers are time critical (Box 38.5) and should proceed immediately with blue light ambulance. Do not delay for interventions that may be done en route, e.g. IV/IO access.

Box 38.5 **Examples of time critical transfer**

Haemorrhage
Eclamptic fit
Cord prolapse
Shoulder dystocia (failed initial management)
Head entrapment with breech presentation
Maternal collapse
Continuing neonatal resuscitation

If birth is imminent prepare for delivery: do not transfer unless birth complications occur. Some common problems are described below with principles of management. Non-obstetric emergencies

are managed with the addition of left lateral tilt if necessary (Box 38.4).

In a secondary survey check the woman's hand-held notes for information. Ensure they accompany the woman throughout.

Aim to transfer to the booked obstetric unit, although if time critical, and another suitable unit is closer then divert. Always inform the accepting unit of impending arrival and clinical condition of woman/baby.

Management of specific obstetric emergencies

Severe pre-eclampsia
Hypertension and proteinuria ≥20 weeks' gestation.
    Features indicating need for time critical transfer:

- headache – severe and frontal
- visual disturbances
- epigastric pain
- right-sided upper abdominal pain (liver capsule)
- muscle twitching or tremor
- nausea, vomiting, confusion.

New systolic BP ≥160 mmHg or diastolic BP ≥110 mmHg requires urgent admission.

Eclampsia
Pre-eclampsia + tonic-clonic fit.
    Can present with no prior signs/symptoms. One-third cases occur in postnatal period.
    Usually self limiting; may be prolonged and repeated.
    Assume a grand mal fit in pregnancy (beyond 20 weeks) is eclampsia until proven otherwise. Epileptic patients have eclamptic fits. Treat a fitting epileptic patient with history of hypertension/pre-eclampsia as eclampsia. If no hypertension/pre-eclampsia treat as epilepsy, but monitor blood pressure until after the postictal phase and discuss with midwife.
    Specific treatment: 4 g of magnesium sulphate IV/IO over 15 minutes (followed by infusion of 1 g/h at hospital). If unavailable and seizure not self-limiting, consider diazemuls 10–20 mg IV/IO or diazepam 10–20 mg PR.
    DO NOT give routine IV fluids due to high risk of acute pulmonary oedema.

Pre-term labour
Before 37 weeks. Very preterm <32 weeks, extreme prematurity <28 weeks.
    May be little or no contraction pain and membranes may rupture before the onset of labour. Malpresentation (e.g. breech) and cord prolapse are more common.
    Pay attention to fundal height – is viability likely?
    Transport without delay unless prehospital birth likely. If so, request midwife and second ambulance, ideally with an incubator. Assemble maternity and paediatric (neonatal) kits, oxygen, Entonox, ALS kit, and warm towels and blankets. Prepare a separate

area for management of the baby and transfer as soon after delivery as possible.

Antepartum haemorrhage

Bleeding prior to delivery (including during labour). Two main causes are placenta praevia (low-lying placenta) and abruption. Differentiating cause does not change pre-hospital management/need for transfer.

A small external bleed may be a massive concealed haemorrhage. Give 250-mL aliquots of crystalloids to maintain SBP at 100 mmHg and analgesia if needed. Maintain nil by mouth.

Postpartum haemorrhage

Blood loss post delivery ≥500 mL. Blood loss >1,500 mL and ongoing needs time critical transfer.

Four Ts as causes of PPH are:

- tone (commonest cause)
- tissue (retained placenta)
- trauma
- thrombin (coagulopathy).

If uterus boggy, 'rub up' a contraction (this may cause discomfort) and give second dose of oxytocic (e.g. IM syntometrine 1 mL or misoprostol 800 µg PR):

1 Gently 'massage' uterus through abdominal wall with your hand.
2 Blood clots may be expelled.
3 Bleeding should reduce and uterus become firm and smaller.
4 May need to continue for several minutes.

If uterus not contracting and haemorrhage increasing, commence bimanual uterine compression (Figure 38.1) to control bleeding during transfer to hospital. Check vulva/perineum for trauma and apply local compression. Catheterise if possible (aids contraction).

Uterine inversion

Post delivery, occurring spontaneously or with incorrect cord traction. Can be incomplete (may feel a 'dimple' in the uterus per abdomen) or complete (uterus visible at or through introitus).

Can be associated with severe bradycardia: treat with 500 µg of atropine titrated to effect (3 mg maximum) and if mass visible attempt to replace inverted uterus (Figure 38.1).

1 Inform patient that you are going to try to replace the womb inside the vagina and that this will be uncomfortable.
2 Sterile gloves.
3 DO NOT remove the placenta if still attached
4 Gently squeeze the part of the uterus nearest the vaginal entrance and gradually ease it back within the vagina.
5 Gradually move your hands to the fundus of the uterus in the same way.
6 Once the uterus is replaced rub up a contraction and gently remove the inserting hand.
7 Time critical transfer in the supine position.

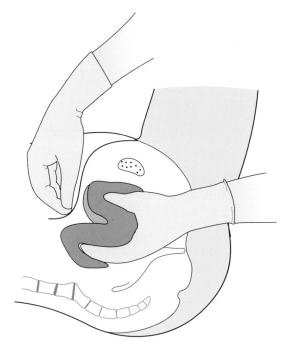

Figure 38.1 How to replace the uterus after inversion. (Source: Manley, K. (2013). Care of Special Groups: The Obstetric Patient. In: Nutbeam, T. and Boylan, M. (eds). ABC of Prehospital Emergency Medicine. John Wiley & Sons Ltd, Oxford, pp. 150–158).

Prolapsed cord

Presenting with absent membranes.

If delivery imminent, encourage pushing. Prepare for neonatal resuscitation.

If delivery not imminent, elevate presenting part of the foetus above pelvic inlet to relieve compression (Box 38.6). Bring trolley as close as possible to patient: do NOT use carry-chair as this increases cord compression. A rescue board with 15–30 degree left lateral tilt and hips raised on blankets can be used.

Box 38.6 **Elevation of the presenting part**

Method 1: Positioning patient kneeling and leaning forward with face near the floor/bed and buttocks raised. This is optimal position whilst preparing for transfer.
Method 2: For transfer 15–30 degree left lateral position and lower the head of trolley below level of pelvis. Secure with seat belts.
Method 3: Cradle loop of cord gently in your palm and use index and middle fingers to apply upward pressure to presenting foetal part. Maintain to hospital.
Method 4: Insert urinary catheter and fill bladder with up to 500 ml fluid & clamp. This replaces need for manual displacement. Ideally perform prior to transfer to the ambulance.

Monitoring before and during transfer

Record routine observations, frequency is dictated by clinical condition. Continuous monitoring in normal labour may not be required.

Fetal heart rate should not be monitored unless a midwife is present; it will not change management. Auscultation should not delay transfer. During transfer it is very difficult due to environmental noise. A history of foetal movements can be obtained as part of the secondary survey and is useful information for the accepting team.

Resuscitation of maternal cardiac arrest

Cardiac arrest in pregnancy is rare (1:30,000 pregnancies). Common causes include haemorrhage, pulmonary embolism, cardiac conditions, stroke, trauma and overdose. The commonest presenting rhythm is PEA.

Management follows standard advanced life support algorithms with the addition of these key principles:

- displace gravid uterus (maintain left lateral tilt)
- Intubation as preferred airway management technique
- consider perimortem Caesarean section and perform within 5 minutes (Box 38.7). Not usually done in the pre-hospital setting
- pre-alert ED/obstetric unit including the neonatal/paediatric team
- continue CPR until further assessment in hospital setting unless there are obvious other signs of non-survivable injury (apply local protocol).

Box 38.7 How to perform a perimortem Caesarean section

Rapid decision to proceed (anaesthesia not needed)

Continue CPR

Wear sterile gloves and apply basic skin preparation

A midline incision provides better access but it may be quicker to perform low transverse incision depending on clinical experience

Open uterus with midline incision or in lower segment depending on clinical experience

Deliver baby, hand over for assessment and resuscitation

Leave placenta *in situ*

Bleeding is minimal because of cardiac arrest

Bimanual 'open' cardiac massage via the diaphragm may be performed

If resuscitation successful, anaesthesia will be required for delivery of placenta and incision closure.

'How to' advice

Normal delivery in the absence of a midwife

- Allow woman to find comfortable position
- Allow spontaneous delivery
- Document time of delivery of head and body
- Dry and wrap baby; assess and treat as per neonatal guidelines
- Clamp and cut cord when stopped pulsating, 15 cm from baby. Keep neonatal fingers and genitalia clear of scissors!
- Keep baby warm (e.g. skin-to-skin)
- Depending on local policy, call for midwife attend or transfer to appropriate unit
- If delay in delivery of the body, instigate shoulder dystocia protocol.

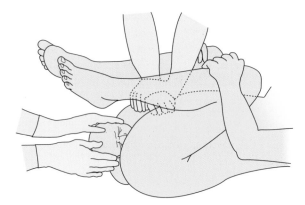

Figure 38.2 McRobert's manoeuvre with suprapubic pressure. (Source: Manley, K. (2013). Care of Special Groups: The Obstetric Patient. In: Nutbeam, T. and Boylan, M. (eds). ABC of Prehospital Emergency Medicine. John Wiley & Sons Ltd, Oxford, pp. 150–158).

Shoulder dystocia protocol

- Do not pull, twist or bend baby's neck
- Do not press on the uterine fundus
- Do not cut cord before baby is delivered
- Attempt to deliver anterior shoulder with gentle downwards traction
- If unsuccessful after two contractions, move on to **McRobert's manoeuvre** (Figure 38.2: McRoberts with suprapubic pressure):
  ◦ lie mother flat with one pillow under her head
  ◦ bring knees towards chest and abduct slightly
  ◦ attempt delivery with gentle traction downwards.
- After 1 minute move on to **suprapubic pressure**:
  ◦ identify foetal back
  ◦ second person stands on the side of the baby's back (if the baby is facing left, stand on the mother's right or vice versa)
  ◦ place heel of hand two finger breadths above symphysis pubis behind baby's shoulder (cf. CPR hand placement)
  ◦ apply moderate pressure across and downwards
  ◦ attempt to deliver with gentle traction and suprapubic pressure.
- After 1 minute move on to:
  ◦ **rocking** suprapubic pressure: gently rock backwards and forwards whilst applying suprapubic pressure
  ◦ attempt to deliver with gentle traction downwards.
- After 1 minute move on to:
  ◦ **all fours' position**: as for cord prolapse (Box 38.6)
  ◦ attempt to deliver posterior shoulder with gentle traction downwards towards the floor.
- If all above manoeuvres fail move on to:
  ◦ **time critical transfer to nearest staffed obstetric unit.**

Breech delivery in the absence of a midwife

- Request urgent attendance of midwife.
- Position woman in semi-recumbent position with buttocks at edge of bed/sofa with legs in lithotomy (support on chairs or she can hold them) or allow her to adopt squatting position or all fours.

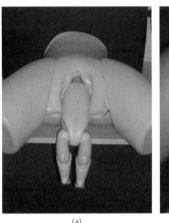
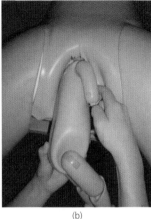

(a)   (b)

Figure 38.3 (a,b) Delivery of the foetal arm. (Source: Manley, K. (2013). Care of Special Groups: The Obstetric Patient. In: Nutbeam, T. and Boylan, M. (eds). ABC of Prehospital Emergency Medicine. John Wiley & Sons Ltd, Oxford, pp. 150–158).

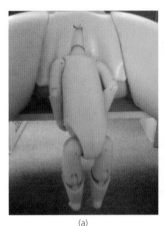
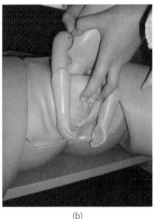

(a)   (b)

Figure 38.4 (a,b) Supporting the baby during spontaneous vaginal delivery. (Source: Manley, K. (2013). Care of Special Groups: The Obstetric Patient. In: Nutbeam, T. and Boylan, M. (eds). ABC of Prehospital Emergency Medicine. John Wiley & Sons Ltd, Oxford, pp. 150–158).

- **Hands off approach**: allow spontaneous delivery.
- Breech should rotate spontaneously so baby's umbilicus points to mother's anus.
- Wrap a towel around the baby's body during the delivery to maintain warmth.
- DO NOT pull on the baby: optimise position and gentle traction only.
- If no spontaneous rotation: hold baby's pelvis & rotate to required position.
- If legs do not deliver: flex at knee joint and abduct hip. Take care not to pull down a loop of cord.
- If arms do not deliver: hold baby's pelvis, gently lift and rotate until one of shoulders is in the anterior position (Figure 38.3). Run finger over shoulder and down to elbow and sweep arm across front of baby. Rotate so baby's umbilicus points to mother's anus. Repeat to free other arm.
- If head does not deliver: support baby's trunk horizontally over your arm and place two fingers of supporting arm into mother's vagina, one on each of baby's cheekbones. With other hand, place index and fourth fingers on baby's shoulders. Use middle finger to flex of head by pressing on occiput (Figure 38.4).
- McRobert's position (see shoulder dystocia) and suprapubic pressure can aid head delivery. If head still does not deliver and midwife has not arrived, obtain most rapid skilled obstetric assistance through the usual channels.
- Be prepared to resuscitate baby.

Further reading

CMACE. Saving Mothers Lives: Reviewing maternal deaths to make motherhood safer 2006-2008. BJOG 118(Suppl 1) March 2011

JRCALC guidelines 2013

Woollard M, Hinshaw K, Simpson H, Wieteska S (eds) *Pre-hospital Emergency Training*. Wiley-Blackwell 2010.

CHAPTER 39

Cardiac Transfers

C. Westrope[1] and C. Harvey[2]

[1]University Hospitals of Leicester NHS Trust, UK
[2]ECMO Department, University Hospitals of Leicester NHS Trust, UK

OVERVIEW

- Temporary devices can be used to support cardiac and respiratory function pending medical or surgical treatment
- Patients may require transfer with these devices *in situ* to tertiary centres
- Transfer and retrieval practitioners should therefore be familiar with these devices and the practicalities of transferring patients supported by them
- Services and stakeholders should work to develop SOPs and specific checklists for these specialist transfers.

Introduction

Those working in transfer and retrieval services should be familiar with the management of acute coronary syndromes and cardiac arrhythmias for which there are well publicised international protocols.

Devices to support acute severe physiological deterioration in cardiac and respiratory function include extracorporeal life support systems and assist devices. While an in-depth review of these devices is beyond the scope of this book, some practical considerations relating to transfer of patients with these devices are considered.

Extracorporeal life support (ECLS) is a general term to describe prolonged but temporary support of heart and lung function using mechanical devices for patients with potentially reversible pathology where conventional therapy is failing. The concept of supporting respiratory function with extracorporeal gas exchange is not new: the first patients were treated in the 1970s. Recent advances in technology coupled with evidence of the efficacy of adult ECMO has led to worldwide increased use.

Extracorporeal life support techniques

All ECLS devices have the following:

ABC of Transfer and Retrieval Medicine, First Edition.
Edited by Adam Low and Jonathan Hulme.
© 2015 John Wiley & Sons, Ltd. Published 2015 by John Wiley & Sons, Ltd.

- vascular access catheters of sufficient sizes to permit desired blood flow
- circuit tubing
- blood pump (centrifugal or roller pump)
- gas exchange device (oxygenator)
- heat exchanger
- MONITORING devices.

To prevent blood clotting in the circuit systemic anticoagulation is also required.

The various subtypes of ECLS (with varying degrees of overlap) include the following.

Extracorporeal membrane oxygenation (ECMO)

The term ECMO is used synonymously with ECLS. Oxygenation and carbon dioxide removal via pumped high blood flow through the device replace lung and/or heart function.

Vascular access may be veno-venous (VV) where support is primarily required for the respiratory system or veno-arterial (VA) providing full cardorespiratory support.

Extracorporeal lung assist (ECLA)

These low flow systems may be used to prevent intubation or minimise ventilation. Blood passes around the circuit and oxygenator due to an extrinsic pump system (e.g. Hemolung RAS) or due to the patient's own blood pressure (e.g. Novalung).

Extracorporeal carbon dioxide removal ($ECCO_2R$), Arteriovenous carbon dioxide removal ($AVCO_2R$) and pumpless ECLA (pECLA) are other terms also describing forms of lung assist.

Extracorporeal cardiopulmonary resuscitation (ECPR)

Emergency cardiac support in refractory cardiac arrest.

Ventricular assist device (VAD)

ECLS undertaken solely for cardiac support using blood pumps is LVAD (left ventricular assist device), RVAD (right ventricular assist device) or BiVAD (biventricular assist device).

ECMO support for adult patients

Indications for adult ECMO

Adult patients with potentially reversible cause(s) for their respiratory and/or cardiovascular failure who are failing maximal conventional ICU therapy, and have:

- less than 10 days total ventilation of which not more than 7 days has been with peak pressure >30 cmH$_2$O and FiO$_2$ >0.8
- no new intracranial haemorrhage
- no contraindication to minimal anticoagulation
- no contraindication to continuation of active treatment.

While not absolute contraindications, the following are often associated with very poor outcomes with ECMO support:

- presence of concomitant advanced comorbidities
- age >65 years
- compromised immune system.

Veno-venous (VV) ECMO

VV ECMO provides oxygenation and carbon dioxide removal. It relies on native cardiac function to pump blood, drained from and returned to the venous system, around the circuit.

Cannulation typically uses a percutaneous Seldinger technique with ultrasound or fluoroscopic guidance. The number and size of cannulae used is governed by the patient's weight and desired flow. Multiple single lumen cannulae (21–28 Fr for adults) or a double lumen cannula (20– 31 Fr) can be used with good outcomes.

The presence of significant inotropic support is not a contraindication to VV support as inotropic requirement often diminishes rapidly once therapy commences.

Veno-arterial (VA) ECMO (Figure 39.1)

VA support in adult patients is reserved for those cases with profound cardiac failure (or cardiac arrest when it is termed as ECPR). Blood is drained from the venous system via a cannula in the right internal jugular/femoral vein, and returned to the arterial system through a femoral artery. Blood is mechanically pumped into the arterial system providing direct cardiac assist.

While possible to cannulate both vein and artery with a Seldinger technique, surgical exposure via femoral cut down can be beneficial. It aids both accurate placement of a correctly sized arterial cannula and also facilitates placement of an additional perfusion cannula to prevent distal ischaemia of the cannulated limb.

Mobile ECMO

Despite advances in conventional intensive care, ECMO used appropriately can significantly improve survival. Although patients can be moved to an ECMO centre with conventional cardiorespiratory support, if they have rapidly become too unstable, it is possible to transport on ECMO to a specialist centre (Box 39.1). Emergency cannulation/ECPR is started in the referring centre either by the referring team or the ECMO retrieval team.

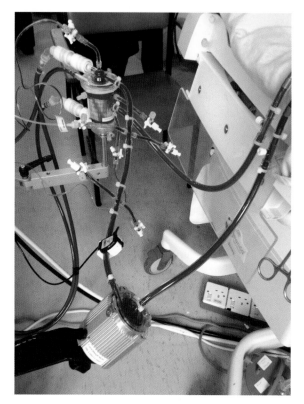

Figure 39.1 Modern centrifugal ECMO system.

Box 39.1 **Considerations for instigating mobile ECMO**

Advantages

ECMO is commenced sooner
Patients are stabilised in the hospital environment prior to transfer
Patients with gross haemodynamic and or respiratory failure can be transported safely

Risks

Procedure often performed with assistance of inexperienced staff
Failure to cannulate
Complications of cannulation
Mechanical failure of the ECMO circuit
Greater movement of patient increases likelihood of inadvertent decannulation or circuit rupture.

ECMO retrieval services

In the UK, mobile ECMO retrieval is a standard part of the national adult ECMO service. Such a service requires medical, nursing and perfusion professionals to be available round the clock and trained both in ECMO and transport medicine. A typical team has between two and four members depending on the skillset. Roles include the following.

Cannulator/transport doctor

The siting of an ECMO cannula into a critically ill patient requires personnel trained in insertion techniques and the ability to manage procedural complications (e.g. haemothorax, cardiac tamponade/rupture, distal leg ischaemia from arterial cannulation).

In established ECMO centres cannulation is usually performed in an operating room with a full theatre team present and fluoroscopy guidance for insertion of a bicaval double lumen line.

For mobile ECMO, the local team will almost certainly have little, if any, experience of extracorporeal life support; time spent briefing the team is essential for the procedure to be performed safely.

Prior to moving a patient from critical care to theatre, the ECMO circuit and essential staff should be ready in case the patient arrests. It may be necessary to take separate critical care and surgical staff especially if VA ECMO is envisaged.

Perfusionist

As the clinical expert in extracorporeal techniques and equipment, the perfusionist builds and primes the circuit and troubleshoots during transport. Some mobile ECMO teams do not take a perfusionist, but this should not be the routine, and reserved only for very experienced centres.

Transport nurse

Responsible for basic nursing care but should also be a qualified ECMO specialist, trained in circuit management and capable of dealing with related emergencies.

Equipment

The transport trolley (Figure 39.2) needs to be adapted to carry the patient, ECMO circuit and standard ICU equipment safely secured and conforming to relevant national standards.

The team must take equipment required to cannulate and maintain the patient on ECMO from referring hospital back to the ECMO centre.

Vehicles

Mobile ECMO can be performed in a road ambulance or, for longer distances, by fixed or rotary wing (Figure 39.3).

Modern ECMO pumps have a low power consumption and run for significant periods (up to 4 hours) on internal batteries. However, the water heater requires mains power to function so ideally the ambulance should be equipped with 240 V power (Figure 39.4). If it does not, it is possible to travel without a heater unit in adults without a clinically significant temperature drop.

Fixed-wing transport is limited by aircraft regulations governing equipment carried, size (particularly door size to enable patient transfer into the aircraft) and weight of the team, patient and equipment. DC power may be available but is often insufficient to power the heater unit.

Intra-aortic balloon pumps and assist devices

Heart failure is associated with increased morbidity and mortality; though some aetiologies portend a better prognosis. Reduction of

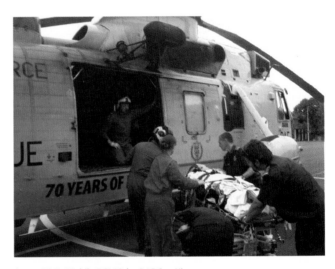

Figure 39.3 Mobile ECMO by RAF Sea King.

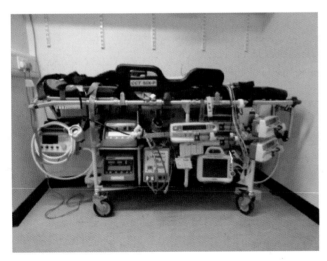

Figure 39.2 Mobile ECMO trolley.

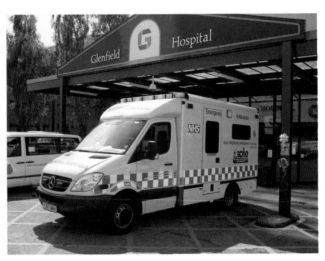

Figure 39.4 Dedicated ECMO Ambulance with 3 kW mains power.

Table 39.1 Summary of cardiac assist devices that may be encountered.

Device	Indication	Contraindications	Special considerations
IABP	Cardiogenic shock Cardiomyopathy Sepsis Unstable angina Acute MR and VSD	Dissection Aortic regurgitation Bilateral fem–pop bypass grafts	See Box 39.1
LVAD	Cardiogenic shock Bridge to transplant	End organ failure Reversible heart failure Metastatic malignancy Severe aortic/mitral valve lesions	Need anti-coagulation and anti-platelets Ensure patient has device details with them, controller and spare battery pack Meticulous attention to fluid balance Maintain sinus rhythm
BiVAD	Cardiogenic shock Destination therapy for end stage heart failure	Severe peripheral vascular disease Aortic regurgitation	Need anti-coagulation and anti-platelets Ensure patient has device details with them, controller and spare battery pack Risk of fluid shifts with gravitational pulls in transfer = decompensation Maintain sinus rhythm

myocardial oxygen demand with mechanical support, can allow time for optimised medical management including revascularisation and be a bridge to transplantation. Table 39.1 provides an overview of devices that may be encountered. It is not uncommon for patients to require secondary/tertiary transfers with these devices in situ and there is accumulating evidence that safe transfer can be undertaken, supported by relevant stakeholders and formalised protocols.

Box 39.2 summarises some practical considerations for transferring patients with intra-aortic balloon pumps. The patient

---

Box 39.2 Considerations for transferring a patient with a IABP *in situ*

Equipment

Retrieval services IABP versus hospital's

Changeover of pumps must be safe with time factored in for these 'handovers'

The service should have access to a 'Perfusionist' for advice

Select 'Autofill Mode' for balloon to allow for pressure changes with altitude if undertaking aeromedical transfer

Ensure adequate supply of helium for transfer

Ensure adequate battery life for duration of transfer (and delays)

Ensure the pump device and helium cylinder are safely secured for transfer

---

Drugs

Ensure adequate anticoagulation (low molecular weight heparins can be used rather than continuous infusions)

Rationalise inotropic infusions and number of syringe drivers

Pump

The referring team should ensure that the timing of the pump is optimised, and reviewed as part of handover to retrieval team

Check and document the balloon position

Change balloon trigger to pressure sensing (some devices will have a transport mode that will safely select pressure vs ECG sensing)

Patient

Check the insertion site for bleeding/haematoma

Check and monitor distal pulses throughout

Check and monitor left radial – changes may suggest balloon movement and warrant prompt review

Compartment syndrome is a rare complication. Assess lower limbs carefully before departure

Monitor haemoglobin and platelet count.

---

must be adequately stabilised before undertaking the transfer, including a risk: benefit assessment. The use of specific checklists is recommended. Staff must have regular training on using the transport IABP.

Conclusions

Extracorporeal life support is an increasing modality of critical care treatment. Mobile ECMO should be a standard part of ECMO service provision.

Established ECMO centres have shown a rapid increase in mobile ECMO transports as they become more adept with the logistics, reflecting the perceived benefit for selected patients of earlier treatment and more stable transport. Advances in ECMO provision and equipment have contributed to making mobile ECMO a reality.

Intra-aortic balloon pumps are more commonly encountered and more likely to be used on transfers of patients effected by non-specialist teams.

Further reading

Berset A, Albrecht R, Ummenhofer W, et al. Air transfer of patients with intra-aortic balloon pump support. Swiss experience and recommendations. Swiss Med Wkly 2012;142:w13552.

Burns B, Reid C, Habiq K. Review of aeromedical intra-aortic balloon pump retrieval in New South Wales. Eur J Emerg Med 2013;20:23–6.

McLean N, Copeland R, Casey N, et al. Successful trans-Atlantic air ambulance transfer of a patient supported by a bi-ventricular assist device. Aviat Space Environ Med 2011; 82:825–8.

CHAPTER 40

Contagious Patients

R. MacDonald[1,2,3]

[1]Emergency Services, Sunnybrook Health Sciences Centre, Canada
[2]Emergency Medicine Fellowship Program, Department of Medicine, University of Toronto, Canada
[3]Quality Care Committee, Ornge Transport Medicine, Canada

OVERVIEW

- Modes of disease transmission
- Commonly encountered disease conditions
- Routine precautions

Introduction

Retrieval specialists and other first responders are often the first healthcare providers to encounter sudden illnesses or other emergencies in the community. Responding to these emergencies puts personnel at risk because the type, extent and severity of this illness are not yet known. A *contagious* disease is one that is spread from one person or organism to another, typically by direct contact. Strictly speaking, this differs from an *infectious* disease, where microorganisms in the air or water transmit infection. However, the risk of the unknown highlights the need to protect personnel against such exposures, whether contagious or infectious. For the purposes of this discussion, and in the interest of provider safety, the two will be considered as one.

The mode of transmission is the way in which an agent is transferred from the source to the host. Modes of transmission and examples of each are outlined in Table 40.1. The most common mode of disease transmission in the pre-hospital setting is by direct contact with an infected or colonised individual. Transmission can, therefore, be effectively prevented with appropriate barrier measures.

The risk of disease is not as apparent as other physical risks. Responding personnel must use the same level of suspicion and precaution when approaching a patient before the risk of communicable disease is known. The use of appropriate personal protective equipment (PPE) is necessary for every patient encounter in order to mitigate this risk.

When making patient contact, personnel can identify the at-risk patient. A rapid history and physical examination can raise

Table 40.1 Modes of disease transmission.

Mode	Description	Examples
Contact	Direct contact between patient and provider or passive transmission through contaminated intermediate	MRSA, VRE, Clostridium difficile, HIV, Norwalk virus
Droplet	Large droplets containing infecting agent (typically virus) generated by respiratory tract propelled and deposited on mucous membranes of others or surfaces in immediate environment	Influenza, rhinovirus, coronavirus (SARS), respiratory syncytial virus (RSV)
Airborne	Very small droplets containing infecting agent, easily dispersed, and remain suspended in air for prolonged periods; inhaled by others	Rubeola (measles), varicella, tuberculosis
Vector-borne	Infection spread by contact with carrier, such as insect or animal; transmission does NOT occur by direct contact with infected person	Malaria, West Nile virus
Vehicle	Spread of infectious agent by a single contaminated source, such as food, water, or other physical item, resulting in large outbreaks of disease.	Water (E coli); food (Salmonella); contaminated medication, equipment, or IV fluids.

suspicion for a contagious disease. The following screening questions help assess if the patient is at risk for a contagious disease:

- new or worsening cough or shortness of breath?
- fever?
- shakes or chills in the past 24 hours?
- abnormal temperature (>38°C)?
- taken medication for fever?
- travel to any location where people were, or have become ill in the past 10–14 days?

A screening physical examination will also identify obvious signs of a contagious disease. They may include any new symptom of infection (fever, headache, muscle ache, cough, sputum, weight loss and exposure history), rash, diarrhoea, skin lesions or changes in colour (jaundice), or draining wounds.

ABC of Transfer and Retrieval Medicine, First Edition.
Edited by Adam Low and Jonathan Hulme.
© 2015 John Wiley & Sons, Ltd. Published 2015 by John Wiley & Sons, Ltd.

Personnel must receive appropriate training to enable them to identify at-risk patients and appropriate PPE use, and take appropriate precautions when a patient presents with any signs or symptoms suspected to be due to a potentially contagious disease (Box 40.1).

Box 40.1 **Indicators of potential contagious disease**

At-risk patient – take precaution if:

- fever, chills, shakes
- new or worsening cough or dyspnoea
- recent travel to at-risk locale
- skin lesions, draining wounds
- body fluids (blood, faeces, vomit).

Commonly encountered disease conditions

Influenza

Influenza classically presents with the abrupt onset of fever, usually 38–40°C, sore throat, non-productive cough, myalgia, headache and chills. Unfortunately, only half of infected persons develop the 'classic' symptoms. Transmission occurs through airborne spread when a person coughs or sneezes, but may also occur through direct contact of surfaces contaminated with respiratory secretions. Handwashing and shielding coughs and sneezes help prevent spread. Influenza is transmissible from 1 day before symptom onset to about 5 days after symptoms begin and may last up to 10 days in children. Time from infection to development of symptoms is 1–4 days. Individuals at high risk of influenza complications include young children, people over age 65, the immunosuppressed and those suffering from chronic medical conditions. Death occurs in about 1 per 1,000 cases of influenza, mainly in people >65 years. Influenza vaccine is the principal means of preventing influenza morbidity and mortality. Healthcare providers should be immunised annually.

Antiviral drugs are available for preventing and treating influenza. When used for prevention of influenza, they can be 70–90% effective. When used for treatment, antivirals can reduce influenza illness duration by one day and attenuate the severity of illness. Antiviral agents should be used as an adjunct to vaccination, not a replacement. If an influenza outbreak is caused by a variant strain of influenza not controlled by vaccination, chemoprophylaxis should be considered for healthcare providers caring for patients at high risk of influenza complications, regardless of their vaccination status. In the setting of an influenza outbreak, pre-hospital systems may opt to restrict duties for providers who are not immunised or who have not yet received prophylactic antiviral therapy in an attempt to prevent spread of the outbreak.

Tuberculosis

The *Mycobacterium tuberculosis* complex causes tuberculosis (TB). The majority of active TB is pulmonary that will typically present with cough, scant amounts of non-purulent sputum and possibly haemoptysis. Systemic signs such as weight loss, anorexia, chills, night sweats, fever and fatigue may be present. It is difficult to distinguish pulmonary TB from other respiratory illness; however, certain risk factors should raise consideration of its possibility. These include immigration from a high-prevalence country, homelessness, exposure to active pulmonary TB, silicosis, HIV infection, chronic renal failure, cancer, transplantation or other immunosuppressed states.

Active pulmonary TB is transmitted via droplet nuclei from infected individuals during coughing, sneezing, speaking or singing. Retrieval procedures such as intubation or deep tracheal suctioning carry high risks of transmission. Respiratory secretions on a surface soon lose the potential for infection. Effective medical therapy eliminates communicability within 2–4 weeks of starting treatment.

The time from infection to active symptoms or positive TB skin test is about 2–10 weeks. If transporting a patient with known or suspected TB, precautions to prevent transmission must include a submicron mask. Patients should cover their mouth when coughing or sneezing, or wear a surgical mask. In the event of suspected exposure to a patient with active pulmonary tuberculosis, report the case and exposure to the pre-hospital system or health system authority. If the retrieval provider or contact develops either active TB with symptoms or latent asymptomatic TB, as diagnosed with a new positive TB skin test, treatment should be sought. A physician skilled in management of TB must initiate and monitor treatment and provide suitable follow-up.

MRSA

Skin infections due to *Staphylococcus aureus* are increasingly common, and the emergence of methicillin-resistant-*Staphylococcal aureus* (MRSA) is a large problem both in hospital and in the community. MRSA also causes severe and invasive infections such as necrotising pneumonia, sepsis and musculoskeletal infections such as osteomyelitis and necrotising fasciitis. MRSA skin infections typically present as necrotic skin lesions, and are often confused with bites. There are no reliable clinical or risk factor criteria to distinguish MRSA skin and soft-tissue infections from those caused by other infectious agents.

About 1% of the population is colonised with MRSA, and transmission is through hand contact from infected skin lesions, such as abscesses or boils. Transmission of infection is prevented by routine precautions, particularly gloves and proper handwashing. Draining wounds should be covered with clean, dry bandages. Contaminated surfaces should be cleaned with disinfectants effective against *Staphylococcus aureus*, such as a solution of dilute bleach or quaternary ammonium compounds. Ambulances have significant degree of MRSA contamination, highlighting the need for proper cleaning and decontamination of all equipment and the vehicle itself after every patient transport. The choice of therapy should be dictated by local susceptibility patterns.

Meningitis

Meningitis refers to inflammation of the meninges covering the brain. It can be caused by infectious and non-infectious causes. It is typically classified as bacterial meningitis versus aseptic meningitis. Aseptic meningitis refers to meningitis with cerebrospinal fluid absent of microorganisms on gram stain and/or routine culture. Viral meningitis is more common, less severe and requires supportive measures with no specific treatment. Bacterial meningitis, though, has a case-fatality rate of 13–37% (as high as 80% in the elderly) despite appropriate antibiotic therapy. Transmission is by droplet spread from respiratory secretions. Respiratory and contact precautions should be undertaken when transporting patients with suspected meningitis. The time from transmission to the development of symptoms depends on the causative organism, and ranges from 1 to 10 days.

In the absence of diagnostic tests such as lumbar puncture, retrieval personnel cannot depend on clinical signs and symptoms alone to distinguish meningitis types. Considering the high morbidity and mortality with untreated bacterial meningitis, all patients with suspected meningitis should be treated as bacterial meningitis until proven otherwise.

Empiric treatment of adult bacterial meningitis is vancomycin plus a third-generation cephalosporin, such as cefotaxime. In neonates, those over age 50, and those with altered immune status or alcoholism, ampicillin is added to cover *Listeria monocytogenes*. Treatment may last 14–21 days depending on the infectious agent. In addition to treating the patient, retrieval teams exposed or in close contact to patients with meningitis may require prophylactic therapy. This is particularly important for personnel exposed to the patient's oral or respiratory secretions. Exposed personnel should contact their employer or healthcare provider immediately. Prophylactic treatment with ciprofloxacin, ceftriaxone or rifampin to prevent infection due to close contact will likely be offered (Box 40.2).

Box 40.2 **Key Indicators for risky infections**

Cough: TB, pneumonia, influenza
Headache: meningitis
Rash: MRSA.

Routine precautions

The concept of 'routine precautions' was developed to protect healthcare workers from bloodborne pathogens, specifically the hepatitis B and human immunodeficiency viruses. The concept includes the following components:

- patient assessment
- hand hygiene
- personal protective equipment
- sharps safety
- patient accommodation and transport considerations
- routine cleaning of equipment
- environmental control, including routine vehicle disinfection.

Routine precautions apply to blood, body fluids containing visible blood and the following fluids:

- CSF (surrounds the brain and spinal cord)
- synovial fluid (found inside joints, i.e. knee)
- pleural fluid (found inside the chest cavity but outside the lung)
- pericardial fluid (surrounds the heart)
- amniotic fluid (surrounds the foetus in the uterus)
- peritoneal fluid (found inside the abdominal cavity).

While routine precautions do not apply to the following body fluids, unless visible blood is present, practitioners may not always be able to tell if blood is present in a body fluid. For this reason, **all body fluids must be considered hazardous:**

- faeces
- nasal secretions
- oral secretions, including vomitus and saliva
- respiratory secretions, including sputum
- sweat
- tears
- urine.

A complete and detailed description of PPE types, indications and use are beyond the scope of this text. Table 40.2 provides

Table 40.2 PPE for common procedures.

Intervention	Gloves	Facial protection	Gowns
Drawing blood	Yes		
Starting an intravenous/ intraosseous access	Yes		
Dressing minor skin wounds	Yes		
Any patient contact where provider has any skin problems on the hands (abrasions, etc.)	Yes		
Measuring temperature	Yes		
IM, SC, finger pokes (i.e. blood glucose monitoring)	Yes		
Controlling minor bleeding with pressure	Yes		
Contact with patient with cough or projectile vomiting	Yes	Yes	Yes (if febrile respiratory illness or vomiting present)
Needle thoracostomy or other invasive thoracic procedure	Yes	Yes	Yes (if febrile respiratory illness present)
Tracheal intubation or other procedure where respiratory secretions are likely encountered	Yes	Yes	Yes (if febrile respiratory illness present)
Oral/nasal suctioning	Yes	Yes	Yes (if febrile respiratory illness or vomiting present)
Controlling arterial or heavy venous haemorrhage	Yes	Yes	Yes
Emergency childbirth	Yes	Yes	Yes
Known infection or colonisation with antibiotic-resistant organism (VRE, MRSA)	Yes	Yes	Yes
Disinfecting or cleaning contaminated equipment or transport vehicle	Yes	Yes	Yes

Table 40.3 PPE for a known contagion.

Level 1	Level 2	Level 3
Abscesses	Chicken Pox	AIDS*
Diarrhoea	Common cold	*Clostridium difficile*
Hepatitis A	Croup	Hepatitis B*
Hepatitis E	Diphtheria	Hepatitis C*
Cytomegalovirus	Epiglotitis	Hepatitis D*
Herpes Simplex	German measles (Rubella)	SARS† and other coronaviruses during known outbreaks or produce rapid person-to-person spread
Herpes zoster	Red measles	Influenza if contact with respiratory secretions is likely
Lice	Herpes zoster	
Viral meningitis	Infectious mononucleosis	
Scabies	Meningitis, meningococcal	
Syphilis	Meningitis, *Haemophilus influenza*	
	Mumps	
	Pharyngitis	
	Pneumonia	
	Tuberculosis	
	Whooping cough	

Level 1: gloves and handwashing.
Level 2: Level 1 plus mask (N95 or equivalent) and safety glasses or full face shield.
Level 3: Level 2 plus disposable plastic gown.
*Level 3 if exposure to blood or body fluid is anticipated; otherwise, Level 1 precautions are appropriate.
†Although transmission of SARS may be considered to be similar to other highly contagious viral agents listed requiring Level 2 precautions, SARS and related viruses requires Level 3 precautions in outbreak situations

examples of situations encountered in the retrieval setting, and the types of PPE indicated. If in doubt, use the maximum PPE possible. Table 40.3 proposes the level of appropriate PPE given specific or known contagious disease threats (Box 40.3).

Box 40.3 **Key points about the use of PPE**

Any body fluid is potentially hazardous
When in doubt, use maximum PPE.

Handwashing is the single most important means of preventing the spread of infection. Waterless handwash solutions are not effective against spore-forming organisms such as *Clostridium difficile*. Waterless handwash solutions are therefore **not** an acceptable form of handwashing when caring for patients with spore-forming organisms.

Problems encountered during transfer

Patients with suspected or proven contagious disease still require the same care as non-infected patients, but additional precautions

Table 40.4 Special precautions for high-risk interventions.

Intervention	Risk to provider	Suggested precaution
Advanced airway management, including intubation, mechanical ventilation, and tracheal suctioning	Droplet formation and/or airborne transmission	Level 3 PPE. Closed ventilator circuit, suction device in-line on ventilator circuit once intubated. Avoid non-invasive ventilation. Appropriate sedation and /or paralysis to prevent upper airway response (cough, gag, etc.) to airway manipulation
Nebulised therapy	Droplet formation and/or airborne transmission	Alternate route of mediation delivery, such as metered-dose inhaler
'Bloody' procedures (needle thoracostomy, emergency childbirth, external haemorrhage)	Blood, body fluids, and respiratory secretions	Minimise number of providers. Use shields, screens, or other barrier devices
Care in aircraft or other enclosed space	Contamination of aircraft	Physical barrier between pilot(s) and air medical crew/patient. Predetermined ventilation system parameters to prevent further spread. Equipment and consumables protected to prevent contamination
Post-response aircraft cleaning	Contaminated aircraft and equipment; risk of contaminating aircraft hangar/ base/maintenance facility	Appropriate PPE for personnel decontaminating aircraft and equipment. Contained location for decontamination. Appropriate disposal of contaminated items, including those used in cleaning

are needed to prevent disease transmission to those providing patient care. Table 40.4 illustrates examples of 'high-risk' interventions that merit close attention.

Intubated and mechanically ventilated patients pose the greatest risk to providers. The process of securing the airway places the provider in close, direct contact with respiratory secretions, and the procedure itself is likely to promote spread of contagion via the airborne or droplet route. This risk was noted during outbreaks of SARS more than a decade ago, where disease transmission was found to be highest during invasive airway procedures such as direct laryngoscopy or bronchoscopy. Providers should carefully consider whether intubation is necessary, use the maximum PPE possible, and consider use of appropriate sedation and paralysis to mitigate the risk of patient response during airway manipulation. Once intubated, the patient should be attached to a mechanical ventilator using a closed circuit. Suctioning should only be performed using a closed suction system, with suction catheter integrated into the ventilator circuit.

Further reading

Centers for Disease Control and Prevention. Workplace health and safety topics: emergency medical service workers. Available at http://www.cdc.gov /niosh/topics/ems/. Accessed 2014 March 13.

Centers for Disease Control and Prevention. Preventing exposures to blood-borne pathogens among paramedics. Available at http://www.cdc.gov /niosh/topics/ems/. Accessed 2014 March 13.

MacDonald RD . Infectious Diseases and Bioterrorism (Chapter 44), in D Cooney (ed.): *EMS Medicine: Physician Practice and Medical Oversight*, 1st edition. New York, NY: McGraw Hill, 2014.

MacDonald RD. Communicable Diseases, in J Brice, D Cone, T Delbridge, B Myers (eds): *Emergency Medical Services: Clinical Practice and Systems Oversight*, 5th edition. Oxford, UK: Wiley and Sons, 2014.

CHAPTER 41

Bariatric Patients

Z. Dempsey and M. Ross

Department of Anaesthesia and Pain Medicine, Royal Infirmary of Edinburgh, UK

OVERVIEW

- Bariatric patients are at increased risk of associated comorbidities which may lead to or complicate critical illness
- Transfer of bariatric patients is challenging due to restrictions on space, crew and equipment
- Physiological effects of obesity are compounded in the transfer environment
- Patient girth and not weight is usually the main restricting factor and difficulties will be encountered transferring patients wider than 65 cm
- Give careful consideration to securing the airway and ventilation strategy prior to transfer and use invasive monitoring.

Introduction

Obesity is a global epidemic with rates predicted to rise significantly in the future. Currently 1:4 adults in the UK are clinically obese, and the prevalence of morbid obesity (defined here as a body mass index (BMI) >40 kg/m^2) is around 3%. Bariatric patients are at increased risk of associated comorbidities which may lead to or complicate critical illness and necessitate transfer to a specialist centre. Challenges in caring for the bariatric patient are compounded in the transfer environment where space, crew and equipment are limited.

Physiological effects

Airway

Bariatric patients have an increased incidence of difficult intubation (Box 41.1). These anatomical changes can impede the view at laryngoscopy. There is also a high incidence of gastro-oesophageal reflux and delayed gastric emptying which increases the risk of aspiration. The airway of all bariatric patients must be carefully assessed, and secured in any patient with the potential for compromise.

When positioning the patient prior to intubation, view at laryngoscopy can be improved by adopting the 'ramped' position. This involves maintaining a 30° head-up tilt during pre-oxygenation

Box 41.1 **Factors associated with difficult rapid sequence induction and intubation in obese individuals**

Airway
Large thoracic fat pad
Large breasts
Decreased neck movement and or C-Spine immobilisation
Excess head and neck soft tissue
Reduced mouth opening
Large tongue and increased intraoral adipose tissue
History of snoring or Obstructive sleep apnoea

Respiratory
Impaired bag mask ventilation
Obesity hypoventilation syndrome
Reduced oxygen reserve
Hypoxia in supine position
Increased carbon dioxide production
Cardiovascular
Difficult IV access
Lack of invasive monitoring
Cardiovascular instability

Others
Altered drug kinetics
Gastro-oesophageal reflux disease
Delayed gastric emptying

and padding under the patient's shoulders and head with additional pillows or blankets until the auditory meatus is in line with the sternal notch (Figure 41.1). Alternatively, the Oxford Head Elevation Laryngoscopy Pillow (HELP, Alma. Medical Oxford, UK) may be used.

If available, access to a difficult airway trolley is advised. Video laryngoscopes can be particularly helpful especially if the cervical spine is immobilised. Uncut endotracheal tubes should be used and tied securely.

Breathing

Patients have increased work of breathing, increased oxygen consumption and increased carbon dioxide production. Functional residual capacity (FRC) is reduced due to excursion of abdominal contents into the chest cavity and diaphragmatic splinting. Ventilation perfusion mismatching results in an increased shunt

---

ABC of Transfer and Retrieval Medicine, First Edition.
Edited by Adam Low and Jonathan Hulme.
© 2015 John Wiley & Sons, Ltd. Published 2015 by John Wiley & Sons, Ltd.

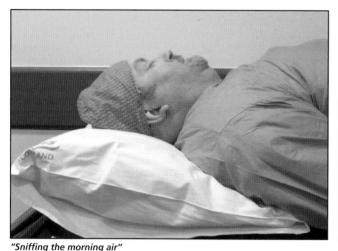

"Sniffing the morning air"

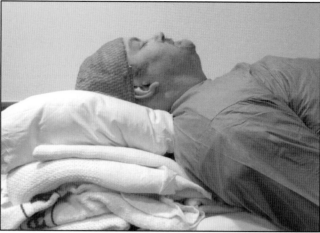

"Ramped Position"

Figure 41.1 Comparison of the 'sniffing the morning air' position and 'ramped position.'

fraction and coupled with the reduced oxygen reservoir, patients can desaturate rapidly. The increased weight of the chest wall and restricted diaphragmatic movement result in reduced compliance and requirement for higher airway pressures. Acceleration and deceleration forces and the supine position during transfer can significantly impair ventilation further.

Bariatric patients should be ventilated with tidal volumes of 6–8 mL/kg based on ideal body weight (IBW) and end tidal carbon dioxide controlled by the respiratory rate. Higher levels of positive end expiratory pressure should be used to promote alveolar recruitment. High airway pressures may be minimised by prolongation of the inspiratory time.

Circulation

An increased circulating blood volume and cardiac output can lead to increased left ventricular workload, hypertension, hypertrophy, ischaemic heart disease and left-sided heart failure. Autoregulation of blood flow to vital organs may be altered and consideration should be given to maintaining a higher mean arterial pressure during transfer.

Blood pressure cuffs may not be large enough to fit around the upper arm and are often inaccurate. An arterial line should be inserted for prolonged transfers and in unstable patients.

Intravenous access may be difficult due to increased soft tissue. Central access may be the only definitive means of establishing a secure intravenous route before departure.

There is also an increased risk of venous thromboembolism aggravated by the cramped conditions and immobility of prolonged transfer.

Drugs

The dose of drugs should not be calculated based on the patient's actual weight. IBW should be used to calculate highly lipid soluble drugs, such as induction agents and synthetic opiates (Box 41.2). This is due to the increased volume of distribution. For water soluble drugs, such as muscle relaxants, lean body mass should be used or IBW plus 20%. Intubated patients should be kept well sedated and paralysed during transfer.

Box 41.2 **Calculating ideal body weight (IBW)**

Males: IBW (kg) = height (cm) − 100
Females: IBW (kg) = height (cm) − 105

Inter-hospital transfer

Often the main limiting factor will be the patient's girth. Transferring a patient wider than 65 cm with standard ambulance equipment will prove challenging. It is useful to measure the patient's maximum width. This will usually be the inter-elbows distance measured with the patient's arms by their side (as they would be in transfer).

Consideration should be given to movement and handing issues with the need for additional staff and specialist bariatric equipment to aid transfer. Conscious patients should be encouraged to move themselves if possible.

All ambulance vehicles and aircraft have absolute weight limitations for compliance with crash regulations and operation of trolley and winching mechanisms. Patients' weights are frequently underestimated by healthcare staff and when considering if a patient exceeds weight limitations you must also include the additional weight of any transfer equipment (Box 41.3).

Box 41.3 **Approximate weights of critical care transfer equipment**

Vacuum mattress	7 kg
Pro paq monitor and cables	7 kg
Oxylog 3000	6 kg
Size D oxygen cylinder	7 kg
ZD oxygen cylinder	5 kg
Syringe driver	1 kg
2 blankets	1 kg
Pillow	0.5 kg
Fluids	1 L = 1 kg

Packaging

Tight restraining straps may cause pressure sores, peripheral nerve damage, impede ventilation and precipitate venous thrombosis. Vacuum mattresses therefore offer several advantages in immobilising and protecting patients. Specific bariatric vacuum mattresses are now available which can safely accommodate larger patients.

Road ambulances

Transfer capability will depend on the type and dimensions of ambulance trolley used. Most standard ambulance trolleys can carry a maximum weight of 300 kg, although the height cannot be adjusted above 200 kg. The CCT6 trolley, specifically developed for critical care transfers, has a maximum weight restriction of 181 kg. These trolleys, however, will not accommodate patients wider than 65 cm.

Specific bariatric ambulances are now available with wider trolleys and moving and handling aids. They may not be suitable for critical care transfers due to inability to secure critical care equipment.

A bariatric critical care transfer trolley, the CCT6-M (Figure 41.2), is available. It has removable side extensions which can accommodate patients' up to 100 cm wide and can take a

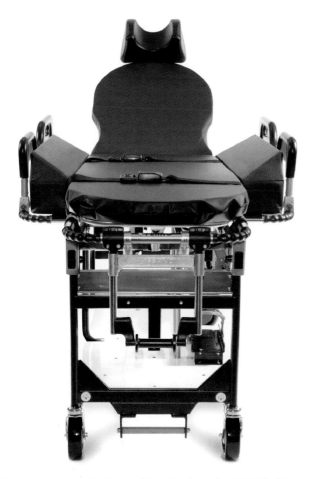

Figure 41.2 Ferno Bariatric Critical Care Transfer trolley, CCT6-M. (Source: www.ferno.co.uk/assets/products/cct_six_m_bariatric_critical_care_trolley /cct-six_m_large_001.jpg. Reproduce with permission of Ferno.co.uk).

patient weight of 250 kg. As the trolley is not collapsible, critical care equipment, including additional oxygen cylinders, can be secured. The CCT6-M can be transferred in any ambulance capable of taking the standard CCT6. Motorised winches to load patients into ambulances can take weights of up to 425 kg.

Aero-medical transfer

Patients will still require transfer to and from the aircraft usually by road. If a patient cannot be secured safely in the ambulance trolley consideration can be given to transferring the patient on the floor of the largest ambulance available. This will only be suitable for very short transfers (within hospital grounds) and is at the discretion of the road ambulance crew.

Air stretchers will generally not accommodate patients wider than 65 cm. In fixed wing aircraft the central aisle must be kept clear and patients wider than 65 cm are at risk of falling into the aisle causing injury and obstruction. Additional personnel will be required to help load and unload non-ambulatory patients. This requires good communication and loading and unloading patients from helicopters should not be done with rotors running. Maximum weight of any winch used to help load a patient into an aircraft should be checked prior to use.

Increasing altitude decreases the partial pressure of oxygen and can worsen patient hypoxia. In rotary wing aircraft, where the cabin is not pressurised, flying altitude should be restricted to less than 2000 feet. In fixed wing aircraft, the cabin should be pressurised to 'sea level'.

Intra-hospital transfer

Trolleys

Standard hospital trolleys have a maximum safe working load of around 180 kg, although some can accommodate up to 250 kg. Specialised bariatric trolleys are wider and can accommodate heavier loads. Electrically powered motors ease mobilisation and minimise staff injury. Glide sheets and boards are used routinely in transferring patients from bed to trolley. Specific bariatric hover mats are advantageous in transferring bariatric patients and further protect staff from harm.

Radiology

Bariatric patients will often require radiological imaging. The latest generation of CT and MRI scanners can accommodate up to 212 kg and 250 kg respectively. The imaging aperture may be the limiting factor as current MRI scanners can permit patients no more than 70 cm wide and CT no more than 78 cm. Open CT and MRI scanners may be an alternative to conventional imaging however they are not widely available.

Conclusion

Despite rising rates of obesity we are currently ill equipped to transfer bariatric patients without specialist equipment, which may not be widely available. Difficulty will be encountered in trying to transfer any patient exceeding 65 cm wide. Physiological effects of obesity are compounded in the transfer environment and successful transfer requires careful planning, teamwork and communication.

Further reading

http://www.noo.org.uk/NOO_about_obesity/morbid_obesity (accessed 18 April 2013)

Collins, Lemmens, et al. Laryngoscopy and morbid obesity: a comparison of the 'sniff' and 'ramped' positions. Obesity surgery 2004; 14; 1171-5

Dempsey Z, Proctor J. Standard operating procedure for bariatric patient transfer. Emergency Medical Retrieval Service. www.emrs.scot.nhs.uk (Accessed 18 April 2013)

London Association of Anaesthetist of Great Britain and Ireland. Peri-operative management of the morbidly obese patient. London Association of Anaesthetist of Great Britain and Ireland 2007

Ri-Li G, Chase PJ, Witkowski S, et al. Obesity: associations with a cute mountain sickness. Ann Intern Med 2003;139:253–7.

CHAPTER 42

Acute Behavioural Disturbances

M. Le Cong

Royal Flying Doctor Service Queensland section, Australia

OVERVIEW

- Underlying principle of involuntary treatment of a disturbed patient is use of minimal restraint
- Formal risk assessment of agitated patients assists adequate planning for retrieval and transfer
- Disturbed patients should receive adequate preparation for transfer including oral sedation, fasting and IV access
- Retrieval sedation should provide balanced effects with a targeted sedation range
- High-risk sedation factors may require tracheal intubation and general anaesthesia.

The retrieval of a disturbed patient is one of the most challenging situations for the pre-hospital and retrieval practitioner. It involves medical, legal and ethical decisions. If aeromedical transport is required, it will likely involve aviation laws and decision-making too. Ultimately the balance must be sought for the needs of the patient but also for the safety of all parties involved in the process.

Medicolegal, aviation and ethical considerations

In most countries, there exist specific laws governing the medical situation whereby a person is suffering from an acute diminished capacity for informed consent, due to either a mental illness, intoxication or physical illness. This often involves the legal process to conduct an involuntary medical assessment and treatment of the person unable to give consent due to their acute incapacity.

A universal guiding principle of such acts involving involuntary detention and assessment is the use of minimal restraint, physical and chemical, to enable adequate completion of the process.

All countries with aviation laws have legislated that the pilot in charge of the safe operation of an aircraft, is empowered to refuse any passengers, deemed to present a risk to such safe operation. In addition pilots in general are empowered to request the assistance of other passengers or emergency services to restrain a disturbed passenger to enable safe conduct of the flight. The principle of minimal restraint is also applied here.

While it is often assumed that the safe operation of an aircraft is paramount, this does not absolve the duty of care and ethical considerations for patient rights and quality care without informed consent.

Decision-making and risk assessment for the disturbed patient retrieval

Clearly the process of planning for such a retrieval is to undertake a formal risk assessment. There exists no validated risk assessment tools for the aeromedical retrieval setting but several do exist for emergency mental health and criminal prison settings.

The elements most useful to identify truly high risk patients, based on expert opinion and extrapolated from psychiatric research are illustrated in the following risk assessment protocol (Figure 42.1).

In the author's experience, the benefit of a formal risk assessment process is in mission planning, well before the retrieval team meets the patient. This allows adequate staffing and planning for restraint measures. Ideally a high-risk patient identified during risk assessment will be assigned a retrieval team of at least two providers, with the non-technical and technical skills in managing a wide range of agitated behaviour.

During handover it is important to reassess the risk based on direct contact and communication with the patient. It is prudent to do a proper handover and risk assessment at the referring facility with referring staff on hand to clarify questions and provide assistance. Essential to any risk assessment of the agitated patient is a proper medical examination and review. Sedation during transport in the unintubated patient is like any other anaesthetic, and should be performed with adequate assessment of airway, medical fitness and risks of complications like aspiration, airway obstruction, etc.

Preparing the disturbed patient for transport

Like all critical care retrievals, the key is in stabilisation and preparation for transport. Treating the agitation (Box 42.1) is incredibly helpful and will often make the difference between using minimal restraint and excessive force.

ABC of Transfer and Retrieval Medicine, First Edition.
Edited by Adam Low and Jonathan Hulme.
© 2015 John Wiley & Sons, Ltd. Published 2015 by John Wiley & Sons, Ltd.

SUBJECT AREA	Y/N	Score	Comments
Any known history of violence to persons or property?		10	
Any expressions of anger, frustration or agitation during course of hospital admission or preceding 24hrs?		5	
Multiple expressions of anger, frustration or agitation during current care, requiring special nursing or security measures or chemical restraint/sedation		20	
Signs of intoxication/withdrawal from drugs or alcohol during course of hospital admission or preceding 24hrs?		10	
Known history of substance abuse (Alcohol, opioids, amphetamines, marijuana)?		5	
Known environmental stressors in last 7 days (personal loss, relationship crisis, financial crisis etc.)		5	

THE RISK ASSESSMENT RESULT IS (Circle one)

HIGH RISK (>25) FN, MO, 1 patient per flight, IV access, patient sedated and restrained, recommended Police or trained attendant, consider intubation and ventilation if failed adequate trial of pre-flight sedation

MEDIUM RISK (6-24) FN, MO, 1 patient per flight, patient sedated and restrained, IV access, may have Police or trained attendant.

LOW RISK (0-5) FN, may require sedation, restrained, IV access, MO or another attendant, may be carried with another patient.

This risk assessment tool is a dynamic instrument and does not replace clinical judgement for a given clinical situation. The risk may change as a result of medical intervention/management prior to transfer. Night flights are to be avoided due to the limited available aviation options should a problem develop and the disorientating effect of night flying in some disturbed patients.

Figure 42.1 Risk assessment management protocol utilised by Royal Flying Doctor Service Queensland Section, Australia. (Source: Royal Flying Doctor Service, Queensland Section. Reproduced with permission of Royal Flying Doctor Service Queensland Section, Australia). FN = flight nurse, MO = medical officer.

Box 42.1 Reversible causes of agitation to be considered

Nicotine withdrawal – this is often neglected but can be readily addressed with early initiation of nicotine replacement therapy, as patches or gum

Fear of flying – it is underestimated the fear of flying and it may well be unethical to subject a truly phobic patient to this stress. Often this can be managed adequately with appropriate sedation and simple communication

Hunger/thirst – it is prudent to keep a patient as fasted as possible however clear fluids are reasonable up until 2 hours from transport time and the use of lollies may help

Toileting – efforts to ensure adequate toileting prior to flight will help reduce agitation related to this

Pain – any acute pain condition will exacerbate underlying agitation from another cause.

Agitated patients, particularly those with chronic substance abuse disorders or are on regular psychiatric medications, often require above average levels of acute sedation to help control their distressing symptoms. The key here is to start regular oral sedation early, well before the time for transport. If this is done early enough in sufficient doses, then the need for retrieval sedation is almost eliminated in the author's experience. Oral benzodiazepines combined with an antipsychotic are sufficient in many cases but need to be given regularly to maintain sufficient plasma levels.

The retrieval must provide the same if not greater level of sedation care than would occur in hospital. This generally dictates having at least two trained clinicians for procedural sedation (Box 42.2). If intubation might be needed to control the airway and afford deep level sedation then at least one of these retrieval team members must be competent in advanced airway management and emergency general anaesthesia.

Box 42.2 The minimum preparations for aeromedical retrieval of a disturbed patient under the involuntary section of the mental health act are:

IV access ×2
Fasted state ideally
Adequate oral sedation for preceding 12 hours
Use of physical restraints
Two person retrieval team with skills for procedural sedation and advanced airway management.

Retrieval sedation

The goal of retrieval sedation is to provide the agitated patient with a calmer and more relaxed state, yet still remain cooperative enough to obey verbal commands from retrieval staff. A safe sedation level must be maintained albeit at times deeper levels of sedation may be required during more distressing parts of the transport e.g. engine start up/take off.

A validated sedation scoring system is a valuable tool in monitoring sedation depth and safety. It is important to aim for a target sedation range and have good reason to go deeper or lighter. All procedural sedation is a type of anaesthesia and so meticulous attention to airway assessment, medical fitness for anaesthesia and a rescue plan in event of complications, is mandatory (Box 42.3).

Box 42.3 When should one just proceed directly to emergency intubation and general anaesthesia?

Intoxicated state – safe sedation in an intoxicated patient is challenging. It is better to err on the safe side of securing airway in these cases

Failed procedural sedation – some patients will fail an adequate sedation trial. There is usually no point in persisting if the patient is clearly not improving. It is much safer to proceed to securing airway and general anaesthesia

Complicating medical/surgical condition – some patients have medical conditions that will make effective and safe sedation difficult. Early airway control and general anaesthesia will facilitate the rapid but safe transport of such patients. Hepatic encephalopathy is a good example.

It is optimal to maintain a steady level of sedation effect and avoid peaks and troughs that may cause under or over sedation. The superior strategy is an intravenous infusion of an agent familiar to the provider. Initiating this pre-flight and waiting five half-lives of the infused sedative to lapse, while observing the effect, is a sensible strategy to achieve steady state for the sedation. For a relatively short transfer, regular titrated boluses of IV sedation is a good strategy using a long IV extension line securely attached.

Physical restraints

Retrieval of the disturbed patient must include the use of approved physical restraints. Even in the intubated patient, there have been occasions of too light sedation, allowing a dramatic self-extubation to occur during flight. There are several types in common use, typically ankle and wrist straps, even a body net. There is no perfect system and unless one wants to use police type restraints with body belts and handcuffs, all medical restraints do is to slow the patient down and allow clinical staff time to control the agitated behaviour, generally by providing some acute sedation.

Further reading

Elbogen E, Johnson S. The intricate link between violence and mental disorder: results from the national epidemiologic survey on alcohol and related conditions. Arch Gen Psych 2009;66:152–61.

Gordon, et al. Air travel by patients with mental disorder. Psychiatr Bull 2004;28:295–7.

Jones DR, Aeromedical transportation of psychiatric patients: Historical review and present management. Aviat Space Environ Med 1980;51: 709–16.

Peterson AL, Baker MT, McCarthy K R. Combat stress casualties in Iraq. Part 2: Psychiatric screening prior to aeromedical evacuation. Perspect Psychiatr Care 2008;44:3, Health Module p. 159.

Rossi J, Swan M, Isaacs E. The violent or agitated patient. Emerg Med Clin N Am 2010;28:235–56.

Wheeler S, Wong B, L'Heureux R. Criteria for sedation of psychiatric patients for air transport in British Columbia. BCMJ 2009;51:346–9.

CHAPTER 43

Considerations Regarding Organ Donation

Anders Aneman[1,2] and William O'Regan[1,3]

[1]Intensive Care Unit, Liverpool Hospital, South Western Sydney Local Health District, Australia
[2]University of New South Wales, Australia
[3]Careflight International Retrieval Service, Sydney, Australia

---

OVERVIEW

- The management of the organ donor needs to be optimised to ensure the best outcomes for organ transplantation
- Organ donation can occur following brain death (DBD) or after cessation of circulation (DCD)
- Transport may occur when the acute history or clinical signs are suggestive of impending brain death
- Medical therapy must be formulated with the patient's best interests
- Circulatory disturbances include autonomic storming manifested as hypertension and decreased end organ perfusion, usually followed by hypotension. Vasopressor support and careful fluid management will be needed with ongoing haemodynamic monitoring. Arrhythmias are common and will need specific treatment
- Ventilatory management aims to maintain alveolar ventilation, normocapnoea and a normal pH
- Electrolyte homeostasis needs to be maintained, with diabetes insipidus occurring commonly. Blood glucose levels need to be maintained in the normal range
- Hypothermia is common and normothermia is the goal to allow clinical brain death testing as well as to avoid further haemodynamic instability.

Organ transplantation remains the most successful and at times only possible therapy for end-stage cardiac, pulmonary, hepatic and gastrointestinal failure. Furthermore, renal transplantation significantly improves the quality of life, reduces morbidity and the risk of mortality in dialysis-dependent patients with end-stage renal failure.

Organ donation and transplantation rates vary considerably in an international perspective with Spain being notably successful in achieving a high rate. The large discrepancy between the limited number of organs available for transplantation and the number of organs actually needed remains a universal issue irrespective of healthcare, ethical and legal context, and many patients still die while being listed for transplantation. Hence, it is crucial that the potential for organ donation is always recognised and that the management of the potential or established organ donor is optimised to ensure the best clinical outcomes possible.

The retrieval of organs for the purpose of transplantation is possible following death either determined by the complete and irreversible cessation of all brain functions (donation after brain death, DBD) or the complete and irreversible cessation of circulation (donation after circulatory death, DCD). While the transport of patients for DCD may indeed be challenging, it only occurs in-hospital and is hence beyond the scope of this chapter. Hence we will only focus on the potential for DBD. First, it would be an exceedingly rare occasion that an organ donor is transported for retrieval surgery since the surgical teams will instead be transported to the site where the donor is managed to maintain organ viability. Second, a patient in whom brain death is suspected but cannot be confirmed using clinical criteria might however be transferred to another healthcare facility where necessary investigations can be performed such as four-vessel angiography or nuclear perfusion scan to establish the absence of circulation to the brain. Third, perhaps the most likely scenario pertinent to transfer and retrieval medicine involves the transport to hospital of a patient in whom the acute history or clinical signs are suggestive of impending or established brain death.

The early management of such patients, even before brain death has been formally diagnosed, can significantly impact on the subsequent potential for DBD. This can be particularly relevant in rural areas where delays in transfer and extended transport times are more likely to be of concern. The consequences and medical management of progressive brainstem herniation that are relevant to these three clinical settings will be discussed in this chapter. With a few additional special considerations, transport when organ donation is considered follows generic principles for the transport of the critically ill patient. At any stage, medical therapy must always be formulated with the patient's best interests as the one and only goal, never to make the patient a means to facilitate organ donation. This ethical principle is covered in extension by the Dead Donor Rule that, while at times debated, remains sacrosanct among medical ethicists and physicians.

Circulation

Progressive brainstem ischaemia during herniation triggers an intense but transient sympathetic activation with markedly

---

ABC of Transfer and Retrieval Medicine, First Edition.
Edited by Adam Low and Jonathan Hulme.
© 2015 John Wiley & Sons, Ltd. Published 2015 by John Wiley & Sons, Ltd.

Box 43.1 **Circulation – summary of key issues and treatment targets**

Progressive brainstem ischaemia can trigger autonomic instability. This can lead to hypertension followed by hypotension

Organ hypoperfusion will occur. Vasopressors such as noradrenaline (norepinephrine) with sometimes added vasopressin are used aiming for a mean arterial pressure above 70 mmHg

Volume loading with balanced crystalloid solutions and albumin is used to optimise perfusion of the splanchnic organs.

Haemodynamic monitoring using invasive arterial and central venous pressures are used with surrogate measures of adequate intravascular volume including base deficit and lactate

Tachy- and bradyarryhthmias may occur. Management includes correction of electrolytes, use of antiarrhythmics and cardioversion.

increased systemic vascular resistance. This leads to arterial and venous hypertension, decreased left ventricular output with risk for end-organ hypoperfusion, pulmonary congestion and increased hydrostatic pulmonary capillary pressure, which may manifest as overt pulmonary oedema. This 'autonomic storm' rarely requires any treatment. Only short-acting antihypertensive agents should be used (e.g. esmolol, sodium nitroprusside), since progressive brainstem herniation will invariably lead to bradycardia and hypotension (Box 43.1). Furthermore, there is no unequivocal evidence that ablating the autonomic storm is cardioprotective. Subsequent cerebral herniation and spinal cord ischaemia are associated with arterial hypotension (in >80% of potential donors) and venous pooling (relative hypovolaemia) that unless treated will result in decreased organ perfusion.

Administration of a vasopressor to support mean arterial pressure is usually required, notwithstanding residual effects of deep sedation for ICP control. A MAP above 70 mmHg is generally sufficient to maintain perfusion of the thoracoabdominal organs. Noradrenaline (norepinephrine) is the most commonly used vasopressor but may be combined with vasopressin to reduce excessive catecholamine doses that are known to be cardiotoxic, and to treat any concomitant development of diabetes insipidus. Infusion of fluids to expand the intravascular compartment is often necessary as a result of previous osmotic diuresis, constricted volume and extravasation during the autonomic storm phase. Later unrecognised or suboptimally treated diabetes insipidus and hyperglycaemia can contribute to hypovolaemia. Literature data support avoiding synthetic colloids, in particular hypdroxyethyl starch, and a balanced administration of crystalloids and albumin is recommended to optimise perfusion of the splanchnic organs in particular. Isotonic, chloride deplete crystalloids with a balanced sodium content are preferable, especially if volume losses due to diabetes insipidus need to be vigorously corrected. A more restrictive approach to volume loading might be necessary when the lungs are considered for retrieval and overzealous volume resuscitation might also impair cardiac function. In such cases, concentrated albumin solutions may be considered. Haemodynamic monitoring is commonly restricted to invasive arterial and central venous pressures, particularly during transport.

Pulse pressure variation can be used as a surrogate marker for preload optimisation if a regular heart rhythm is present, with the aim to give fluids to reduce pulse pressure variation below 13% (Murugan). Additional surrogate markers of an adequate intravascular volume include base deficit, lactate, central venous oxygen saturation and arterial-central venous PCO_2 gradient. Central venous pressure has a very limited role if any in assessing volume status and should not be specifically targeted, unless definitely low (<2 mmHg). Urine output is unreliable as a measure of intravascular volume status due to diabetes insipidus being commonplace, but most organ procurement guidelines recommend targeting 0.5–3 mL/kg/h.

Tachy- and bradyarrhythmias may occur related to acute changes in autonomic activity and blood pressure early on, and are often refractory to treatment, while later changes in intravascular volume, electrolyte balance and temperature following established brain death can also be arrhythmogenic. Atrial and ventricular tachyarrhythmias can be managed with amiodarone and/or cardioversion while bradyarrhythmias are typically resistant to atropine (loss of brainstem vagal modulation) and should be treated with adrenaline (norepinephrine), isoprenaline or temporary cardiac pacing.

Respiration

If neuroprotective ventilation is no longer required, ventilatory management should be aimed at maintaining alveolar aeration whilst avoiding ventilator induced injury. Typical settings on the ventilator are PEEP 8–10 cmH2O and a tidal volume of 6–8 mL/kg if possible with a peak (plateau) pressure <30 cmH2O. The respiratory rate should be adjusted to maintain normocapnia and a pH of 7.40–7.45, using an inspiratory to expiratory ratio (I:E) of 1:1 as long as dynamic hyperinflation is not present. Normoxia is targeted and S_aO_2 maintained above 95% with the least inspiratory fraction of oxygen. Recruitment manoeuvres should be performed, once normovolaemia has been established, to maintain functional residual capacity, improve oxygenation and whenever the breathing circuit has been disconnected. A head-up tilt of 30–45 degrees should always be maintained (Box 43.2).

Box 43.2 **Respiration – summary of treatment aims**

Maintain alveolar aeration whilst avoiding ventilator induced injury using tidal volumes of 6–8 mL/kg with PEEP 8–10 cmH2O and tidal volumes 6–8 mL/kg with a peak (plateau) pressure <30 cmH2O

Maintain normocapnoea and a pH 7.40–7.45

Aim SaO2 > 95%

Recruitment manoeuvres can be used following establishment of normovolaemia to maintain FRC

Head-up 30–45 degrees should aim to be maintained

Electrolytes, metabolism and hormones (Box 43.3)

Electrolyte homeostasis should be maintained in the potential organ donor. Hypokalaemia is common as a result of polyuria and insulin administration. Hypothermia and should be corrected to avoid arrhythmias. A sudden increase in sodium is common as a sign of unrecognised/untreated diabetes insipidus and should be normalised, since evidence suggests an association between hypernatraemia (>155 mmol/L) and poor hepatic function post transplantation. Magnesium, phosphate and calcium should be kept within normal ranges. Blood sugar levels should be kept within 6–10 mmol/L with the addition of short-acting insulin if necessary. Enteral feeding in progress prior to transport should ideally be continued to maintain glucose levels and given evidence suggesting a protective effect on the gastrointestinal mucosa.

Central diabetes insipidus responds well to desmopressin or vasopressin. The synthetic analogue desmopressin has an excellent antidiuretic effect lasting up to 10–12 hours, while the pressor activity is only 0.1% of that of vasopressin. Desmopressin might therefore be preferred in haemodynamically stable potential donors. Vasopressin has significant vasopressor activity that makes it the drug of choice in haemodynamically unstable patients with hypotension related to vasodilatation. Any pre-existing hypovolaemia must be corrected before commencing vasopressin due to its potent coronary and splanchnic vasoconstrictive properties. Administration of vasopressin should be viewed as a replacement therapy rather than as a vasopressor titrated to effect. Any other hormone replacement therapy such as thyroxine and methylprednisolone should either have been initiated prior to transport or can be deferred until final management in the intensive care unit.

Hypothermia is common as part of acquired poikilothermia following brain death and as a result of body exposure and infusion of fluids at room temperature. Active warming is frequently needed and body exposure should be kept at a minimum to maintain normothermia (aim >36°C), keeping in mind that normothermia is a prerequisite to perform clinical brain death testing.

Many of the strategies discussed above for the management of the potential donor have been discussed in recent reviews, to which the reader is referred for further detail (see Further reading).

As with other aspects of retrieval medicine, the use of checklists is encouraged (Appendix 4). Box 43.4 summarises the additional considerations for potential organ donors.

Further reading

Bernat JL. Controversies in defining and determining death in critical care. Nat Rev Neurol 2013;9:164–73.

Delmonico FL, Domínguez-Gil B, Matesanz, R, Noel L. A call for government accountability to achieve national self-sufficiency in organ donation and transplantation. Lancet 2011;378:1414–18.

Dictus C, Vienenkotter B, Esmaeilzadeh M, et al. Critical care management of potential organ donors: our current standard. Clin Transplant 2009;23: 2–9.

Murugan R, Venkataraman R, Wahed AS, et al. Preload responsiveness is associated with increased interleukin-6 and lower organ yield from brain-dead donors. Crit Care Med 2009;37:2387–93.

McKeown DW, Bonser RS, Kellum JA. Management of the heartbeating brain-dead organ donor. Br J Anaesth 2012;108:96–107.

Framework for Radiology Interpretation

Imaging may form part of the primary survey in acute trauma, or follow interventional procedures that you as the retrieval team undertake as part of the stabilisation process (e.g. central line insertion). Having a systematic approach to imaging interpretation will therefore help to ensure major abnormalities are not missed. Taking the time to thoroughly review imaging will help reduce risk to the patient in transfer (failure to spot a pneumothorax in a ventilated patient may result in tension pneumothorax en route). Remember that on X-rays high-density tissues are radio-opaque, appearing white on the images (e.g. bone), low-density tissues are radiolucent, appearing black (e.g. air) and fluid, fat and connective tissue will be between the two (grey). The following structure provides a systematic framework to the interpretation of CT and plain film images:

Is this the image for the correct patient, taken at the expected time on the expected date?

Adequacy: does the film include all aspects required for full assessment (e.g. lung bases and apices on CXR, C7/T1 on lateral cervical spine x-ray)?
Is the film rotated?
Is the film under or over penetrated? (This is less of an issue on e-film viewers as the contrast can be manipulated).

Bones: are there any breaks in the cortex suggestive of fracture?
Check for alignment?
Compare like with like where possible (e.g. if reviewing films of the pelvis).

Cartilage and connective tissues: check for any obvious swelling. Depending on image type will determine specifics – e.g. on chest X-ray check trachea, hilums, heart shadow, lung fields and diaphragm at this stage. Is there any obvious abnormality or asymmetry? Remember to check the lung apices on chest x-rays for subtle pneumothoraces and surrounding soft tissues for surgical emphysema.
On CT heads, look for symmetry on each side and for any abnormal opacity. Extradural blood will appear concave as it collects between the cranium and dura, pushing the cerebral cortex inwards (biconvex appearance). Subdural blood on the other hand will appear crescent shaped and concave away from the bone.

Drains: check the position of endotracheal tubes (especially in neonates) relative to the carina, chest drains and central lines. A central line tip within the right atrium may predispose to arrhythmias during transfer.

Everything else: think about why the X-ray was ordered or taken in the first place. Interpret this alongside the clinical condition of the patient (physiological parameters) and the mechanism of injury.

ABC of Transfer and Retrieval Medicine, First Edition.
Edited by Adam Low and Jonathan Hulme.
© 2015 John Wiley & Sons, Ltd. Published 2015 by John Wiley & Sons, Ltd.

Framework for Interpretation of Arterial Blood Gases

An in-depth review of how to interpret a blood gas is beyond the scope of this text. Blood gas interpretation should be a part of most practitioner's scope of practice in the retrieval setting. It is worth considering the following points as part of the resuscitation and stabilisation process, irrespective of the transfer type.

Is the patient hypoxic?

If the patient has a PO_2 less than 8 kP then they are in either type 1 or type 2 respiratory failure (depending upon the pCO_2). Take into account the inspired concentration of oxygen that the patient is on (subtract this by 10 to provide a rough guide to what the predicted pO_2 should be). Use this information together with predicted clinical course to plan safe transfer – should the patient be intubated?

Is the pCO_2 normal?

This will need to be considered in the clinical context and the reason the blood gas was taken. A high pCO_2 may be normal for a patient with COPD, which will be indicated by the pH and bicarbonate level (a high bicarbonate to give a relatively normal pH). However a high or rising pCO_2 with worsening acidaemia may indicate ventilatory insufficiency, prompting intubation and ventilation. In the ventilated patient, the arterial pCO2 will allow the clinician to gauge or mentally calibrate the difference between end tidal CO_2 and arterial levels. This will allow ventilator parameters to be altered during the transfer if portable blood gas analysis is not available. In the context of traumatic brain injury, the aim will be for a normal pCO2 initially (4.5–5.5 kPa). However, evidence of raised ICP may prompt medical management including hyperventilation.

What is the acid base status?

As part of this assessment you will need to assess the pCO_2, bicarbonate/lactate and base excess.

This will place the patient into one of three categories:

1 Normal: check the pCO_2 and bicarbonate to assess whether there is any compensation.
2 Acidaemia: high pCO_2 suggests a respiratory cause (type 2 respiratory failure). Low bicarbonate suggests a metabolic cause.
3 Alkalaemia: low pCo_2 suggests a respiratory cause, high bicarbonate a metabolic cause.

Base excess is the amount of strong acid that would need to be added to a litre of the patient's blood to return it to a pH of 7.4 at normal temperature (37°C) and normal pCO_2. This gives an idea of the extent of metabolic disturbance. Generally, the more negative the base excess, the worse the acidaemia, the more positive the worse the alkalaemia. This will allow the clinician to make decisions on fluid resuscitation and ventilatory parameters.

What is the lactate?

Lactate is a byproduct of anaerobic metabolism of glucose at a cellular level. It is important to us as it indicates inadequate delivery of oxygen to cells to maintain aerobic metabolism of glucose. This needs to be urgently addressed. In the context of the critically ill patient, elevated lactate over 4.5 is associated with increased mortality. You need to assess the patient in the context of the history and optimise ventilation or haemodynamics. NEVER ignore a rising lactate.

Additional useful information on arterial blood gas analysers

Most blood gas analysis with also provide information on saturations, haemoglobin/haematocrit (useful to monitor in fluid resuscitation in acute burns), electrolytes (used to determine the anion gap to determine if an acidaemia is due to addition of extrinsic anions), blood sugar and carboxyhaemoglobin.

ABC of Transfer and Retrieval Medicine, First Edition.
Edited by Adam Low and Jonathan Hulme.
© 2015 John Wiley & Sons, Ltd. Published 2015 by John Wiley & Sons, Ltd.

Example of a Triage Sieve

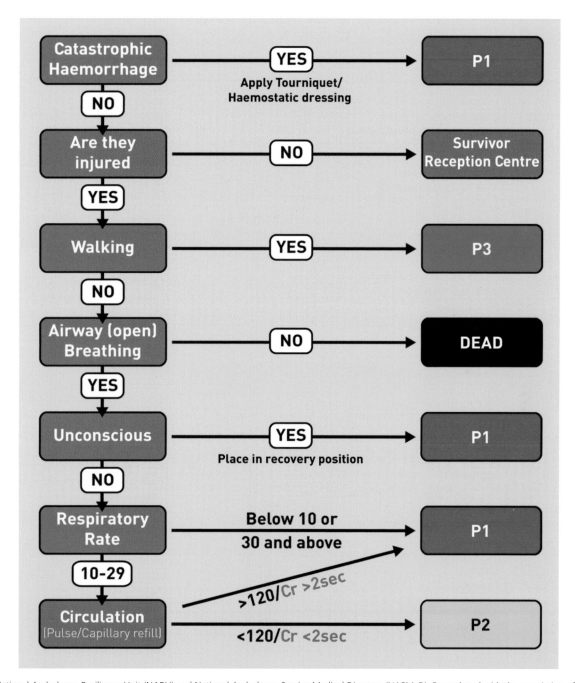

Source: National Ambulance Resilience Unit (NARU) and National Ambulance Service Medical Directors (NASMeD). Reproduced with the permission of the National Ambulance Resilience Unit (NARU) and National Ambulance Service Medical Directors (NASMeD).

ABC of Transfer and Retrieval Medicine, First Edition.
Edited by Adam Low and Jonathan Hulme.
© 2015 John Wiley & Sons, Ltd. Published 2015 by John Wiley & Sons, Ltd.

APPENDIX 4

Example of a Transfer Checklist

ASSESSMENT		./
CATASTROPHIC INJURY	Sufficiently stable for transfer	
	Damage control surgery completed	
AIRWAY	ETT secured	
	Appropriate size & length	
	ETT tip satisfactory on CXR	
	NGT/OGT position (CXR below diaphragm or pH <5.5)	
	Any difficulties to be known (e.g. difficult view)	
BREATHING	$SpO_2 \geq 95\%$ (PaO_2 >13 kPa)	
	Bilateral breath sounds	
	Pneumothorax	RL
	Chest drain (mandatory if IPPV)	RL
	$PaCO_2$ <5 kPa	
	Capnograph trace	
	V_t 6–8 mL/kg, P_{max} <30 cm H_2O	
CIRCULATION	ECG	
	Minimum venous access ×2	
	IV fluid connected	
	Arterial line *in situ*	
	(Zeroed, transducer fixed, pressure bag, flushes)	
	CVC *in situ* (mandatory for vasoactive agent infusion)	
	Obvious blood loss controlled	
	Hb adequate	
	Blood being transported (and forms filled)	
	TXA required	
DISABILITY	C-spine immobilised	
	Pre-anaesthesia GCS noted	
	Propofol and morphine (adult) for adequate sedation	

ASSESSMENT		./
	Midazolam and morphine (paeds) for adequate sedation	
	Paralysis adequate (NDMB)	
	BM >4 mmol/L	
	Pupils: size and responsiveness noted	
	ICP management confirmed	
EXPOSURE	Heat loss measures in place	
	Urinary catheter	
	Fractures splinted	
	Eyes taped	
	Potassium < 6 mmol/L	
	Ionised calcium >1 mmol/L	
	Acid-base acceptable	
ADMINISTRATION	Case notes	
	Radiology (copies or image linked)	
	Blood results	
	Transfer chart prepared?	
	Referring consultant known & recorded in notes	
	Accepting consultant known & recorded in notes	
	Bed confirmed at destination	
	Destination known (MTU & ED, ICU, theatre, etc.)	
	Receiving unit advised of departure time and ETA	
	Patient aware? If not, record in notes why not	
	Relatives aware? If not, record in notes why not	
DEPARTURE (in ambulance)	Stable on transport trolley	
	Infusions running & secured	
	Patient trolley secured	
	Electrical equipment plugged into power supply	
	Ventilator transferred to ambulance oxygen supply	
	All equipment safely mounted & stored	
	Staff wearing seatbelts	

ABC of Transfer and Retrieval Medicine, First Edition.
Edited by Adam Low and Jonathan Hulme.
© 2015 John Wiley & Sons, Ltd. Published 2015 by John Wiley & Sons, Ltd.

Example of Equipment Inventory

Bag 1: Front Pouch (Upper)

Doctors Drug Pack	20-ml syringe
Ketamine 200 mg in 20 ml	10-ml syringe
Thiopentone 500 mg of powder	5-ml syringe
Etomidate 20 mg in 10 mL	2.5-ml syringe
Suxamethonium 100 mg in 2 mL	1-ml syringe
Rocuronium 50 mg in 5 mL	Filter Straws
Midazolam 5 mg in 5 mL	Needles 21G
Ondansetron 4 mg in 2 mL	Needles 23G
Ephedrine 30 mg/mL in 1 mL	Needles 25G
Flumazenil 500 µg in 5 mL	Drawing Up Needles
Naloxone 400 µg in 1 mL	Drug Labels – each drug
Cefotaxime 1-g vial	Luer Slip Caps
Metaraminol 10 mg in 1 mL	RSI Checklist
Lignocaine 1% – 10 mL	MAD (mucosal atomiser device)
Bupivicaine 0.5% – 10 mL	Intranasal Dosing Chart
Tranexamic acid 500 mg in 5 mL	Bag 1: Front Pouch (Lower)
Water for Injection – 10 mL	ALS Drug Pack
Saline prefilled flush – 5 mL	Adrenaline 1:10 000
	Atropine 1 mg mini-jet
	Pelvic stability
	SAM Pelvic Splint

Bag 1: Top Pouch

Miscellaneous	**Bag 1: Side Pouch 2 (Handle side)**
	Adult Ventilation
Clinical waste bags	Adult BVM + reservoir + tubing
Sharps Bin (small)	Face mask size 4
Tuffcuts (sterile)	Face mask size 5
Transpore tape 2.5 cm	Easycap CO2 Detector (adult)
Bag 1: Side Pouch 1	Adult HME filter
Paediatric Ventilation	Handheld Suction Unit

Bag 1: Top Pouch / Bag 1: Side Pouch 2 (Handle side)

Bag 1: Top Pouch	Bag 1: Side Pouch 2 (Handle side)
Paediatric BVM + Reservoir + Tubing	Suction Catheter
Face Mask Size 0	Suction Reservoir
Face Mask Size 1	Trauma facemask (non-rebreathe) - adult
Face Mask Size 2	
Face Mask Size 3	
Easycap CO_2 detector (paed)	
Paediatric HME filter	
Trauma facemask (non-rebreathe) - paed	
Mapelson –F Breathing Circuit	

Bag 1: Main Compartment

Bag 1: Main Compartment	Bag 1: Main Compartment
Bougie holder	Paediatric Airway Pouch
15Ch Bougie –Adult	ETT size 2.5
10Ch Bougie -Paed	ETT size 3.0
5Ch Bougie - infant	ETT size 3.5
Adult Airway Roll	ETT size 4.0
ETT size 9.0	ETT size 4.5
ETT size 8.0	ETT Size 5.0
ETT size 7.0	ETT Size 5.5
ETT size 6.0	ETT Size 6.0
OPA size 4	Magills Forceps - Infant
OPA size 3	Magills Forceps - Child
OPA size 2	Mil Blade 0
NPA size 7	Mil Blade 1
NPA size 6	Mac Blade 2
Adult Laryngoscope Handle (with batteries)	Paediatric Laryngoscope Handle (with batteries)
Mac 4 blade	KY jelly Sachet
Mac 3 blade	Paediatric Thomas Tube Holder
McCoy 4 blade	1″ Micropore Tape
Magills Adult	OPA 008
Catheter mount	OPA 007
HME filter	OPA 006

ABC of Transfer and Retrieval Medicine, First Edition.
Edited by Adam Low and Jonathan Hulme.
© 2015 John Wiley & Sons, Ltd. Published 2015 by John Wiley & Sons, Ltd.

Bag 1: Main Compartment	Bag 1: Main Compartment
Easi-cap adult	iGel 1
20-mL syringe	iGel 1.5
Tube tie	iGel 2
Thomas tube holder	iGel 2.5
Lubricating jelly (sachet)	iGel 3.0
Oxygen	Syringe 10 mL
1 litre MGS O2 cylinder (340 Litres) with integral regulator/therapy head	Syringe 20 mL
	Catheter mount (Extendable)
	Cannulation Pouch
Failed Intubation Pouch	Cannula 14g
Scalpel 22 blade	Cannula 16g
Scalpel 15 blade	Cannula 18g
Tracheal dilating forceps	Cannula 20g
Cuffed tracheotomy tube size 6.0	Cannula 22g
	Cannula 24g
20-mL syringe	10-mL syringe
iGel 3	5-mL syringe
iGel 4	IV dressing pack
iGel 5	0.9% saline flush (5 mL)
Gauze Swabs (pack of 5)	Filter Straw
Cricothyroidotomy kit	1″ tape (Micropore)
Haemorrhage control pouch	Tourniquet
CAT Tourniquet	EZ-IO Pouch
Olaes bandage 4″	EZ IO Power Driver
Blast bandage 4″	Manual IO
Nightingale dressing 6″ × 8″	Adult IO needles (Blue)
Gauze Dressings (×5)	Paediatric IO needles (Pink)
Celox gauze dressing	LD IO needles (Yellow)
	3-way tap extension (Long)
	3-way tap extension (Short)
	EZ Connect extension
	50-mL syringe (Luer lock)
	EZ-IO stabiliser set
	EZ-IO Labels
	0.9% saline flush (5 mL)
	Sterets

Bag 2: Front Pouch	
Miscellaneous	Paramedic Drug pouch
Thermal Blanket (Mediwrap)	Adrenaline 1:10 000
First Aid Pouch	Atropine 1 mg mini-jet
Clinical Waste Bags	Amiodarone 300 mg
Gauze Swabs (Pack)	Frusemide 20 mg
Small Dressing	Hydrocortisone 100 mg
Medium Dressing	Aspirin 300 mg (strip)
Large Dressing	Buccal Gtn (strip)
Betadine (sterile pot)	GTN spray
Transpore (1″)	Salbutamol 2.5 mg
Transpore (2″)	Salbutamol 5 mg
Tuffcuts (sterile)	Atrovent 250 µg
Bag 2: Side Pouch 1	Hypostop

Bag 2: Front Pouch	
Diagnostics	Glucagon
Stethoscope	Benzylpenicillin
Thermometer & Disposable Covers	Chlorpheniramine 10 mg
Peak Flow Meter & Disposable Tubes	Adrenaline 1:1000
	Calpol (paracetamol) sachets
BM kit (includes lancets, strips, monitor, Hypostop)	Naloxone 400 µg
	Metoclopramide 10 mg
NONIN Monitor (with capnography lead, airway adapter and SpO2 cable)	Water for Injection 10 mL
	1-mL syringe
	2-mL syringe
Bag 2: Side Pouch 2	5-mL syringe
Traction	10-mL syringe
Kendrick Traction Device	Filter straws
	Drawing up needle
	0.9% saline flush (5 mL)
	Luer slip caps

Bag 2: Main Compartment	Bag 2: Main Compartment
Collars and Additional Splintage	Surgical kit
Ambu Perfit ACE collar - Adult	Sterile Tuffcuts
Ambu Mini Perfit ACE collar – Paediatric	Scalpel Size 22
	Spencer Wells (8 inch Straight)
Prometheus (adjustable) pelvic splint	Mosquito Artery Forceps (curved 125 mm sterile)
Fluid Pouch	Satinsky Clamp (small)
0.9% Saline (500 mL)	Gigli Saw (2 handles, 1 blade)
0.9% Saline (250 mL)	Finochietto Rib Spreader
Giving set	MerSilk 0 suture on colt hand-held needle – W792
Glucose 10% (500 mL)	
Chest Drainage	Foley Catheter 14Ch Female (with sterile water)
Ambulatory Chest Drainage Set	
Chest Seal	Chlorhexidine Spray
Sterile Gloves Size S, M & L	Sterile Swabs (Pack of 5)
Spencer Wells (6 inch)	Sterile Gloves Size 6
Scalpel Size 22	Sterile Gloves Size 7
Betadine	Sterile Gloves Size 8
Oxygen Therapy Pouch	Sterile Drape
Adult Venturi mask(s)	Cling Film Roll
Paediatric venture mask(s)	
Nebuliser Mask (Adult)	
Nebuliser Mask (Paed)	

Bag 3: Front Pouch	Bag 3: Front Pouch
Clamps for syringe drivers	Spares
12V DC Charging cable	Arterial lines (BD Floswitch)
Link cable (triple adapter to connect pumps to charger)	Arterial lines (Vygon Laedercath)
	Bungs
Thermal blanket (Mediwrap)	Syringes – 20 mL
Miscellaneous	Syringes – 10 mL

Bag 3: Front Pouch	Bag 3: Front Pouch
IV dressing pack	Syringes – 5 mL
Gauze swabs	Syringes – 2 mL
Spencer wells (6″)	Drawing up needles
Side Pouch 1	Tape (1″ Transpore)
Monitoring	Drug Delivery Consumables
Invasive pressure monitoring cable (for Lifepak)	Syringes – 50-mL luer-lock
Transducer set for invasive pressure monitoring	Infusion lines
	3-way taps
Pressure bag	Drug Additive Labels
	Side Pouch 2
	Diagnostics
	Stethoscope
	Thermometer & Disposable Covers
	BM kit (includes lancets, strips, monitor, Hypostop®)
	Spare LifePak batteries - charged

Bag 3: Main Compartment	Bag 3: Main Compartment
Paperwork	Syringe Driver Pouch ×2
PRF	Syringe driver
Transfer Paperwork	Fluids
Blood transfusion paperwork, infusion guide, transfer checklist, BNFs (adult, paed)	0.9% Saline (500 mL)
	Blood giving-sets
Aintree Intubation Catheter	10% Dextrose
Transfer drug Pouch	5% Dextrose – 100 mL
Noradrenaline (4 mg in 4 mL) – box of 5	Mannitol 10% - 500 mL
Adrenaline (1 mg in 1 mL) – box of 10	
Propofol 1% 20-mL vials - boxes of 5	
Tranexamic Acid (500 mg in 5 mL) - box of 10	
Midazolam 5 mg in 5 mL	
Drug additive labels	
Drug labels (each)	

Additional Items
Controlled Drugs Pack (Vehicle Safe)
Oromorph & Oral Syringe
Diazemuls
Stesolid Rectal Diazepam 5 mg
Stesolid Rectal Diazepam 2.5 mg
Doctors Personal Issue Drug pouch (Vehicle Safe)
Morphine 10 mg in 1 mL

Diamorphine 10 mg
Personal issue CD's
PARAMEDIC - Morphine 10 mg in 1 mL (×2)
LifePak Carry Case
Standard Monitoring set (coiled NIBP hose, 4-lead ECG, Pulse oximeter)
Disposable BP Cuff Adult
Disposable BP Cuff Adult – Extra large (side pocket)
ECG Dots (pack)
Defibrillator therapy cable attached
Adult Defibrillator therapy pads
Paediatric defibrillator therapy pads
Disposable BP Cuff Child (Top pouch)
Disposable BP Cuff Infant (top pouch)
SPO2 Finger Probe Paediatric (single use) - (top pouch)
Capnography airway adapter (adult) - side pocket defib side
Capnography airway adapter (infant) - (top pouch)
Nasal capnography (adult) - side pocket defib side
Nasal capnography (paed) - (top pouch)
Printer paper spare - (top pouch)
12-lead adapter cable (defib therapy pouch)
Ventilator Bag
ParaPAC plus 310 ventilator
Ventilator circuit
CPAP circuit (if available)
Oxygen cylinder
PRF Folder
PRF
Cardiac PRF
Hyperacute Transfer Policy
Cardiac Pathway (PCI)
Triage Tool
Stroke Pathway
Entonox Bag
Entonox Cylinder & regulator
Mouthpieces
Suction
Suction Unit
Suction tubing
Yankaur sucker
Endotracheal suction catheter – 10
Endotracheal suction catheter – 12
Endotracheal suction catheter – 14
Endotracheal suction catheter – 16
Navigation Bag
AtoZ maps (for region)
Vacuum Mattress (with pump)
Vacuum splints (small, medium, large and pump)
Sager traction splint
Burns Pack
Maternity Pack
Spare Airway Roll (adult)

SMART Triage Kit

CBRN Kit

Gloves – Small/Medium/Large/X-Large

RTC Helmets

Cleaning Wipes – Large Tub

Sharps Bin

Infection Control Pack

ARP Spare Batteries in charger

Trolley Cart for Bag 3

Fuel card

APPENDIX 6

Summary of useful National Guidelines

AAGBI: Inter Hospital Transfer (2009)

The need for transfer of critically ill patients is likely to increase, and decision to do so should be made at a senior level (and not undertaken lightly as exposes the patient and the transfer team to risk). There should be no reason, however why transfer cannot occur safely, even in the extremely ill patient. Protocols, documentation (a legal requirement) and equipment should be standardised, and administrative delays minimised. Appropriate training and support must be available. A professional, dedicated transfer service has many advantages with this respect and if often the safest option where available, with less impact on the workforce of transferring hospital. Air transfers have additional risks and expense that should be considered, and require additional training.

In most cases, the transfer should not be attempted until the patient is resuscitated and stabilised (which may take several hours). Treatments must not be delayed and specialist advice should be sought from the receiving hospital where appropriate. The patient should be established on transfer ventilator and monitors for a period of time before they are moved. The transfer team should consist of a minimum of two people (who have undergone competency based training and are adequately insured), depending on the type and complexity of the case, and agreed by the senior clinician who has arranged the transfer. The use of pre-departure checklists is encouraged.

Equipment should be mounted at the level of/below the patient, allowing unhindered access and a stable trolley. It should be robust and durable, with adequate battery life. Alarms should be set to appropriate parameters, suitably audible and visible. Ventilators should have as a minimum disconnect and high pressure alarms.

A core dataset should be captured in documentation to allow audit, with processes in place to review delays and critical incidents. Handover of care is not complete until the receiving team have received: a verbal update including incidents en route, documentation, copies of relevant investigations and access to imaging.

ABC of Transfer and Retrieval Medicine, First Edition.
Edited by Adam Low and Jonathan Hulme.
© 2015 John Wiley & Sons, Ltd. Published 2015 by John Wiley & Sons, Ltd.

Recommendations for the Safe Transfer of patients with brain injury (AAGBI 2006)

Patients with acute brain injury often present to medical facilities without a neurosciences unit. Local guidelines should be agreed between hospitals and neurosciences units regarding the transfer of such patients, and be subject to regular audit and review. High quality transfer of patients with acute brain injury improves outcome and should occur within 4 hours in patients with an expanding haematoma (earlier evacuation = better outcome). Such transfers are potentially risky if poorly conducted (adequate training of transfer personnel is therefore vital). Avoiding secondary brain injury is key by avoiding surges in intracranial pressure, hypotension (MAP >80 mmHg), hypoxia (PaO$_2$ >13 kPa), hypercarbia (PaCO$_2$ 4.5–5 kPa), cardiovascular instability and hyperpyrexia, while adhering to the key principles of safe transfer. The following are indications for intubation following acute brain injury:

- GCS <8
- fall in motor score >2 points
- loss of protective laryngeal reflexes
- hypoxaemia
- hypercarbia
- copious bleeding into mouth/airway soiling/base of skull fracture
- spontaneous hyperventilation (PaCO$_2$ <4 kPa)
- seizures.

Thorough resuscitation and stabilisation (even in time critical cases) will minimise complications en route. Consideration should be given to associated trauma/other likely injuries (e.g. cervical spine). Control of major haemorrhage takes precedence over transfer, and hypotension investigated to exclude all possible cause pre departure, and inotropes started if required.

The following should be specifically monitored throughout transfer (the patient should receive the same standards of physiological monitoring as they would on an intensive care unit): pupil size/reactivity, capnograpghy, urine output, central venous pressure (where appropriate), invasive blood pressure and temperature (core and peripheral). Ideally the patient should be positioned 20° head-up (trolleys should be developed that allow for this with concurrent spinal immobilisation).

Ample supply of the following classes of drugs should be available throughout: hypnotics, muscle relaxants, analgesics, anticonvulsants, mannitol/hypertonic saline/furosemide, vasoactive drugs, resuscitation drugs and intravenous fluids.

The ability to communicate with receiving and hospital of origin throughout the transfer is vital – mobile phones normally suffice. Relatives should be informed of the transfer and if possible/appropriate accompany the patient.

AAGBI Infection Control in Anaesthesia (2008)

Precautions against the transfer of infection between patients, or patient to practitioner should be a routine part of practice. Individual patients should be risk assessed for need for additional precautions. Good hand hygiene is central to the prevention of health care associated infections. Gloves should be used as single use items, and judgement for sterile versus non-sterile based on procedure being performed and likely contact with mucous membranes. Gloves should be removed before handling case notes, pens or telephones and after each patient contact. Single use equipment should be used wherever possible (especially in transfer medicine as practicalities of decontamination and sterilisation may be difficult).

All equipment for managing the airway should be single use and filters should be used in all ventilator circuits (also single use). Facility for the safe disposal of sharps should be readily available throughout, needle protection devices considered and blunt aspirating needles used for drawing up intravenous medications. An aseptic technique should be used for drawing up all intravenous infusions. Maximal barrier precautions (full hand washing, sterile surgical gown, sterile gloves, mask, hat, drapes and skin disinfection) should be used for invasive procedures (e.g. central line insertion).

ANZCA Minimum Standards for Intrahospital Transport of Critically Ill Patients

Physiological changes occurring during transfer may have a significant impact on morbidity and mortality, especially in the ventilated patient. The benefits of transfer must outweigh the risks and follow hospital protocol. The transfer team must be appropriately trained (new practitioners adequately supervised until competent), familiar with the equipment and performing any emergency procedures that may be required. Equipment utilised should reflect the diagnosis, severity of illness, predicted duration of transfer and level of intervention required, balanced against weight considerations. Specialist equipment is needed for paediatric/neonatal transfers. Equipment must be checked pre-departure and functioning monitored throughout. It should be durable and securely stowed (not resting on the patient) throughout and allow minimum standards of clinical monitoring (end tidal capnometry in all ventilated patients).

Mode of transport depends upon: clinical requirements, vehicle availability and weather conditions. Coordination of services should be centralised wherever possible.

The patient must be stable and continually reassessed throughout transfer. Pre-departure checklists should be utilised. The team must

ensure adequate communication facilities are available throughout and closely liaise with receiving facility. The transfer team should remain with the patient until the receiving team is fully ready to take over care. The transfer, including physiological variables should be accurately recorded in the case notes. The quality of transfers should be critically appraised to address system faults and improve the service.

Initial Care and Transfer of Patients with spinal cord injuries. British Orthopaedic Association 2006.

Spinal cord injuries have a significant impact on the patient, their family and society as a whole. In the UK the incidence of traumatic cord injury is approximately 19 per million (50% cervical injuries). They require specialist care and rehabilitation, but the early management has a significant impact. Early transfer (ideally from presenting ED) to regional Spinal Cord Injuries centre improves outcome. This will depend upon patient clinical stability and bed availability, but advice is always available from the centres.

Resuscitation: consider spinal injury depending on mechanism of injury and patient factors (e.g. pain/guarding on neck or back examination). Follow standard protocols (e.g. ATLS) for resuscitation and stabilisation.

Secondary injury from extension of ischaemic injury from the directly injured cord may worsen neurological outcome. Maintain adequate oxygenation and spinal cord perfusion pressure. Nurse spinal cord injury patients flat initially and monitor neurological level (extension may occur with oedema). A standardized examination/recording chart is useful (e.g. ASIA chart).

Spinal shock occurs in injuries above/at the level of T6 and may last from several hours to several weeks. Associated bradycardia may be worsened by intubation, leading to cardiac arrest. Maintain SBP 90-100 mmHg and adequate U/O. Be wary of concurrent hypovolaemia. Have a low threshold for inserting a central line.

High cervical injuries are associated with a high risk of respiratory failure and infection due to poor cough. Consider invasive ventilation pre-transfer or if vital capacity is <1 litre (voluntary VC >15 mL/kg).

Other important considerations: deep vein thrombosis prevention measures, pressure care and skin breakage (high risk – active planning for prevention required), paralytic ileus is common which should be actively managed as can adversely impact upon ventilatory adequacy and the patients are at risk of GI stress ulceration. In the case of priapism, a suprapubic catheter must be sited to avoid bladder over-distension. Monitor urine output.

Transfer may be requested for decompression (risk vs benefit) or spinal stabilisation (reduced complications, improved analgesia, reduced length of stay and overall costs). Anaesthesia is challenging as autonomic dysfunction may result in significantly labile blood pressure.

The use of high dose steroids in spinal cord injury is not recommended.

Use of a pre-departure checklist is advised (example given). Maintain steady speed en route, avoiding sudden acceleration/deceleration.

Index

ABC of Transfer and Retrieval Medicine, First Edition.
Edited by Adam Low and Jonathan Hulme.
© 2015 John Wiley & Sons, Ltd. Published 2015 by John Wiley & Sons, Ltd.